INTRODUCTION TO HEALTH PROMOTION & BEHAVIORAL SCIENCE IN PUBLIC HEALTH

INTRODUCTION TO HEALTH PROMOTION & BEHAVIORAL SCIENCE IN PUBLIC HEALTH

PUBLIC HEALTH BASICS

Hala Madanat ▪ Elva M. Arredondo ▪ Guadalupe X. Ayala

Series Editor: Carleen H. Stoskopf

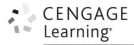

CENGAGE
Learning·

Australia • Brazil • Mexico • Singapore • United Kingdom • United States

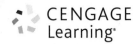

**Introduction to Health Promotion &
Behavioral Science in Public Health**
Hala Madanat, Elva M. Arredondo,
Guadalupe X. Ayala

SVP, GM Skills & Global Product Management:
Dawn Gerrain

Product Manager: Jadin Kavanaugh

Senior Director, Development: Marah
Bellegarde

Senior Product Development Manager:
Juliet Steiner

Content Developer: Lauren Whalen

Product Assistant: Mark Turner

Vice President, Marketing Services:
Jennifer Ann Baker

Marketing Manager: Erica Glisson

Senior Director, Production: Wendy Troeger

Director, Production: Andrew Crouth

Media Producer: Jessica Peragine

Content Project Management and
Art Direction: Lumina Datamatics, Inc.

Cover image(s): ©iStock.com/Mlesna

Library of Congress Control Number: 2014947852

ISBN: 978-1-133-69367-3

Cengage Learning
20 Channel Center Street
Boston, MA 02210
USA

Cengage Learning is a leading provider of customized learning solutions
with office locations around the globe, including Singapore, the United
Kingdom, Australia, Mexico, Brazil, and Japan. Locate your local office at:
www.cengage.com/global

Cengage Learning products are represented in Canada by Nelson Education, Ltd.

To learn more about Cengage Learning, visit **www.cengage.com**

Purchase any of our products at your local college store or at our preferred
online store **www.cengagebrain.com**

Printed in the United States of America
Print Number: 01   Print Year: 2014

Contents

CHAPTER 3   THEORY IN HEALTH PROMOTION   54

CHAPTER 6   TOBACCO   167

CHAPTER 7   CHRONIC DISEASE MANAGEMENT   198

Preface

INTRODUCTION

Introduction to Health Promotion & Behavioral Science in Public Health, First Edition is a text developed for students with some exposure to public health who want to gain a better understanding of the subdiscipline of health promotion and behavioral science. Although many students may be familiar with community health education or program planning, this book provides a more in-depth look at the science of health promotion and how research is informing best practices for promoting health among individuals, families, and communities.

WHY WE WROTE THIS TEXT

We love health promotion and behavioral science research! We wrote this book to share this passion with others and to help students better understand the importance of taking a rigorous approach to studying health behaviors and how to change them. This text fills a gap on the bookshelf by breaking down complex concepts, models, and theories used in health promotion and behavioral science research by illustrating their application to some of the most important health behaviors of our time. In addition to highlighting the importance of working at multiple levels of influence to create lasting changes in the health of individuals and communities, we share with students the various methods that researchers use to measure these behaviors (see Chapter 5 on physical activity for a great example of how to measure this behavior observationally, through self-report, and objectively using technology). In short, we wrote this text to excite and guide students to conduct meaningful health promotion and behavioral science research.

ORGANIZATION OF THE TEXT

This text is organized into three parts. Part 1 (Chapters 1–3) introduces the student to the field of health promotion, including its terminology, models for guiding health promotion efforts, and the theories that underlie the selection of change strategies. Chapter 1 presents a thoughtful discussion of five dimensions important to the study of health promotion and behavioral science in public health, including the universality of concepts across cultures and differences between inductive and deductive reasoning. The chapter challenges students to consider how research might look different when communities are recipients versus active participants in the change process. In Chapter 2, we present a comprehensive yet easy-to-follow program planning and evaluation model. It could be applied to a group assignment during which students prepare a written program plan as a final project and present it to fellow students. The chapter ends with examples of well-known program planning and evaluation models to expose students to models they may read about and apply in the future. Our review of theories in Chapter 3 is organized according to the Change to Social Ecological Framework, a theme that is carried into Part 2. Our review of theories is comprehensive and includes theories that are relevant for individual change, family and other social-factor change, organizational change, and community change. Although our focus is on how to change factors to promote health, we also acknowledge the appropriateness of these theories for understanding what factors are associated with these behaviors. A notable feature of this section is the use of case studies. This helps students digest often complex material through presentation of interesting, real-world examples.

Part 2 (Chapters 4–9) brings these concepts, models, and theories together and applies them to the top leading causes of early morbidity and mortality, including lifestyle behaviors and the health conditions associated with them. Nutrition and physical activity are presented first, behaviors important for preventing and controlling obesity, one of the leading epidemics of our time. Tobacco use is presented next, a behavior with major individual and public health consequences that is increasing in developing countries. We then move to discussing chronic disease management and how behavioral science public health approaches are needed to help individuals manage their disease and attain a good quality of life. Chapters 8 and 9 move the student into the realm of infectious diseases, including HIV/AIDS. Students can be encouraged to obtain more information about a current outbreak in the world, turning to various sources of social media and other news outlets for understanding how diseases are spread. Importantly, the goal of these chapters is not to achieve mastery in any of the behaviors; rather, the behaviors are used as illustrations of how to apply the concepts, models, and theories to behaviors that they may face later as health promotion specialists in the field or as graduate students.

Part 3 (Chapters 10 and 11) brings all of this together and discusses the relevance of health promotion and behavioral science research for meeting Healthy People 2020 guidelines and where more research is needed, including how to move research to practice.

ANCILLARY PACKAGE

The complete supplement package for *Introduction to Health Promotion & Behavioral Science in Public Health* was developed to achieve two goals:

1. To assist students in learning and applying the information presented in the text, and

2. To assist instructors in planning and implementing their courses in the most efficient manner and provide exceptional resources to enhance their students' experience.

Instructor Companion Website

ISBN 13: 978-1-133-78788-4

Spend less time planning and more time teaching with Cengage Learning's Instructor Resources to accompany *Introduction to Health Promotion & Behavioral Science in Public Health*. The Instructor Companion Website can be accessed by going to http://www.cengage.com/login to create a unique user login. The password-protected Instructor Resources include the following:

Instructor's Manual

An electronic Instructor's Manual provides instructors with invaluable tools for preparing class lectures and examinations. Following the text chapter by chapter, the Instructor's Manual reiterates objectives, provides a synthesized recap of each chapter's main points and goals, and houses the answers to each chapter's review questions.

Online Cognero Test Bank

An electronic test bank generates tests and quizzes in an instant. With a variety of question types, including multiple choice, true or false, and matching exercises, creating challenging exams will be no barrier in your classroom. This test bank includes a rich bank of more than 250 questions that test students on retention and application of what they have learned in the course. Answers are provided for all questions so instructors can focus on teaching, not grading.

Instructor PowerPoint Slides

A comprehensive offering of more than 250 instructor support slides created in Microsoft® PowerPoint outlines concepts and objectives to assist instructors with lectures.

About the Authors

Dr. Hala Madanat is an associate professor in the Division of Health Promotion and associate director for the Graduate School of Public Health at San Diego State University. She is also deputy director of the San Diego Prevention Research Center and a core investigator with the Institute for Behavioral and Community Health. Her research examines the nutrition transition among immigrants and implications for intervention research, including interventions to foster intuitive eating.

Dr. Elva M. Arredondo is an associate professor in the Division of Health Promotion and co-director of the Joint Doctoral Program in Health Behavior Sciences in the Graduate School of Public Health at San Diego State University. She is also a senior core investigator with the Institute for Behavioral and Community Health. Her research examines sociocultural, behavioral, familial, and environmental influences on physical activity and cancer screening behaviors and implications for multilevel interventions to promote an active lifestyle and cancer screening.

Dr. Guadalupe X. "Suchi" Ayala is a professor in the Division of Health Promotion in the Graduate School of Public Health at San Diego State University. She is a codirector of the Institute for Behavioral and Community Health and the San Diego Prevention Research Center. Her research examines sociocultural, behavioral, familial, organizational, and environmental influences on diet and physical activity and implications for multilevel, multisector interventions to prevent and control obesity and associated chronic diseases.

About the Public Health Basics Series

Lead by series editor Dr. Carleen Stoskopf, PUBLIC HEALTH BASICS is a series that brings to life the interdisciplinary nature of public health and the integration of multiple scientific approaches to public health problem solving through surveillance, critical data analysis, planning and implementation of interventions and programs, evaluation, and management of constrained resources. Through this book series, students will grapple with the major public health issues we are facing locally and globally while learning and putting to practice the principles of public health.

Acknowledgments

The editorial team would like to thank all of the students and faculty members who contributed to this book, including those named in chapters, and also individuals who have guided our thinking and writing. The team would also like to thank the blind reviewers who provided excellent critiques and suggestions for improving the contents of this book.

Contributors

Chapter 1
John P. Elder, PhD, MPH and Alexandra Hidalgo-Sotelo, MA

Chapter 2
Emily Schmied, PhD(c), MPH and Hala Madanat, PhD

Chapter 3
Kyle Gutzmer, MA, Guadalupe X. Ayala, PhD, MPH and Elva M. Arredondo, PhD

Chapter 4
Jennifer A. Emond, PhD and Guadalupe X. Ayala, PhD, MPH

Chapter 5
Ernesto Ramirez, MS and Elva M. Arredondo, PhD

Chapter 6
Reem Daffa, MPH and Hala Madanat, PhD

Chapter 7
Sheila F. Casteneda, PhD, Jessica T. Holscher, MPH and Gregory A. Talavera, MD, MPH

Chapter 8
Maria Luisa Zúñiga, PhD and Isela Martinez, BA

Chapter 9
Joe Smyser, PhD, MSPH and John P. Elder, PhD, MPH

Chapter 10
John Pierce, PhD and Sheila Kealey, MPH, Bsc

Chapter 11: Conclusion
John Pierce, PhD

Reviewers

David Brown, EdD, MCHES
Assistant Professor
Jackson State University
Jackson, MS

Shae Lee Donham-Foutch, PhD, CHES
Coordinator, Health Care Administration
Northeastern State University
Tahlequah, OK

Michael A. Melchior, PhD, MPH
Operations Manager
International Health Connection, Inc.
Miami, FL

Carolyn M. Springer, MA, MPhil, PhD
Associate Professor
Adelphi University
Garden City, NY

How to Use This Text

A GUIDED WALKTHROUGH

Key Terms

action	delivery system design	messages
appraisal support	dramatic relief	model
attitude	early adopters	observability
audience segmentation	early majority	observational learning
behavior	emotional arousal	outcome expectancies
behavioral capability	management	outcome expectations
behavioral intentions	emotional support	perceived barriers
clinical information	environmental	perceived behavioral
systems	reevaluation	control
community resources	equivalence	perceived benefits
and policies	exchange	perceived severity
compatibility	framework	perceived susceptibility
complexity	generalization	physical structures
conceptual models	health care	

KEY TERMS: The Key Terms listing introduces important terminology covered in the chapter. Definitions of these terms appear in the margins closest to where they are first presented in the chapter. This provides a quick and easy way to familiarize yourself with important terms and concepts.

Learning Objectives

Upon completion of this chapter, you should be able to:

1. Describe the field of health promotion and the basic strategies involved.
2. Identify the constructs that are essential to the definition of health education.
3. Describe the knowledge-attitude-behavior (K-A-B) approach and how health education embodies its assumptions.
4. Identify the fundamental aspects of positivism and how positivists view subjective information.
5. Explain inductive and deductive reasoning and how they relate to measures of health promotion and education.
6. Describe the evolution of community involvement in regard to health promotion and education.

LEARNING OBJECTIVES: Learning Objectives are presented at the beginning of each chapter and introduce the core concepts you should be able to master after reading and studying each chapter. These can be a great review tool as well.

Chapter Outline

Theoretical Foundations of Health Promotion
 Importance of Theory to Health Promotion
 Conceptual Models in Health Promotion
Social Ecological Framework
 Application of the Social Ecological Framework
Individual-Level Theories
 The Health Belief Model
 The Transtheoretical Model
 The Theory of Reasoned Action
 The Theory of Planned Behavior
 Behavior Analysis
Interpersonal-Level Theories
 Social Cognitive Theory
 Social Support
 Social Influence
Organizational-Level Theories
 Chronic Care Model
 Diffusion of Innovations

CHAPTER OUTLINE: Use the Chapter Outline as an excellent reference guide to direct your learning and to ensure that you are competent and knowledgeable about each section of the chapter.

SPOTLIGHT

Health promotion researchers often employ community members to deliver interventions to other community members. These types of interventions are often called community health worker (or lay health advisor, or promotor) models (Ayala et al., 2010, Cherrington et al., 2008). They are based on the assumption that the person who can provide the best type of support to someone learning to manage a chronic disease such as diabetes or helping to prevent one like obesity is someone who is like the individual and thus can relate to the challenges that the person might face. Community health workers are often naturally supportive individuals who are then trained to provide a specific type of support.

SPOTLIGHT: The Spotlight feature highlights need-to-know information in each chapter.

Model for Understanding

A case in point revolves around the assessment of physical activity (PA), which has challenged researchers in health education and health promotion for decades. Typically, PA has been measured through self-report instruments such as physical activity recalls and diaries and related scales examining confidence and other attitudes. Knowledge, attitude, and related data derived from recall and introspection ruled the day in PA research for some time. Dr. Thom McKenzie's approach, in contrast, involves the direct observation of active and sedentary behaviors, as well as the objectively measured elements of the environment that may facilitate or impede those behaviors. Dr. McKenzie supplements these observations with contextual variables, such as the size of a playground or the structure and leadership of physical education classes (McKenzie, 2002).

MODEL FOR UNDERSTANDING: Models for Understanding go deeper into the concepts discussed in each chapter by providing real-world examples of how those concepts can be applied to improving specific health behaviors.

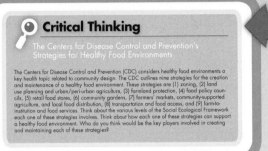

Critical Thinking

The Centers for Disease Control and Prevention's Strategies for Healthy Food Environments

The Centers for Disease Control and Prevention (CDC) considers healthy food environments a key health topic related to community design. The CDC outlines nine strategies for the creation and maintenance of a healthy food environment. These strategies are (1) zoning, (2) land use planning and urban/peri-urban agriculture, (3) farmland protection, (4) food policy councils, (5) retail food stores, (6) community gardens, (7) farmers' markets, community-supported agriculture, and local food distribution, (8) transportation and food access, and (9) farm-to-institution and food services. Think about the various levels of the Social Ecological Framework each one of these strategies involves. Think about how each one of these strategies can support a healthy food environment. Who do you think would be the key players involved in creating and maintaining each of these strategies?

CRITICAL THINKING: The Critical Thinking boxes encourage you to think more deeply about chapter concepts and apply your knowledge to real-life challenges.

CASE STUDY: The Case Studies present real examples of research into health behaviors and health promotion. Thought Questions are posed along with the case study that require you to evaluate and think critically about the research described.

4-1 CASE STUDY — Nutritional Education and Dietary Behaviors of WIC Enrollees

The Special Supplemental Nutrition Program for Women, Infants and Children (WIC) is a federally funded program to help low-income individuals purchase healthy food items. Those eligible include women who are pregnant, breastfeeding, or recently gave birth and children under the age of 5. The WIC program provides enrollees with money to purchase food; the food purchased must be from a list of specific items called the WIC food package. In October 2009, the WIC food package underwent a major revision. For the first time, the food package included fresh fruits and vegetables, whole grains, and lower-fat milk. These changes were made so that the WIC food package better agreed with the USDA Dietary Guidelines for Americans.

Review Questions

1. True or False: The Jakarta Declaration provides the most-cited definition of health promotion.

2. A primary goal of health education outlined in the WHO 1998 definition includes improving:
   a. Patient costs
   b. Ecological health
   c. Health literacy
   d. Community involvement

3. Which is a dimension proposed by the authors to add to the K-A-B approach?
   a. Costs
   b. Choices
   c. Expectations

REVIEW QUESTIONS: Test your understanding of the information presented in the chapter with a variety of review-style questions, including critical thinking questions. Use this practice to identify areas in the chapter that you may need to go back and reread until you are confident in answering those questions.

Web Resources

Visit the following websites to learn more about some of the topics presented in this chapter.

American Public Health Association—Public Health Education and Health Promotion: http://www.apl .org/membergroups/sections/aphasections/phehp/

American Alliance for Health, Physical Education, Recreation, and Dance http://www.aahperd.org/

World Health Organization—Health promotion resources: http://www.who.int/healthpromotion/en/

WEB RESOURCES: Utilize the Web Resources section at the end of the chapter for further learning and networking opportunities.

PART 1

PROMOTION, PLANNING, AND THEORIES

Chapter 1

John P. Elder, PhD and Alexandra Hidalgo-Sotelo, MA

DISTINCTIONS BETWEEN HEALTH PROMOTION AND HEALTH EDUCATION

Key Terms

health belief model
health education
health promotion

knowledge-attitude-
behavior (K-A-B)
approach

patient education
positivism

Learning Objectives

Upon completion of this chapter, you should be able to:

1. Describe the field of health promotion and the basic strategies involved.
2. Identify the constructs that are essential to the definition of health education.
3. Describe the knowledge-attitude-behavior (K-A-B) approach and how health education embodies its assumptions.
4. Identify the fundamental aspects of *positivism* and how positivists view subjective information.
5. Explain inductive and deductive reasoning and how they relate to measures of health promotion and education.
6. Describe the evolution of community involvement in regard to health promotion and education.

7. Describe the historical context of researching high-risk populations and how the use of patient education has been involved.
8. Explain the influence culture can have on society's approach to public health research and practice.

Chapter Outline

Dimension #1: Introspection vs. Positivism
Dimension #2: Deductive vs. Inductive Reasoning
Dimension #3: Community as a Recipient or Active Participant
Dimension #4: High-Risk vs. General Population
Dimension #5: Western Culture vs. Traditional Values vs. Universalism

INTRODUCTION

health promotion Health promotion is a process of enabling others to improve their health (World Health Organization, 1986).

The field of health promotion has evolved over the past four decades but is still largely based on that of its forbearer: health education. Numerous definitions exist for health promotion, but the most widely used was presented by the World Health Organization (WHO) in its Ottawa Charter for Health Promotion in 1986 (WHO, 1986). According to the Ottawa Charter, **health promotion** involves a set of comprehensive social and political processes that strengthen the health-promoting skills and capabilities of individuals as well as processes that improve the social, environmental, and economic conditions that impact the public's health. Health promotion is, therefore, a process of empowering communities to increase control over their own health and the factors that influence it. Participation is essential to sustained health promotion actions.

The Ottawa Charter sets forth five priority action areas for health promotion: (1) building public health policy, (2) creating supportive environments, (3) strengthening community action, (4) developing personal skills, and (5) reorienting health services. To accomplish these, the Charter defines three basic strategies to promote health: enabling and empowering individuals to control the determinants of health, advocating for improved essential conditions that affect health, and mediating between and collaborating with different groups and interests across society. The 1997 Jakarta Declaration (WHO, 1997) refined these five priorities to include (1) promoting social responsibility for health, (2) increasing investments for health and development, (3) expanding partnerships for health promotion, (4) increasing community capacity and empowering the individual, and (5) securing an infrastructure for health promotion. In their 1998 *Health Promotion Glossary*, the WHO goes on to further articulate the concept of health promotion, which they label ecological public health (WHO, 1998) given its focus on change at multiple levels of influence.

Ecological public health refers to the interaction among society (including international society) as a whole, individuals and their health status, and the many factors in between at both macro-environmental (e.g., economic, cultural, political) and micro-environmental (e.g., neighborhood, family) levels. This very broad conceptual basis is reflected in the recent popularity of socio-ecological models (see Chapter 3), which, like the transition from health education to health promotion, implies a movement away from an individually oriented approach to community health research and practice. The WHO contrasts this very broad concept of health promotion to that of disease prevention, specifically emphasizing disease prevention through risk factor reduction, as well as reducing the worsening consequences of a disease once it is established. Health promotion is meant to prevent disease in the first place.

Health education, in contrast, comprises the traditional approach to community, organizational, and even individual health protection and promotion through specific efforts to modify the knowledge, attitudes, and health behaviors of individuals. According to the WHO, **health education** comprises consciously constructed opportunities for learning involving some form of communication designed to improve health literacy, including improving knowledge and developing life skills that are conducive to the promotion of individual and community health.

> **health education** Health education is a combination of planned learning experiences based on theories that provide individuals, groups, and communities the opportunity to acquire information and the skills needed to make informed health decisions (Modeste & Tamayose, 2004).

Health education encompasses not only the communication of information but also the motivation, skills, and confidence a person needs to improve health. The WHO health education definition implies but does not stress changing social, economic, and environmental factors that impact health as well as individual risk factors and risk behaviors. Though not common to many other definitions, the WHO definition of health education holds that it may be broadly defined as including social mobilization and advocacy.

Problematic for these two WHO definitions (especially health promotion) is their breadth. They seem to include nearly any public health action while not being specific to any one activity or set of activities. As these definitions have evolved over time, there seems to be less of a distinction between them, let alone between these two and other endeavors in public health, such as environmental health, health services management, maternal and child health, and general chronic and infectious disease prevention and control.

The current chapter does not propose a new and improved definition of either health promotion or health education. Rather, this chapter provides a summary of the various definitions that have been proposed by international organizations and leading authors in the field (see Tables 1-1 and 1-2) and discusses five dimensions on which they may be distinguished. This information is intended to provide a firmer conceptual basis that is both sensitive to health education and health promotion's overall position in public health as well as specific to endeavors that do not overlap with other aspects of public health.

TABLE 1-1 Definitions of Health Promotion

Health Promotion Definition	Source
"Educational, political, environmental, regulatory or organizational mechanisms that prompt and reinforce health-promoting actions and environmental conditions."	Joint Committee on Terminology. (2012). Report of the 2011 Joint Committee on Health Education and Promotion Terminology. *American Journal of Health Education, 43*(2), 101.
"The process of enabling people to improve their health."	World Health Organization. (1986, November). Ottawa Charter for Health Promotion. An International Conference on Health Promotion, Ottawa, Canada.
"The science and art of helping people change their lifestyle to move toward a state of optimal health."	O'Donnell, M. P. (1986). Definition of health promotion. *American Journal of Health Promotion: Premier Issue, 1*(1), 4–5.
"Seeks the development of community and individual measures which can help... [people] to develop lifestyles that can maintain and enhance the state of well-being."	Department of Health, Education and Welfare. (1979). *Healthy people: The Surgeon General's report on health promotion and disease prevention.* Washington, DC: U.S. Dept. of Health, Education and Welfare.

DIMENSION #1: INTROSPECTION VS. POSITIVISM

patient education Patient education is a process of improving patients' knowledge and skills with the purpose of influencing specific attitudes and behaviors required to maintain or improve health (Rankin & Stallings, 2001).

health belief model The HBM theorizes that health-related behavior change depends on having sufficient motivation, a belief of a perceived health threat, and belief that the intended behavior will reduce the perceived threat (Rosenstock, 1974).

K-A-B approach The knowledge-attitude-behavior approach assumes that either on an individual level or via mass communication, changing knowledge and attitudes may result in risk factor reduction and other forms of behavior change (Bettinghaus, 1986).

Historically, health education and its theretofore previously better-known counterpart **patient education** rested on the assumption that individuals or patients, when presented with the negative consequences of a current course of action (or, alternatively, lack of action) and the potential benefit of changing that action, would respond in such a way as to protect their health. Research and development in health education was contextualized within the **Health Belief Model** (Becker, 1974; Rosenstock, 1974), which still has important parallels in popular theories in the field (such as the notion of outcome expectations in social cognitive theory; see Chapter 3). Thus, health education largely embodied a knowledge-attitude-behavior or **K-A-B approach** to improving public health. The K-A-B assumption is that, either on an individual level or via mass communication, changing knowledge and in many cases corresponding attitudes would result in risk factor reduction and other forms of behavior change. By arriving at the correct facts and feelings through introspection, the logical individual would arrive at a healthy choice. As a result, the field of health education emphasized unobservable mental constructs such as knowledge, emotions, and attitudes. The primary emphasis of health education was to modify these mental processes in a way that would result in corresponding behavior change, with the corollary of this assumption being that

TABLE 1-2 Definitions of Health Education

Health Education Definition	Source
"[Any] combination of planned learning experiences based on sound theories that provide individuals, groups, and communities the opportunity to acquire information and the skills needed to make quality health decisions."	Joint Committee on Terminology. (2012). Report of the 2011 Joint Committee on Health Education and Promotion Terminology. *American Journal of Health Education, 43*(2), 17.
"[The] profession of educating people about health. Areas within this profession encompass environmental health, physical health, social health, emotional health, intellectual health, and spiritual health. It can be defined as the principle by which individuals and groups of people learn to behave in a manner conducive to the promotion, maintenance, or restoration of health."	McKenzie, J., Neiger, B., & Thackeray, R. (2009). Health education and health promotion. In J. McKenzie, B. Beiger, & R. Thackery (Eds.), *Planning, implementing, & evaluating health promotion programs* (5th ed., pp. 3–4). San Francisco, CA: Pearson Education, Inc.
"An educational process concerned with providing a combination of approaches to lifestyle change that can assist individuals, families, and communities in making informed decisions on matters that affect the restoration, achievement, and maintenance of health."	Modeste, N. N., & Tamayose, T. S. (2004). *Dictionary of public health promotion and education: Terms and concepts* (2nd ed.). San Francisco, CA: Jossey-Bass.
"[Health education] is comprised of consciously constructed opportunities for learning involving some form of communication designed to improve health literacy, including improving knowledge, and developing life skills which are conducive to individual and community health."	World Health Organization. (1998). *Health promotion glossary*. Geneva: World Health Organization.

one then could measure both preexisting cognitive processes and changes in those processes through self-report instruments asking individuals to think about what they knew and felt. Knowledge and feelings are assessed either directly through surveys or indirectly through projective techniques (Wiehagen et al., 2007).

In the past two centuries, the relevance of these mentalistic assumptions (those that rely on posited but unobservable cognitive processes) came to be challenged by philosophers. For example, in the school of thought known as **positivism**, it is held that only phenomena that can be directly and reliably assessed through sensory observation (seeing, hearing, etc.) are of interest to science. Positivists do not deny the existence of cognitive processes, but they question the extent to which they are relevant given that they are unique to the person who is thinking or feeling and are experienced only by that person. Thus, the validity of measuring constructs such as self-efficacy or health knowledge, central to health education in its traditional

Model for Understanding

A case in point revolves around the assessment of physical activity (PA), which has challenged researchers in health education and health promotion for decades. Typically, PA has been measured through self-report instruments such as physical activity recalls and diaries and related scales examining confidence and other attitudes. Knowledge, attitude, and related data derived from recall and introspection ruled the day in PA research for some time. Dr. Thom McKenzie's approach, in contrast, involves the direct observation of active and sedentary behaviors, as well as the objectively measured elements of the environment that may facilitate or impede those behaviors. Dr. McKenzie supplements these observations with contextual variables, such as the size of a playground or the structure and leadership of physical education classes (McKenzie, 2002).

positivism Positivism is the branch of the philosophy of science that holds that objective empirical verification is the only manner through which we can establish scientific validity. 'Verification' means that two or more individuals must be able to see, hear or otherwise objectively sense the same phenomenon in the same way. It is thus the opposite of introspection and subjectivity. In applied terms, positivists rely on direct observation, are skeptical about self-report measures, and reject inferences that scientists and practitioners make about mental causes of behavior that they observe rather than simply describing the behavior. Positivism is often associated with the work of Comte and Mach in the 19th Century.

form, is challenged by this position. Positivists do not argue that the subjective personal experiences of one's actions and the environment in which they occur do not exist, nor are they unimportant in the grand scheme of life. Instead, positivists assert that only behaviors, physical or physiological outcomes, or other actions or their consequences that can be publicly observed in a reliable fashion are of interest to scientific inquiry. Health education theories that rely heavily on inferred psychological processes implicitly reject a positivistic approach, one that could contribute to their scientific quality and generalizability.

To shed light on the dialectic that surfaces between the positivistic and mentalistic perspectives, we should revisit the aforementioned K-A-B approach and add an environmental element. The physical and social consequences that the actor encounters after a behavior occurs will make that behavior more likely (if the consequences are favorable) or less likely (if they are disagreeable) to occur in the future. Given the powerful ways in which positive and negative reinforcement, punishment, and other consequences influence one's behavior, we propose adding "consequence" to the current three-element K-A-B approach to promoting health behavior change, rendering the sequence K-A-B-C. Those emphasizing the individual's subjective experience and relying on data from introspection would stress the first two (K-A) elements of this four-step process, whereas positivists would be more likely to begin with objectively measured behavior-consequence (B-C) measures.

DIMENSION #2: DEDUCTIVE VS. INDUCTIVE REASONING

In his analysis of the field of psychology, Kurt Lewin famously noted that "there is nothing more useful than a good theory" (1951). In keeping with this tenet, the health behavior field has tended to approach community health promotion through the application of one or more specific psychological or pedagogical theories such as the Health Belief Model (Becker, 1974; Rosenstock, 1974). Health behavior theories evolve over years of research and tend to be contextualized within a worldview or model of the human condition in order to structure health promotion and/or health education. This process involves a model of logic referred to as deductive reasoning, whereby one starts with such models or worldviews and works down to specific examples and applications. We may assume that social cognitive theory (Bandura, 1989) or other theories current in the field will inform the development of interventions that result in behavior change if applied correctly.

With inductive reasoning (more recently referred to as "Grounded Theory"; Strauss & Corbin, 1994), the opposite approach is taken. Through the process of inductive reasoning, the scientist views the human experience phenomenologically through a variety of experiences and observations that are then gradually developed into a conceptual model. The model may then be applied to other examples, or scientists may start anew with every new experience. In applied science, inductive reasoning is represented in a variety of efforts. Of interest for our purpose are the time series design and qualitative research. In time series methodology, rather than simply having posttest comparisons of groups or pre-post examinations of group differences, behaviors or other activities are defined and observations of these phenomena are taken over a long period of time at frequent or at least regular intervals. Thus, the scientist is able to objectively observe the occurrences and nonoccurrences of a specific behavior or other action and may make some inferences with respect to the association of these occurrences with environmental events. Intervention strategies may then be developed that reflect these inferences whereby a type of environmental or other influence is brought to bear to bring about positive health outcomes.

Techniques associated with anthropology and the field of marketing, both of which rely extensively on qualitative research to build knowledge bases, present other examples of inductive reasoning. Through qualitative research, individuals or groups (through techniques known as in-depth interviews, focus groups, etc.) are brought together to speak of their various experiences and how they view these experiences in terms of both objective and subjective memories and reflections. Compiling evidence from a series of qualitative research efforts, scientists are able to develop ideas for specific strategies that may lead to better community health programs. Again, applications to new communities, groups, or societies may require repeating the process of qualitative research and building inductive cases for such work. Thus, a broader health promotion approach must consider previously developed theories based in health education and behavioral sciences but at the same time be able to explore new ground that may ultimately entail radical challenges to and modifications of these theories.

Finally, the very act of defining the "field" of health promotion as though it were a theory-driven academic discipline in the tradition of arts and sciences may be misleading. As noted in the list of important historical developments in health promotion over the past 50 years (Table 1-3), major initiatives that have improved the health of populations have been launched with limited or no input

TABLE 1-3	Important Dates in the History of Health Promotion

Year	Event
1964	First United States Surgeon General's Report on Smoking and Health (by Dr. Luther Terry) clearly linked smoking to disease and death and was the first governmentally sanctioned statement to do so. The report launched decades of state, federal, and international efforts to reduce smoking and tobacco use in general.
1972	The Stanford 3-City Project employed mass media campaigns via television, radio, newspapers, and other efforts to reduce heart disease risk in entire cities (Farquhar et al., 1977).
1974	The Lalonde Report issued by the Canadian Minister of National Health and Welfare distinguished a broader ecological view of health as distinct from medicine and medical care and encouraged public health efforts to target those segments of the population most vulnerable to hazards in physical and social environments. It is considered to represent a key step in the evolution of the concept of health promotion.
1978	Originally developed by social psychologist William McGuire, the concept of "social inoculation" was applied to cigarette smoking prevention by researchers at the University of Houston and elsewhere. Instead of simply acquiring knowledge and attitudes against acquiring the smoking habit, young adolescents were given specific skills needed to resist peer pressure to use cigarettes (Evans et al., 1978).
1980	Thirteen-year-old Cari Lightner was killed by a repeat drunk driver in California. Her mother Candice established Mothers Against Drunk Driving (MADD), which gets a great deal of credit for the subsequent major drop in DUI–caused vehicle fatalities through media and advocacy and policy development and enforcement.
1988	In the face of massive campaign advertising by the tobacco industry, the voters of California passed "Proposition 99," which raised the price of cigarettes by $0.25/pack and dedicated much of the revenue raised to antismoking campaigns and local policy enactment. This effort demonstrated that multifaceted approaches including innovative mass-media ads and clean indoor air regulations led to substantial reductions in tobacco use across the entire state, as did simply raising the price of cigarettes themselves.

from the health professions, the organization of the Prop 99 campaign in California and the rise of the Mothers Against Drunk Drivers advocacy movement being prime examples. Advances in our field are often made because we are able recognize important social changes that can be built on and extended, regardless of who generates them.

DIMENSION #3: COMMUNITY AS A RECIPIENT OR ACTIVE PARTICIPANT

Being able to build on successful social change, however, requires a view of the community as a partner in this effort. Within traditional public health, including what has heretofore been defined as health education, individuals and communities have been looked at largely as passive participants in the health promotion process. Thus, patient education was conducted largely to complement the work of the expert physician or other health care provider. Immunization, vector control, clean water, and other similar efforts were carried out by professionals, while individual citizens were expected to do little or nothing on their own behalf.

Over time, and as implied in the WHO definitions of health education and health promotion, the concept of community health is characterized increasingly by active involvement of a community in its own health challenges and advocacy for community improvement and social justice. As a result, individually oriented research on patient education and risk factor reduction evolved into a broader approach that gives equal emphasis to physical and social environments. Recent work has added the concept of social capital to the mix, whereby individuals' health is viewed as the product not only of their risk factors but also of their integration and involvement in the social and political life of their community. As shown in the gradual evolution of definitions of health education in Table 1-2, communities were initially to be helped by health education professionals, with the communities themselves being passive recipients of the service. In later definitions of health promotion, the community is recognized as more of a partner in the process, for example, through the "process of enabling people to increase control over their health and its determinants, and thereby improve their health" as described in the 2005 Bangkok Charter (WHO, 2006).

DIMENSION #4: HIGH-RISK VS. GENERAL POPULATION

More than a half century ago, the field of medicine perceived a problem. Patients were leaving the primary care setting or being discharged from the hospital and yet not following through with prescribed actions that could maintain the health gains they experienced from their treatment. Forerunners of health promotion, patient educators came on the scene to address this problem, often in the form of auxiliary medical personnel who devoted at least part of their time to patient education. By definition, patient education addressed a higher-risk population, individuals who were seen specifically to remediate an illness or at least lessen the impact of the disorder on daily functioning.

During this time period (1950s–1980s), chronic disease epidemiologists were examining the health of populations in new ways, seeking to find out what heart disease and other risk factors were prevalent and whether individuals were under medical care or not. Much of health promotion today owes its focus to the Framingham, Seven Country, and Honolulu studies (Ho, Pinsky, Kannel, & Levy,

1993; Keys, 1980; Yano, Reed, & McGee, 1984) that documented the extent to which chronic disease develops before symptomatic stages and what behavioral and other risks put individuals at especially high risk for heart disease, stroke, and cancer.

The impact of these studies comprises some of Western health promotion's greatest success. For example, the National High Blood Pressure Education campaign (Chobanian et al., 2003) conducted in the 1970s determined that individuals with dangerously high blood pressure (HBP) were not getting proper (if any) care. The National Institutes of Health launched a nationwide effort to bring patients and physicians together to diagnose and treat HBP and maintain the treatment over the patient's lifetime. The smoking epidemic, sedentary behavior, and diets high in fat and cholesterol were also addressed, though with more complex and resource-intensive efforts (and with less of a dramatic impact). By bringing individuals with relatively high risk profiles into compliance with medical and behavior-change prescriptions, the United States and other industrialized countries realized important gains in chronic disease control, particularly in the area of coronary heart disease. Large community trials such as the Stanford 5-City Project and the Minnesota and Pawtucket Heart Health Programs were launched to accelerate these changes in community as well as clinical settings (Shea & Basch, 1990).

Whether through patient education or community heart health promotion, the typical participants evidenced some sort of risks that would need to be reduced in order for them to achieve optimal health. The resulting public health promotion modality can thus be referred to as a "risk-reduction" approach and characterizes much of health promotion research and practice today. As such, we seek to conserve our resources for those who are not physically fit, smoke, or weigh too much while not being too concerned with others who are relatively healthy. This public health promotion approach is characterized in Figure 1-1.

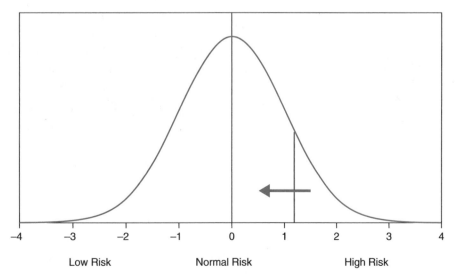

FIGURE 1-1 The public health promotion approach emphasizing reducing risk factors among those at relatively high risk (moving them from right [higher risk] to left [lower risk]) and thus reshaping the overall population curve.

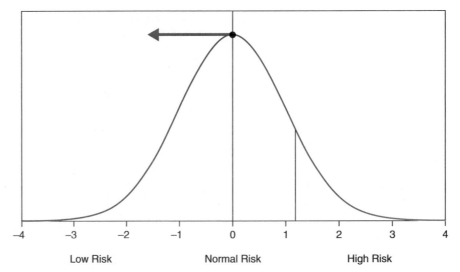

FIGURE 1-2 The Population Attributable Risk approach, entailing moving an entire population from generally higher to generally lower risk.

However, Geoffrey Rose (1981) and others have challenged this high-risk perspective. In examining concurrent heart disease risk patterns among many industrialized countries, these researchers have shown that nations and societies evidence relatively healthy and unhealthy profiles that cannot be fully explained by aggregate individual risks. These risk differentials are known as Population Attributable Risk (PAR), and the public health promotion implications are quite distinct from those of the high-risk approach. As shown in Figure 1-2, working within the context of the PAR, we seek not just to identify and treat high-risk individuals but instead to change entire communities and (implicitly) their social and physical environments to reduce the risk of future disease.

By way of illustration, let us examine the case of HIV/AIDS prevention and control. Many public health efforts, especially earlier ones, correctly identified that (in Western countries) men who had unprotected sex with men were at high risk for HIV infection. Thus, communication campaigns, condom distribution efforts, and other initiatives were launched in gay communities in an effort to stem the rapidly spreading epidemic. These efforts epitomized a high-risk approach to public health promotion. Over time, however, the HIV/AIDS pattern became far more complex, spreading quickly through Sub-Saharan Africa and Southeast Asia, and among heterosexuals. With the identification of additional risks through blood transfusions and vertical (mother-to-neonate) transmission, it became clear that most people and not just a small segment of communities and societies were at some risk. A striking contrast can now be found between HIV/AIDS control efforts of 25 years ago and those of today. Although communication efforts do not tend to target those at very low risk of infection (e.g., elementary school children, elderly couples), elements of current PAR–based promotion include destigmatization campaigns, the promotion of screening and treatment adherence, and empowering women to demand that they be protected from potentially infected partners. In Uganda and other countries with aggressive control campaigns, virtually everyone is exposed to the "ABC" message (abstinence, be faithful, use a condom), regardless of their risk profile.

DIMENSION #5: WESTERN CULTURE VS. TRADITIONAL VALUES VS. UNIVERSALISM

Although often sanctioned by such multilateral institutions such as WHO and United Nations International Children's Emergency Fund (UNICEF), much of the research and writing produced about health promotion consists of the work of North American, European, and other "Western" academics and officials. This derives not from a lack of interest among researchers and practitioners in non-Western countries nor in their potential for enormous contributions to the field but instead from the reality of the wealth of nations, which in turn defines their ability to afford support for these efforts. We are far less likely to be exposed to writings from India or Nigeria, even though they have enormous populations and their language of instruction is English, than, for example, to work from Scandinavian or Benelux nations, where neither of these is true.

Why is this important? Without this awareness, we are unable to examine the degree to which American society and culture and that of nations most similar to us influence our approach to public health research and practice. For example, most health behavior theories are predicated on the individual as the center of his or her own universe, weighing through various health options and learning to choose those that seem most fitting. Witness the numerous terms that characterize that emphasis and the popular theories from which they derive: self-efficacy, outcome expectations, and decisional balance. Families and friends matter to some extent, communities less, and broader physical and social environments little at all. This emphasis on the individual is fairly recent in history and not universally held. Judeo-Christian traditions transformed by the Protestant Reformation and later the Enlightenment appealed to the potential of the individual to a greater extent than had been the case in the Middle Ages and before, but this was primarily in Western Europe. The advent of the middle class transformed feudal societies into more urbanized ones, loosening traditional ties to land and older belief systems.

American capitalism extended this transition by providing an opportunity for many to acquire wealth and even more to be mired in poverty, with the assumption held by many (especially those in power) that personal worth accounted for the difference. Great social changes through legislative and judicial accomplishments accelerated decade after decade in the middle of the 20th century, beginning with Social Security in the 1930s, followed by the GI Bill (1940s), the desegregation of schools and public places (1950s), and Medicare, Medicaid, Head Start, and related programs (1960s into the early 1970s). More accepting views of race, gender, and culture developed and spread through much of society. However, beginning in the late 1970s, conservative political trends in the United States and the rapidly widening gap between rich and poor accompanied a diminished sense of collective responsibility for the health, education, and welfare of all people. The relatively tepid health care reform (the Affordable Care Act) barely survived state challenges and a Supreme Court vote. Ironically, the overall conservative shift in American politics has accented differences between the United States and its Western counterparts (NATO and EU countries, Japan and South Korea, etc.), all of whom provide greater access to primary care and generally more generous benefits to their citizens than does the United States.

At the same time, the world's underdeveloped countries in Sub-Saharan Africa, South Asia, and elsewhere, as well as many of its recently developed ones (e.g., Thailand, Mexico) are urbanizing very rapidly, with rural communities shrinking and losing their impact on traditional values and social norms. Electronic interconnectedness has challenged some very fundamental questions on how a community itself can be defined. In all, these rapid demographic, political, economic, and health sector transitions, as well as the distinctions between societies and communities within them, will have a strong impact on how individuals are viewed vis-à-vis their personal responsibility for their own health. These changes in turn will continue to shape our working definitions of health promotion and health education.

Summary

The fields of health promotion and health education are very closely related and encompass virtually all public health actions involving individuals, communities, and organizations. Health promotion, as described in the Ottawa Charter, is the process of improving health by enabling individuals to increase control over specific health factors—the person's social and economic contexts, physical environment, and behaviors—with the aim of preventing serious health risks before they occur. Health education encompasses efforts to disseminate health-related knowledge, with the goal of increasing a person's motivation to change his health behaviors and attitudes.

Effective communication of health information is the primary tool in health education, and this effort relies on an individual's ability to introspect about the desired behavior change; here improved health results from the modification of mental processes. The approach to health promotion has evolved from being individually focused to being focused on changing organizations, communities, and policies. In addition, the role of the individual as a passive participant in the health promotion process has evolved into one in which individuals are involved in the process of organizational, community, and policy change through advocacy and community engagement. Educated community members play essential roles in health promotion interventions by disseminating their knowledge to other members within their communities. Individually focused health education and risk-factor reduction are slowly becoming obsolete.

Reliance on qualitative measures such as subjective experiences and self-report can make it difficult to observe cognitive outcomes such as self-efficacy or planned behavior. As earlier explained, positivists argue for the development of observable quantifiable measures of objectively observed experiences using deductive reasoning, forming conclusions based on data by applying rules of logic and premise. Through the use of inductive and deductive reasoning in health promotion and education, operationally defined actions and behaviors can be evaluated with respect to environmental influences. This method helps identify consistent patterns that apply to behavioral phenomena, which can then be studied and used to construct and evaluate a theory or even demonstrate evidence of a community health program's efficacy.

When intervening with vulnerable populations, health promotion often involves a more population-based approach and does so through community and organizational development. Health education also has the capacity to reach high-risk populations but, in contrast, offers dissemination opportunities to the general population, such as through physician–patient and teacher–student contacts or, at a larger scale, through public service announcements (PSAs). When focusing on higher-risk populations, the primary focus is on empowerment over personal health, whereas efforts targeting the general population strive to increase public awareness of a health issue.

Theories and models that presently inform health education curricula and influence health promotion interventions tend to be grounded in Western ideals and fail to acknowledge limitations of applicability, relevance, and acceptability to non-Western cultures. Individualism and changing personal attitudes as a route to improving health behaviors are concepts commonly accepted in Western societies. Interventions rooted in individualism will be almost irrelevant for collectivistically oriented cultures that stress human interdependence and whose focus is on the group's goals rather than an individual's. When attempting to transfer Western-derived, theory-driven health programs to non-Western cultures, not only will there be numerous potential barriers to dissemination, but intervention acceptability and efficacy are also at risk.

Review Questions

1. True or False: The Jakarta Declaration provides the most-cited definition of health promotion.

2. A primary goal of health education outlined in the WHO 1998 definition includes improving:
    a. Patient costs
    b. Ecological health
    c. Health literacy
    d. Community involvement

3. Which is a dimension proposed by the authors to add to the K-A-B approach?
    a. Costs
    b. Choices
    c. Expectations
    d. Consequences

4. Fill in the blank: _____ is a top-down process that begins with models and worldviews and works down to understanding specific applications.

    a. Inductive reasoning
    b. Deductive reasoning
    c. Probabilistic reasoning
    d. Observational reasoning

5. True or False: Health behavior theories in Western cultures place more value on the individual compared to societies that hold more collectivistic views.

6. Short answer: How is a Population Attributable Risk different than a high-risk approach to improving public health?

7. Which theoretical construct demonstrates the current emphasis on the individual in health behavior theories?

    a. Self-efficacy
    b. Outcome expectations
    c. Social environment
    d. Decisional balance
    e. All of the above
    f. a, b, & d
    g. a, c, & d

8. True or False: In science, "positivism" refers to the emphasis on health rather than on illness.

9. Which acronym refers to national HIV/AIDS–control campaigns?

    a. ABC
    b. PSA
    c. K-A-B

10. Which of the below is NOT a type of behavioral consequence?

    a. Positive reinforcement
    b. Negative attitude
    c. Negative reinforcement
    d. Punishment

Web Resources

Visit the following websites to learn more about some of the topics presented in this chapter.

American Public Health Association—Public Health Education and Health Promotion: http://www.apha .org/membergroups/sections/aphasections/phehp/

American Alliance for Health, Physical Education, Recreation, and Dance http://www.aahperd.org/

World Health Organization—Health promotion resources: http://www.who.int/healthpromotion/en/

References

Bandura, A. (1989). Social cognitive theory. In R. Vasta (Ed.), *Annals of child development. Volume 6. Six theories of child development* (pp. 1–60). Greenwich, CT: JAI Press.

Becker, M. H. (1974). The Health Belief Model and sick-role behavior. *Health Education Monographs, 2,* 409–419.

Bettinghaus, E. P. (1986). Health promotion and the knowledge-attitude-behavior continuum. *Preventive Medicine, 15*(5), 475–491.

Chobanian, A. V., Bakris, G. L., Black, H. R., Cushman, W. C., Green, L. A., Izzo, J. L., Jones, D. W., et al. (2003). Seventh report of the Joint National Committee on Prevention, Detection, Evaluation, and Treatment of High Blood Pressure. *Hypertension, 42*(6), 1206–1252.

Department of Health, Education and Welfare. (1979). *Healthy people: The Surgeon General's report on health promotion and disease prevention.* Washington, DC: U.S. Dept. of Health, Education and Welfare.

Evans, R. I., Rozelle, R. M., Mittelmark, M. B., Hansen, W. B., Bane, A. L., & Havis, J. (1978). Deterring the onset of smoking in children: Knowledge of immediate physiological effects and coping with peer pressure, media pressure, and parent modeling. *Journal of Applied Social Psychology, 8,* 126–135.

Farquhar, J. W., Wood, P. D., Breitrose, H., Haskell, W. L., Meyer, A. J., Maccoby, N., Alexander, J . K., Brown, B. W., McAlister, A. L., Nash, J. D., & Stern, M. P. (1977). Community education for cardiovascular health. *The Lancet, 1* (8023), 1192–1195.

Ho, K. K., Pinsky, J. L., Kannel, W. B., & Levy D. (1993). The epidemiology of heart failure: the Framingham Study. *The Journal of American College of Cardiology, 22,* 6A–13A.

Joint Committee on Health Education Terminology. (2012). *Report of the 2011 Joint Committee on Health Education and Promotion Terminology.* Reston, VA: American Association for Health Education.

Keys, A. (1980). *Seven countries. A multivariate analysis of death and coronary heart disease.* Cambridge/ London: Harvard University Press.

Lewin, K. (1951). *Field theory in social science; selected theoretical papers.* D. Cartwright (ed.). New York: Harper & Row.

McKenzie, J., Neiger, B., & Thackeray, R. (2009). Health education and health promotion. In J. McKenzie, B. Neiger, & R. Thackeray (Eds.), *Planning, implementing, & evaluating health promotion programs* (5th ed., pp. 3–4). San Francisco, CA: Pearson Education, Inc.

McKenzie, T. L. (2002). Use of direct observation to assess physical activity. In G. J. Welk (Ed.), *Physical activity assessments for health-related research.* (pp. 179–195). Champaign, IL: Human Kinetics Publisher, Inc.

Modeste, N. N., & Tamayose, T. S. (2004). *Dictionary of public health promotion and education: Terms and concepts* (2nd ed.). San Francisco, CA: Jossey-Bass.

O'Donnell, M. P. (1986). Definition of health promotion. *American Journal of Health Promotion: Premier Issue, 1*(1), 4–5.

Rankin, S. H., & Stallings, K. D. (2001). *Patient education, principles, and practice.* (4th ed.). Philadelphia, PA: Lippincott, Williams, and Wilkins.

Rose, G. (1981). Strategy of prevention: Lessons from cardiovascular disease. *British Medical Journal, 282* (6279), 1847–1851.

Rosenstock, I. M. (1974). Historical origins of the Health Belief Model. *Health Education Monographs, 2,* 328–335.

Shea, S., & Basch, C. E. (1990). A review of five major community-based cardiovascular disease prevention programs. Part I: Rationale, design, and theoretical framework. *American Journal of Health Promotion, 4*(3), 203–213.

Strauss, A., & Corbin J. (1994). Grounded theory methodology: An overview. In N. K. Denzin & Y. S. Lincoln (Eds.), *Handbook of qualitative research* (pp. 273–285). Thousand Oaks, CA: Sage Publications, Inc.

Wiehagen, T., Caito, N., Sanders Thompson, V. F., Casey, C., Jupka, K., Weaver, N., & Kreuter, M. W. (2007). Applying projective techniques to formative research in health communication development. *Health Promotion Practice, 8*(2), 164–172.

World Health Organization. (1986, November). Ottawa Charter for Health Promotion, An International Conference on Health Promotion. Ottawa, Canada.

World Health Organization. (1997) *Jakarta declaration on leading health promotion into the 21st century.* Geneva: World Health Organization.

World Health Organization. (1998). *Health promotion glossary.* Geneva: World Health Organization.

World Health Organization. (2006). *The Bangkok charter for health promotion in a globalized world.* Geneva: World Health Organization.

Yano, K., Reed, D. M., & McGee, D. L. (1984). Ten-year incidence of coronary heart disease in the Honolulu Heart Program: Relationship to biologic and lifestyle characteristics. *American Journal of Epidemiology, 119*(5), 653–666.

Chapter 2

Emily Schmied, PhD(c), MPH and Hala Madanat, PhD

PROGRAM PLANNING MODELS: AN APPROACH TO INTERVENTION DESIGN

Key Terms

baseline measure

community mobilization strategies

comparison group

cost objectives

environmental change strategies

evaluation

experimental design

goal

health communication strategies

health education strategies

health policy/ enforcement strategies

health-related community service strategies

healthy people 2020

impact evaluation

impact objective

in-kind contributions

learning objective

marketing

needs assessment

objective

observational design

outcome evaluation

outcome objective

pilot testing

primary data

priority setting

process evaluation

process objective

program management

program planning

quasi-experimental design

resource development

secondary data

segmentation

target

visioning

Learning Objectives

Upon completion of this chapter, you should be able to:

1. Describe a general model for health promotion program planning.
2. Describe the process of conducting a needs assessment.
3. Explain how health priorities are identified.
4. List some of the main health promotion intervention strategies.
5. Explain the difference between process, outcome, and impact evaluations.
6. Identify some of the most commonly used program planning models.

Chapter Outline

General Program Planning Model
    Needs Assessment
    Priority Setting
    Goals and Objectives
    Methods and Implementation
    Evaluation
    Budget
PRECEDE-PROCEED Model
    Phases of the PRECEDE-PROCEED Model
    The PRECEDE-PROCEED Model in Action
PATCH Model
    Phases of the PATCH Model
APEX-PH Model
    Phases of the APEX-PH Model
    The APEX-PH Model in Action
MAPP Model
    Phases of the MAPP Model
    The MAPP Model in Action
CDCynergy Model
    Phases of the CDCynergy Model
Logic Models
    Key Components of Logic Models
    Logic Models in Action

INTRODUCTION

program planning is the process of designing a public health program through implementation and evaluation.

This chapter addresses **program planning** and evaluation. To efficiently implement an intervention, program planners must first allocate a substantial amount of time and effort to planning the intervention and its subsequent evaluation. The planning phase of a program is a multifaceted process designed to tailor the intervention to the unique needs of the target community. Numerous systematic models have

TABLE 2-1 Special Considerations for Selecting a Program Planning Model

Consideration	Details
Purpose of the model	As this chapter demonstrates, each program planning model is designed to serve a unique purpose. For example, PATCH was designed for use by state or local health departments to strengthen their infrastructure and capabilities, whereas CDCynergy was designed as a tool for developing health communication programs. As such, it would not be appropriate to apply PATCH to a health communication program or vice versa. Planners must take into consideration the purpose of the planning model and determine if it is appropriate for their project.
Resources	Time and funding. Different planning models require different amounts of time and money to utilize. Planners must consider the resources needed to use each planning model and make a selection based on what is feasible.
Stakeholder preference	Often program planners work with organizations or communities that already have experience participating in public health program development. These groups, referred to as stakeholders, may have a preference for a particular planning model based on past use. Because stakeholders play an integral role in program planning and implementation and are often responsible for sustaining programs, planners must take into consideration the stakeholder preference when selecting a planning model.

been developed to provide a framework for program planning, each varying in the terminology used, components included, and intended application. In this chapter, we will introduce a general model of program planning and then six models that are commonly used in the field of health promotion. These include PRECEDE-PROCEED, PATCH, APEX-PH, MAPP, CDCynergy, and logic models. Table 2-1 describes considerations for selecting the most appropriate planning model.

GENERAL PROGRAM PLANNING MODEL

Although there are many well-established program planning models available, it is not always feasible to apply a comprehensive model to a program due to time constraints or planning committee member preferences. For example, later in this chapter, the PRECEDE-PROCEED model is discussed, which can require an extensive period of time to complete. When it is not possible to use a more comprehensive program planning model, a general planning model, composed of six steps critical to program planning, can be utilized instead. These six steps—needs assessment, priority setting, goals and objectives, methods and implementation, evaluation, and budgeting—represent the basic components of program planning and are shown in Figure 2-1. It is important to note that many of the steps included in the general model do overlap with more comprehensive program planning models.

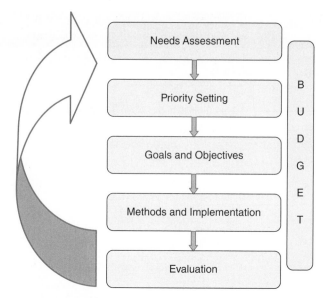

FIGURE 2–1 Health promotion program planning general model.

Needs Assessment

A **needs assessment** is the initial step in program planning in which the priority population and the health issues within the population are identified to determine what is needed to improve health outcomes.

The first step in developing a public health program or intervention is to conduct a needs assessment. A **needs assessment** is the process through which planners determine who the priority population is, what issues they face, and what can be done to improve health outcomes. The purpose of conducting a needs assessment is to acquire enough information to allow planners to identify what the program should provide and ultimately establish the program goals (see Table 2-1).

To complete the needs assessment, planners must first collect enough relevant data to define the population and the issues. Specifically, demographic (i.e., age, ethnicity, gender, income), employment, health (i.e., morbidity and mortality), and environmental data (i.e., crime, political, health care access) are needed. Data can and should be acquired through a variety of sources so that all questions can be answered. Primary sources of data, or data that are collected directly by the planners to answer their specific questions, can be useful tools for determining the needs and wants of the community. **Primary data** sources include original surveys, key informant interviews, community forums, and focus groups. More specifically, a planner who develops an original written survey and administers it to members of the community of interest is collecting primary data. In these surveys and interviews, it is important to assess what the community feels is most needed and how community members feel about issues specifically related to their health. Given the variety of sources from which primary data are derived, they often yield both qualitative and quantitative data. Conversely, secondary sources of data, obtained from preexisting records, usually provide more quantitative data. **Secondary data** sources include Census data (United States Census Bureau, 2011), state and local health department data, unemployment records, and national sources of data (e.g., Behavioral Risk Factor Surveillance System, or BRFSS, data; CDC, 2014a). Although acquiring secondary data may necessitate fewer resources, it often lacks key information on the

primary data are information collected via direct observation, interviews, or surveys from the priority population to inform a health program.

secondary data are preexisting information not collected for the priority program.

norms, opinions, and beliefs of the community that can be acquired only through primary data collection. Also, because secondary data have often been collected for a different purpose, such as general health surveillance, it may not be sufficient to answer the planner's specific questions about the community or subpopulations within the community. For example, a planner may be interested in learning about the risk factors for head injuries among adolescents between the ages of 12 and 16 and the preexisting secondary data may only have information for children ages 2 to 10 years old.

It is important to consider the potential discordance between the community's perceived needs and actual needs when conducting a needs assessment. For example, community members may perceive a great need for a certain program or service, such as a pedestrian walkway, but other data sources may indicate the community would benefit more from better lighting. The priority setting models in the following section can help to weigh the balance between a perceived and actual need.

Following data collection, the data are analyzed to identify trends in behaviors and health outcomes. The analysis may only require simple descriptive statistics or complicated computations, depending on the types of data available. Results of the data analysis will reveal the magnitude of the problems within the community, potential hindrances in attempting to solve the problem, and the necessity of solving the problem. More specifically, planners will learn how much of an impact certain issues have on the population and what barriers may exist to addressing the issues such as lack of community support or resources. At the conclusion of the data collection and analysis, program planners should have a comprehensive understanding of the health problem affecting the target community, thus concluding the needs assessment.

Priority Setting

priority setting involves selecting the key health issue the program will target based on the importance and changeability of that health issue.

Priority setting is the process of selecting the key issues the program will focus based on the information gathered during the needs assessment. The process of identifying a priority health issue is conducted systematically through one or more methods. Often priority setting is performed in a group setting, called the nominal technique. In the nominal technique, key members of the planning group collectively list and rank the issues identified in the needs assessment, discussing the merits or disadvantages of each. The group setting is advantageous in that it can generate or eliminate new ideas in a short amount of time.

Another common procedure for selecting priorities is the Basic Priority Rating process (BPR), also known as the Hanlon Method (Neiger, Thackeray, & Fagan, 2011; Pickett & Hanlon, 1984). The BPR process consists of four components, A, B, C, and D, where A = size of the problem, B = seriousness of the problem, C = effectiveness of the intervention, and D = PEARL, which stands for propriety, economics, acceptability, resources, and legality (described below). Each component is given a numeric score and then inserted into the following formula:

$$BPR = \frac{(A + B)C}{3} \times D$$

The issue with the highest total score is identified as the priority of the program. Once priorities are established, they serve as the guiding force behind the intervention and the remaining steps of program planning. Using the example of a program with an overall goal of improving health in a university population, we will examine each component of the BPR.

Component A is the size of the problem. The size of the problem refers to the number or percentage of individuals within the community who are directly affected by the problem. It is usually scored on a scale from 0 to 10. To assess this issue in a university population, planners would likely look to the campus's student health center for information on the most common health issues being treated. Based on this information, planners can determine the percentage of students who are affected by each health issue and score them accordingly.

Component B is the seriousness of the problem. The seriousness of the problem is determined by looking at several factors: the urgency, severity, economic loss, and impact on others. Urgency is generally defined as the risk of continued harm as a result of the problem and is assessed using incidence rates or community opinion. Economic loss is the amount the problem costs individuals, families, and the community. The impact on others refers to the probability that the problem will begin to affect people other than those initially affected. Each area of urgency is scored from 0 to 5, making 20 the maximum score for urgency.

Keeping with the example of targeting a university population, the seriousness of the problem could also be derived from student health services data. In assessing the size of the problem, planners will know what types of health issues the population faces. They can then examine which of those issues results in the greatest economic costs and also which present the greatest threat to overall health. For example, if the leading causes of illness, determined from student health center data, are influenza, mental health disorders, and the sexually transmitted disease Herpes simplex virus (HSV-2), planners can compare the respective seriousness of each and assign an appropriate score.

Component C is the effectiveness of the intervention and is measured according to the success of prior interventions and the degree to which the priority population is likely to engage in the intervention activities. If no similar interventions have been implemented to address the health issue at hand, planners must gather as much information as possible on related interventions and hypothesize how effective the program will be and how the audience will respond. Component C is arguably the most time consuming part of the BPR process. The effectiveness of the intervention is scored from 0 to 10.

During the previous step of the BPR, we discovered that influenza, mental health disorders, and HSV-2 were the most common causes of illness at our hypothetical university student health center. Component C requires that planners now look to past research to identify previous interventions targeting these issues in similar populations. Based on the results of this search, planners will assign each health issue a score, taking into consideration the success and adoption rates of the previous efforts.

Component D, or PEARL, is the final step of the BPR process and determines the overall feasibility of the program. PEARL includes five critical factors: propriety, economics, acceptability, resources, and legality. Propriety assesses whether the planners' organization is well suited to address the problem. Economics determine if it is worthwhile to invest resources to target the problem. Acceptability considers whether the community will accept the program. Resources consider if sufficient funding is available to complete the program. Lastly, the legality of the program and the organization's authority to implement it are considered. Each factor is scored as either a 0 or 1. Because the other three component scores are multiplied by D, if PEARL is equal to 0, the factor being rated will no longer be considered as a priority. Thus, planners often start with PEARL to exclude those health problems that do not meet this criterion and focus on prioritizing those which may be most important or relevant.

Completing PEARL in our example requires planners to evaluate their organization's own capabilities. They must ask, can our organization successfully address this issue with the resources we have or can acquire? If the answer is no, planners must eliminate the issue from their list of priorities.

A prioritization matrix offers a simpler method of prioritizing the issues experienced by a community (Green & Kreuter, 1999). The matrix is a visual tool with four quadrants (Figure 2-2). The columns represent the importance of the issue, and the rows represent the changeability. This prioritization matrix is a commonly used tool among planners because it is completed via a much less time- and resource-intensive process than the BPR model. It allows planners to make decisions fairly quickly, but still with a high level of objectivity.

Another step in priority setting is determining the specific audience that will be targeted. After describing the community with data, planners can identify subgroups within the population through a process called **segmentation**. Segmentation is necessary to ensure that the program is designed appropriately for the audience so it can be maximally effective. For example, if a program is designed to increase condom use among students at a university, planners must recognize that male and female students will respond to the same messages. Therefore, students are segmented based on similar characteristics (e.g., lack of knowledge of the topic, age group, gender, race/ethnicity). Variables used to identify subgroups include geographic, demographic, behavioral, and social factors. Segmentation is valuable because it often identifies the subgroup with the highest need for the program.

> **segmentation** is a process of dividing a large population into smaller subgroups based on personal characteristics such as ethnicity, religion, age, or education.

		Importance	
		High	Low
Changeability	High	Highest priority	Moderate priority
	Low	Moderate priority	Lowest priority

Adapted from Green & Kreuter, 1999

FIGURE 2-2 Prioritization matrix.

Goals and Objectives

A **goal** is a broad statement of intention that describes the expected effects of a program.

An **objective** is a specific statement that describes incremental effects of a program or intervention leading toward achieving the program goal.

Program goals and objectives are the cornerstone of health promotion programs. The goals and objectives are based upon the identified priorities and determine every aspect of the program itself. While goals and objectives are related, they are not interchangeable. A **goal** is a broad statement of intention (CDC, 2003). It is a short and concise declarative statement that describes the expected long-term effect of the health promotion program. A goal is typically not achieved during the course of the program and may take several years to reach. An example of a goal is, "To reduce the rate of skateboarding-related musculoskeletal injuries among students".

Conversely, **objectives** are narrow and concrete steps directed toward achieving the goal. Objectives describe the incremental changes in the priority population as the program is implemented. An example of a program objective is, "By January 1, 2016, 50% of students at Hope University will be screened for depression." A frequently used guide for developing program objectives is SMART, which is an acronym for specific, measureable, appropriate, realistic, and time-phased (CDC, 2003). The objective must specify who will be affected and what will change (i.e., "*students* attending *Hope University* "). Additionally, objectives must be measurable in that they state how much or what kind of change will occur (i.e., increase, decrease) and also be realistic, or not beyond the scope of the program. Ensuring that objectives are not beyond the scope involves considering many factors, including program budgets, the number of participants involved, and how difficult it is to change the target behavior or health issue. Lastly, objectives set specific timelines for when they will be met (i.e., "*by January 1, 2020* "). Developing well-written objectives is imperative; program objectives form the foundation of the intervention and evaluation activities.

There are four levels of objectives used in program planning that cumulatively bring the program toward achieving its goal. The four levels of objectives are process, learning, impact, and outcome. Each level is specific and includes a target timeframe for completion.

Process Objectives

A **process objective** is a statement that describes the completion of program tasks during the implementation of a program.

The **process objectives** guide the program and are the means by which the other objectives are achieved. Process objectives focus on the details of running the program and include such factors as resource allocation, materials, appropriateness of the program activities, and priority audience attendance. An example of a process objective is, "Conduct four skateboard safety training sessions for students within 3 months of program initiation."

Learning Objectives

A **learning objective** is a statement that describes the changes in knowledge, attitudes, skills, or awareness as a result of a program or intervention within 1 year of program initiation.

Learning objectives address the process of educating the priority audience about the issue so that they can eventually change their behavior. Learning objectives include changes in awareness, knowledge, attitudes, and skills of the priority population. An example of a learning objective is, "Seventy percent of students will know how to prevent skateboarding wrist injuries within 6 months of program initiation."

Impact Objectives

*An **impact objective** is a statement that describes the effect of a program or intervention on behavior within 1 to 5 years following program initiation.*

*An **outcome objective** is a statement relating to the long-term effect of the program on the target health problem, usually achieved 5 to 10 years following program initiation.*

Impact objectives set targets for how much the behavior or knowledge of the priority audience will change throughout the program. An impact objective is, "Sixty percent of students will use wrist-protective equipment while skateboarding within 1 year of program initiation." As you can see, if this objective is achieved then the program will likely achieve the goal of reducing skateboarding-related injuries.

Outcome Objectives

Outcome objectives are the final objectives of the program. These objectives describe the outcomes of the program and are long term. Generally, if a program meets its outcome objectives, it will also achieve its goals. An outcome objective is, "The number of new wrist injuries due to skateboarding among students will be reduced by 50% within 5 years following program initiation." As you can see, if this objective is achieved then the program will likely achieve the goal of reducing skateboarding-related injuries.

Healthy People 2020

healthy people 2020 is a set of goals and objectives with 10-year targets designed to guide the public health efforts of the United States.

The Department of Health and Human Services' (USDHHS) Healthy People initiatives provide an excellent example for how to select and develop goals and objectives (www.healthypeople.gov). The criteria for proposing **Healthy People 2020** objectives placed high importance on achievability, importance, and measurability (USDHHS, 2014a). Also, the objectives were to be data driven, using only the most valid and reliable data derived from currently established and, where possible, nationally representative data systems, such as National Health Interview Survey, CDC, and National Center for Health Statistics (NCHS) data (USDHHS, 2014a). Each of the more than 400 objectives in Healthy People 2020 includes a baseline, target, target setting method, and data source. The **baseline measures**, derived from the preexisting data sources, are used to determine an appropriate target. A **target** is comparable to an impact objective; it specifies the amount of change the program seeks to reach on its way toward achieving the objective. A target setting method refers to the amount of change from the baseline measure the target intends to attain. A data source is where the program received the baseline data. An example of a Healthy People 2020 objective, Objective PA-1, is, "Reduce the proportion of adults who engage in no leisure-time physical activity" (USDHHS, 2014b). The *baseline* is, "36.2% of adults engaged in no leisure-time physical activity." The *target* is 32.6% and the *target setting method* is 10% improvement. The *data sources* are the National Health Interview Survey, CDC, and NCHS. Each objective pertains to one of the four overarching goals of Healthy People 2020: (1) attain high-quality, longer lives free of preventable disease, disability, injury, and premature death, (2) achieve health equity, eliminate disparities, and improve the health of all groups, (3) create social and physical environments that promote good health for all, and (4) promote quality of life, healthy development, and healthy behaviors across all life stages (USDHHS, 2014c).

*A **baseline measure** is the initial measure of a behavior or health outcome at the start of a health program. Put simply, it provides information about the health problem at the beginning of the program.*

*The **target** is the final measure of a behavior or health outcome a health promotion program aims to reach. Put simply: where we want to be at the end of the program.*

Methods and Implementation

Once program goals and objectives are established, program planners must plan an intervention that is designed to achieve these goals and objectives. An intervention is composed of all program activities and can include a wide variety of activities.

There are several different intervention strategies, which have been categorized by the CDC into the following seven groups (CDC, 2003): health communication, health education, health policy/enforcement, health engineering, health-related community service, community mobilization, and other. The intervention strategies used are not always mutually exclusive; rather, some activities could be a combination of several strategies.

It is important to consider numerous factors when choosing the intervention strategy and accompanying components to be used in a health promotion program. One of the most important factors to consider is how well the intervention design corresponds with the program goals and objectives. Planners must ask themselves, "How will this intervention help us to reach our goals?" Other key factors are the logistics of the intervention: what resources are available, the expected program length, and the feasibility of conducting the planned activities. Finally, it is necessary to determine the scientific basis for all program components. Activities that do not originate from an established theory or model may be unsuccessful and unappealing to stakeholders, the individuals or organizations that have a vested interest in the program results.

pilot testing is the process of trying out certain components of a study, such as surveys or written materials, on a small group of people before using them to make sure that they work for the target population.

Once an intervention has been selected and designed, planners must conduct a pilot test within the priority community. **Pilot testing** is a process in which various components—or, if time permits, the intervention in its entirety—are implemented within a subset of the priority audience for the purpose of receiving feedback. The results of pilot testing are used to adjust any parts of the intervention that were found to be unsuccessful or unfavorable to the subset of the community who received it. Once the intervention strategies are finalized, planners can finalize formal protocols for implementation and begin the implementation.

resource development is the identification and organization of program components.

There are several elements in intervention implementation. Three such elements include resource development, program management, and marketing. **Resource development** is a key to maximizing available funds, materials, and other resources necessary to facilitate program implementation. Planners must not only assess the funds that are currently available to them but also determine preexisting programs and assets they can access. Also, part of resource management is identifying individuals or materials that can be mobilized for use in the current program. Organizing and utilizing every available resource increases the success of the intervention.

program management is the continuous organization of program resources including staff, materials, and funds throughout a program.

Program management is also crucial to the success of a program. There are several components within program management. Human management is the organization of the people involved in the program in a way that is most efficient. Task management is the tracking and completion of each program component to ensure that the plan is followed and adheres to the planned timeline. Fiscal management is the management of program funds to ensure that the program remains within the available budget. Lastly, risk management ensures that the program is implemented in a safe manner and that human protection protocols are followed.

marketing involves publicizing the program to raise awareness and is performed prior to and during program implementation.

Another key component of program implementation is marketing. **Marketing** involves generating awareness of the program. Marketing is initiated prior to program implementation and also often throughout the duration of the program. The purpose of marketing is twofold. First, it increases the likelihood of participation because individuals are alerted to the presence of the program. Second, it provides an opportunity to establish credibility within the target population by offering an explanation of the goals of the program and advertising that it is for the benefit of the people. Marketing must be planned well in advance of the start of the program so that advertising materials can be designed and distributed. It must be noted that marketing strategies are informed by results of the needs assessment and priority setting processes. As you may recall from earlier in the chapter, it is during these prior steps that planners develop an understanding of how supportive or accepting of the program a community will be. A community that expresses strong enthusiasm for a program may require a different marketing approach from one that has reservations about it.

Health Communication Strategies

Health communication is defined as "The study and use of communication strategies to inform and influence individual and community decisions that enhance health" (National Cancer Institute, 1989). Health communication strategies serve as the vehicle for educating audiences about health. **Health communication strategies**, which include both verbal and written communication, are the most commonly used intervention strategies in public health for several reasons. First, the number of individuals who can be reached by a single form of communication is substantial. Also, health communication is an appropriate means of achieving many types of program goals and objectives such as those that seek to increase awareness, knowledge, attitudes, and skills among the priority audience. Furthermore, many forms of health communication can be completed with relatively few resources, such as basic printed materials.

health communication strategies are a set of techniques used to inform individuals or groups of topics pertaining to health.

Health communication strategies can be grouped by the type of communication channel employed and the population level it is applied to. A communication channel is the method used to deliver the health message such as in-person communication, print media, telephone, Internet, radio, or television. The communication channel used determines the number of people the messages will reach. Communication strategies can be received via interpersonal, community, or mass media messages. Historically, interpersonal, or person-to-person, health communication has been most commonly used within the health care setting in which a health professional is educating a patient. An exception to this is the emergence of the *promotora* or community health worker model, which includes a trained community health worker making one-on-one visits with participants. The downside to using interpersonal communication is that it is extremely time consuming and limited in the number of people who can be reached, even when delivered in group settings such as meetings, classes, and workshops. However, with the rapid increase of computer and telephone availability in the general public, personalized electronic, video, and telephone messages have gained popularity among health promotion planners.

Community-level communication offers a means of efficiently reaching a specific priority audience. Community communication occurs at commonly visited locations such as churches and offices and through community-specific media such as newsletters or bulletin boards. Mass media communication reaches the largest number of people through print and electronic media such as billboards, newspapers, television commercials, radio advertisements, and public Internet sites. Mass media messages can be very expensive and also very difficult to control as far as who is reached.

Health Education Strategies

health education strategies are formal scholastic techniques used to increase the knowledge and skills of an individual or group pertaining to a health topic.

Health education strategies typically involve formally organized educational workshops, classes, or lectures in which participants are provided information about a particular issue. Such sessions are often composed of health communication components such as print materials, like pamphlets and worksheets, or verbal lectures. What is unique about health education is that it also offers hands-on learning activities and encourages participant engagement.

Health Policy/Enforcement Strategies

health policy/enforcement strategies are the application and enforcement of mandated regulations pertaining to health behaviors or factors that could influence health such as laws banning smoking in public areas to protect nonsmokers from second-hand smoke.

Health policy/enforcement strategies are those that mandate and control certain health behaviors. These strategies include laws, policies, rules, regulations, and executive orders. The use of health policy/enforcement strategies is both controversial and difficult. The concept of mandating a behavior, such as seat belt use or cell phone usage while driving, offends some individuals who believe it is a violation of their personal rights. Also, to put a policy in place can require a tremendous amount of time and resources, particularly if it is to be regulated by a local, state, or government agency. In spite of the difficulties, health policy/enforcement strategies allow program planners to reach groups that have been resistant to change.

Environmental Change Strategies

environmental change strategies are techniques used to alter factors external to an individual or in the community.

Environmental change strategies, also known as health engineering strategies, are those that change factors external to an individual and improve health. Some examples of these strategies that could be used to make university campuses safer for students include installing lampposts on an outdoor running path, putting handrails on stairways to prevent falls, and putting up "no smoking" signs to ensure nonsmokers are not exposed to second-hand smoke. Such strategies are effective because they frequently do not require individuals to change their behaviors, or they provide cues for behavior change such as the "no smoking" signs. However, environmental change strategies can also be difficult and costly to use.

Health-Related Community Service Strategies

health-related community service strategies include health-related services, tests, and programs offered to the community.

Health-related community service strategies are services, tests, or treatments aimed at improving health (CDC, 2003). These strategies include such activities as mammogram screening or flu shots. Health-related community service strategies are frequently employed in public areas visited by members of the priority population such as grocery stores, churches, and schools and are even sometimes run out of mobile vehicles. This is done in order to make the service, test, or treatment as accessible as possible to the audience so that individuals do not have to go out of their way to seek the service. Planners who wish to use community service strategies must also consider the affordability of the service being offered.

Community Mobilization Strategies

Community mobilization strategies are those that are part of a "capacity-building process through which community members, groups, or organizations plan, carry out, and evaluate activities on a participatory and sustained basis to improve their health" (Howard-Graham & Snetro, 2003). Community mobilization involves a process of researching the community to identify values, beliefs, and behaviors that may affect the health issue, gaining the trust and support of the community, and working directly with community members to create a plan for improving health outcomes. When successful, community mobilization efforts create long-term changes by increasing the community's ownership of the issue, thereby motivating the group to sustain the actions responsible for change. Community member participation is vital to such strategies, and there are many levels of participation from cooption, in which local members are involved but have no real power, to collective action, in which community members create their own agenda and mobilize without outside assistance (Howard-Graham & Snetro, 2003).

Other Strategies

Finally, other intervention strategies are those that do not fit in the previously discussed categories. Such strategies include the use of incentives and disincentives, social activities, and behavioral modification. The use of incentives as a means of inspiring participation and/or behavior change is sometimes quite challenging. The type of incentive offered must be appealing to the participants, and even within a specific segment of the audience, there may be great variations in the wants and needs of individuals. Some guidelines for the use of incentives include ensuring that each member of the group can receive one and that everyone has an equal opportunity for earning one (Kendall, 1984). Disincentives can be used in the same ways as incentives; however, the aim is to decrease or eliminate certain behaviors.

Social activities are another intervention strategy and are grounded in the knowledge that social support is a correlate of numerous positive health outcomes (Frasure-Smith, et al., 2000; Thoits, 1995; Uchino, 2004). Such activities as support groups, social networking, and gatherings can be used to connect individuals attempting to make similar behavior changes or facing similar health problems. These meetings can be centered on the health issue at hand or an unrelated issue, but providing individuals with a system of support during the intervention may increase compliance and success.

Role of Theory in Intervention Development

One factor to consider when selecting a planning model and throughout the planning process is the role of theory in the program. As you will learn in the following chapters, there are a wealth of health theories that explain the mechanism of human behavior change from a number of different perspectives. The theory that a program is based upon will greatly impact the types of data that are needed during planning and the intervention activities that are appropriate.

Evaluation

evaluation is the process of assessing the quality and effectiveness of a program.

To run a successful program, planners must evaluate at every step of the process. **Evaluation** is the process of assessing the quality and effectiveness of a program. It is a necessity because it allows planners to recognize which program components are and are not effective so that they can adjust the current and future components (and entire programs) accordingly. Evaluation also holds planners and public health practitioners accountable to stakeholders. The evaluation techniques for all stages of the implementation process should be determined during the program planning stage. This allows planners to match appropriate evaluation techniques with each program activity and allocate resources toward completing the evaluations.

The CDC has created a framework for evaluation that enables planners to design effective evaluation plans using techniques that are "useful, feasible, ethical, and accurate" (CDC, 1999). The framework is composed of six steps, which can be completed in various sequences. Step 1 is to engage stakeholders, including those individuals who are part of the program and those who are affected by the program. Because stakeholders have a vested interest in the program, it is important to receive specific feedback as to what results they are expecting and how the results can be best presented. Step 2 is describing the program in a way that clearly communicates the goals and objectives of the program. The program description is extremely detailed and includes information regarding the need for the program, the expected effects, activities, resources, stage of development, context, and logic model. Step 3 is focusing the evaluation design, which involves directing evaluation activities toward the needs of the stakeholders. To focus an evaluation design, a planner considers the evaluation's purpose, users, uses, questions, methods, and agreements. For example, the planner must take into consideration who will be receiving the results of the evaluation and who will be applying the results to future programs. The evaluation design must be conducive to producing results that can be understood and used.

An **experimental design** is a study design in which participants are randomly assigned to one or more study groups, usually referred to as case and control groups.

A **quasi-experimental design** is a study design in which participants are assigned to one of two or more study groups, referred to as case and comparison groups.

A **comparison group** is the group of participants in a study who receive a different health intervention than the one received by cases.

An **observational design** is a study design in which no intervention or program is taking place.

In Step 3 in the CDC's evaluation planning framework, researchers should determine the evaluation design. The three categories of evaluation design are experimental, quasi-experimental, and observational (Bickman & Rog, 1998). **Experimental design** is considered the gold standard because it involves random assignment of participants with similar characteristics into two study groups, the case and control groups. The case group receives the intervention and the control group does not. Though there are many types of experimental designs, the hallmark feature across all designs is the randomization of participants; this technique minimizes the potential for bias. **Quasi-experimental design** also includes two groups, but there is no randomization and the experimental group is measured against a **comparison group** or **control group**. **Observational designs** involve studying a phenomenon of interest without intervening or introducing a program. The type of evaluation design often relies on the stakeholders' preferences and the availability of funds or time. There are three types of evaluation: process, impact, and outcome evaluation, which will be described in detail later in the chapter.

Step 4 in the framework for evaluation is gathering credible evidence, which involves making sure the information obtained during the evaluation is completed using scientifically sound techniques and quality sources. Step 5 is justifying conclusions. Conclusions can be justified only if they are drawn from proper interpretation of sound evidence and analysis and if they meet the standards set by the stakeholders. Step 6 is ensuring use and sharing lessons learned. This entails making certain that the results of the evaluation are disseminated in an objective manner that reaches the intended audience. The importance of Step 6 should not be overlooked; the results of past programs inform the development of future programs and should be shared with the public.

Process Evaluation

process evaluation provides information on whether the program was implemented the way it was originally proposed.

Process evaluation is an ongoing assessment of the delivery of the program while it is being implemented, through activities such as keeping records of the number of program materials delivered and how many people attend program events. It assesses how well the program is adhering to the original plan, which is referred to as intervention fidelity, and identifies the gaps between what was planned and what was actually delivered. Process evaluation is important for numerous reasons. The information provides evidence of how closely the procedure is being followed, which helps to hold the program accountable to stakeholders, highlights areas of the program that need to be adjusted, and clarifies the relationships between program components and outcomes. For example, if the original program plan called for the delivery of 10 educational courses and 1,000 educational pamphlets, the results of a process evaluation would include how many courses were actually conducted and how many pamphlets were actually distributed. If there is a discrepancy between the planned and actual program, planners must determine why and if these deviations from the original plan affected the program results in a negative or positive way.

Some basic measures used in a process evaluation are participant attendance, demographics, satisfaction, and status of program activities. Participant attendance records can show the number of individuals in the priority audience that are being reached. Demographic information of the individuals attending program activities determine if the correct audience is being reached and will show if certain subgroups are participating at higher rates than others. Informal surveys of program satisfaction will identify any issue the audience has with the program. For example, if the audience feels the meetings are too long, the planners can reassess the content to see how future meetings could be shortened. Assessing the program activities, specifically what is happening at the sessions, who is leading the activities, and what materials are being used, provides details on intervention fidelity.

Impact Evaluation

impact evaluation involves assessing the short-term effects of a program on behavior change.

Impact evaluation measures the program's immediate effects. An impact evaluation begins by establishing evaluation objectives, asking, "What needs to be assessed?" Establishing impact evaluation objectives requires planners to work forward from the program's original impact objectives and activities and determine what changes occurred as a result of those activities. As we know, impact objectives are statements about the changes that occur as a result of program activities, and program activities are created to accomplish the objective. Thus, impact evaluation objectives assess if the activity was successful in achieving the objective. For example, a program impact objective could be "increase daily physical activity by 10% in 4 weeks" and have a corresponding program activity of a weekly meeting teaching participants how to incorporate physical activity into their daily lives. The impact objective would be to determine if the weekly sessions did increase physical activity 10% during the timeframe of interest.

Three typical methods for conducting impact evaluation are pre-post comparison, case-control comparison, and repeated-cross section comparison. Pre-post comparison is most commonly used due to its low cost and simplicity. In pre-post comparison, baseline levels of knowledge, skills, or behaviors are compared with post-intervention levels. This is usually completed via surveys, interviews, and skills testing. As previously described, during case-control comparisons, the intervention participants (i.e., cases) are compared to individuals who did not receive the intervention (e.g., control or comparison). This is more difficult than pre-post testing for several reasons. First, the comparison group must have similar characteristics to the intervention group. For instance, a program with a priority audience of high school students could not use a sample of senior citizens for the control group. Second, it may be difficult to find individuals who are willing to be a part of the control group, especially given the laws that protect human subjects in research settings. These laws are mandated by the Institutional Review Board (IRB), which is a formally organized committee of researchers that reviews all research programs that involve humans.

Repeated cross-section comparison is based on changes at the individual level. It is similar to pre-post testing in that it collects before- and after-intervention data; however, repeated cross-section comparison does not always collect data from the same group of people each time. Also, sometimes there are more than two points at which are is collected; they are often collected at numerous, regular intervals throughout the program. Many examples of repeated cross-section comparisons use different groups of people each time, such as census data and political polls. These data can be used to measure overall change in the priority audience over time.

Outcome Evaluation

outcome evaluation
involves assessing the long-term effect of a program on the target health issue.

Outcome evaluation assesses the overall effectiveness of the intervention in achieving the program goal upon its completion. Outcome evaluation is a longer-term process that can be measured in terms of behaviors, health outcomes, or even morbidity and mortality. It is highly data centered, and the data are usually obtained from a cohort that is followed over time. Outcome data are compared to baseline data. The type of data analysis used is specific to the data available.

Budget

A final crucial component of health promotion program planning is budgeting. Budgeting is the process of determining how to balance the funds available for running the program with the program costs. Like program evaluation, this is an ongoing process that begins in the earliest stages of program planning and continues through the evaluation. Budgeting often begins prior to program development during the process of applying for funding. Most funding applications require applicants to provide a budget justification for the general program costs including staff salaries, travel expenses, and materials (Leutzinger, 2005).

At the start of the intervention, planners must determine the type of budget plan most appropriate for the program (USDHHS, 2012). Many factors are considered when creating a budget plan such as the length, scope, and goals of the program, the source and type of funding, and the preference of stakeholders. One commonly used type of budget is line-item budgeting, which is a relatively simple and generalized system in which all expenditures for a program activity are totaled and used to determine future fund allocation. Line-item budgets assume that all program activities are necessary and are often disconnected from program performance. Line-item budgets are best suited for programs that do not anticipate significant expenditure changes throughout the program.

Activity-based budgeting is another option for health promotion programs (USDHHS, 1998). Activity-based budgeting is often a more practical option for programs expecting growth or change, although it is time consuming because it can require constant revisions. Activity-based budgets divide activities into primary and secondary costs to make certain the activities most vital to achieving program goals are fully funded. This type of budget can identify areas in which costs should be reduced or increased and provides a link between costs and program performance.

One factor to remember when completing a budget is in-kind contributions.

In-kind contributions are nonmonetary donations made to the program from outside sources. Programs often receive support from community organizations that are unrelated to the funding sponsor. Examples include space that is provided for free to hold events or classes, or someone's time that is not compensated. This is a typical resource in public health programs and requires special treatment in a budget. Specifically, many funding agencies require documentation, including an estimated dollar value, of all in-kind services.

in-kind contributions are nonmonetary support, such as goods and services, provided by external sources.

Regardless of the type of budget plan being utilized, programs must establish cost objectives based on each program expense and how it relates to the program goals. More specifically, cost objectives identify and quantify the resources needed to successfully implement each program activity. **Cost objectives** are often determined using historical accounting data, but if it is not available, planners must carefully research the costs of the activity. When developing cost objectives, planners must consider all required resources, including person hours, materials, advertisements, and meeting space. Cost objectives must also anticipate future costs and prepare for the possibility of reduced funding or programming changes. Setting cost objectives at the start of a program enables the activities to be appropriately funded so that they can be completed.

cost objectives include a predetermined budget set for each program component.

Once the budget has been established, the program must be continuously monitored to ensure adherence. Depending on the size of the staff, there is sometimes a designated financial officer, but the program planner must be familiar with the process, alert to the program plan, and aware of how well the program is adhering to the budget. Programs also often use sophisticated computer software designed for tracking program expenses in relation to the budget. Whatever the method for monitoring the budget, it should be established at the start of the program.

As you have seen, each of the six steps in the general program planning model plays a critical role in program development. The remainder of this chapter will describe six other specific program planning models. You will recognize the steps from the general model in many of them.

PRECEDE-PROCEED MODEL

Developed in a series of iterations spanning nearly 40 years, the PRECEDE-PROCEED model is presently the most recognizable and most frequently used model in program planning (Green, 1974; Green & Kreuter, 1991, 1999, 2005; Green, Kreuter, Deeds, & Partridge, 1980). The words PRECEDE and PROCEED are acronyms for "predisposing, reinforcing, and enabling constructs in educational/ecological diagnosis and evaluation" (PRECEDE; Green, Kreuter, Deeds, & Partridge, 1980) and "policy, regulatory, and organizational constructs in educational and environmental development" (PROCEED; Green & Kreuter, 1991, 1992). The model provides a unique and comprehensive framework for program planning by executing a thorough assessment, or diagnosis, of the priority population and its health concerns prior to designing the intervention, essentially working backward toward the development of an intervention. PRECEDE-PROCEED emphasizes the multidimensionality of health by distinguishing among the behavioral, educational, and environmental barriers impeding health outcomes.

The PRECEDE portion of the model was first published in 1974 in response to the increasing demand for health programs to evaluate their own cost-effectiveness (Green, 1974). Over time, the model transitioned into a program planning tool after being applied successfully in various settings. In the third edition of the model, the word "diagnosis" was replaced with "assessment" to move away from the clinical terminology, although the terms are often still used interchangeably by the authors (Green & Kreuter, 1999). PROCEED was developed in the 1980s to meet the need for an efficient framework for evaluation (Green & Kreuter, 1991, 1992). Also, it was at that time that the field of public health began to acknowledge the importance of the environment–health relationship (Glanz, Rimer, & Viswanath, 2008).

Phases of the PRECEDE-PROCEED Model

PRECEDE-PROCEED is composed of eight phases encompassing assessment, implementation, and evaluation (Green & Kreuter, 2005). All phases are shown in Figure 2-3. PRECEDE includes the first four phases, or the assessment, and PROCEED includes the last four phases of the implementation and evaluation. Phase I, the social assessment, participatory planning, and situational analysis, surveys the target community itself to determine the citizens' desired health outcome. Designed to assess the overall quality of life in the community, this phase calls for community participation to identify and rank the wants and needs of people. This

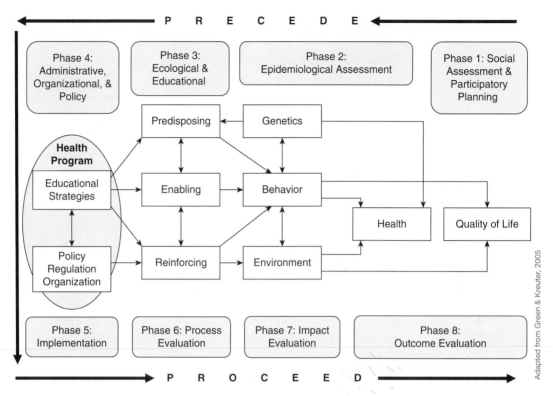

FIGURE 2-3 PRECEDE-PROCEED model.

is performed by collecting basic demographic information and administering surveys or conducting interviews and focus groups with community members. Some examples of the social variables assessed in this phase are unemployment, crime, and self-esteem.

Phase II, the epidemiological assessment, includes health, behavioral, genetic, and environmental assessments. This phase seeks to identify the issue that the program will concentrate on. Health is often assessed through preexisting databases such as the National Center for Health Statistics (http://www.cdc.gov/nchs; CDC, 2014), local health department records, or survey data. Health statistics include disability and mortality. Behavioral determinants refer to human actions that contribute to the health problem and can refer to the actions of an individual, a group, or a community. For example, purchasing and consuming fast food directly influences an individual's health. If a spouse or family member purchases fast food for the individual or he is served fast food at a corporate event, they are also affected directly. Environmental determinants of health refer to factors outside an individual that can influence behavior and include the physical, social, political, and economic environment (Green & Kreuter, 1999). Contributing factors in the physical environment could include the air quality of the region or the condition of the sidewalks. A social determinant of health is the community's attitude toward the issue at large. A political determinant could be the laws that regulate risky or unhealthy behavior such as seat belt usage. Finally, economic determinants include such factors as the average annual income in the community or the affordability of health insurance. Once the epidemiological assessment is complete, the planners can rank the factors to determine where the program should focus its efforts. Ranking criteria include both the size of contribution to the problem and the feasibility of altering or eliminating it.

The educational and ecological assessment in Phase III identifies and classifies factors that influence the issue identified in the previous phases. The factors are classified as predisposing, reinforcing, or enabling. Predisposing factors are preexisting traits that affect an individual or community's motivation to engage in or avoid certain behaviors. Such traits include knowledge, attitudes, beliefs, and values. Enabling factors are the external conditions that influence the ability of individuals and communities to adopt and maintain certain behaviors or environmental conditions. Enabling factors also precede the behavior, including access to care, availability of resources, and laws pertaining to the issue. Reinforcing factors are those that follow a behavior and "provide continuing reward or incentive for the persistence or repetition of the behavior" such as peer support or tangible benefits (Green & Kreuter, 2005). En masse, these factors greatly influence the probability that the behavior or environmental change will be adopted and therefore become the cornerstone of the intervention and the basis of the program goals and objectives. As in Phase II, these factors are ranked by impact and changeability.

The administrative and policy assessment and intervention alignment is Phase IV, the final phase in the assessment portion of the model. It is during this phase that the intervention components are selected using a process of "matching, mapping, pooling, and patching" (D'Onofrio, 2001; Green & Kreuter, 2005; Simons-Morton, Greene, & Gottlieb, 1995). The intervention components are matched to the determinants of the issue and then mapped to preexisting theories and knowledge. Prior interventions are pooled and reviewed for successful components; then the successful components are used to identify and patch any gaps in the current program plan.

Also during Phase IV, the existing administrative issues, policies, and regulations that may influence the success of the intervention are identified, as well as those that may be needed to facilitate the implementation and longevity of the intervention. Administrative issues refer to the internal structure and culture of the organization developing the intervention. The organization must be well suited for the particular intervention, meaning the beliefs and capabilities must align with the goals and components of the intervention. The policy and regulatory issues can be either internal or external to the organization. Internal policies such as the set procedures for collecting data or interacting with participants may hinder the effectiveness of the intervention. External policies or regulations include state or local laws that could interfere with the intervention, such as smoking regulations. These steps collectively ensure the intervention is in alignment with the goals of the program and the resources available. Once the intervention is in place, the project budget and timeline can be solidified.

Implementation occurs in Phase V of the model. The evaluation is performed throughout the duration of the intervention and following its completion. Phase VI, the process evaluation, assesses the intervention as it is occurring to monitor whether the initial plan is being followed. Information collected during this phase can be used to make immediate adjustments such as changing the time and location of meetings. The impact evaluation in Phase VII assesses the immediate effect of the intervention, or the objectives. For example, an intervention with the goal of reducing low back injuries in a moving company would assess improved heavy lifting technique during the impact evaluation. The eighth and final phase of the PRECEDE-PROCEED model is the outcome evaluation, during which the effect of the intervention on the ultimate issue identified in Phase I is assessed. In the example of the low back injury intervention, the outcome evaluation would determine the number of low back injury diagnoses or surgeries within the priority population and determine if the rates were reduced.

The PRECEDE-PROCEED Model in Action

Due to its versatility and theoretical foundation, the PRECEDE-PROCEED model has been used in nearly 1,000 published programs. One such program is the My Body Knows When dietary intervention (Cole & Horacek, 2009, 2010). Aimed at teaching military spouses the principles of intuitive eating and physical activity as a means of improving diet and reducing body weight, the program used the PRECEDE-PROCEED model to design, implement, and evaluate the intervention. During the PRECEDE phase, the researchers used surveys to assess the social, epidemiological, behavioral and environmental, educational and organizational, and administrative and policy measures and determinants (Cole & Horacek, 2009). Additional epidemiologic information was collected using anthropometric measures such as BMI. The researchers ranked the determinants identified during the five assessment phases and were then able to establish the program objectives and choose intervention components to correspond with the objectives. For example, during the social assessment (Phase I), it was discovered that the top two life stressors reported by participants related to body image and weight concerns. Therefore, a program objective and corresponding intervention activity were designed to improve body image.

In the PROCEED portion of the model, the intervention was implemented and evaluated (Cole & Horacek, 2010). During the process evaluation, participant attrition and satisfaction were assessed, and the information was used to adjust the program accordingly. For example, participants reported they could not attend the intervention sessions because of child-care issues, so the researchers began offering free child-care services during the times of the intervention meetings. The impact evaluation assessed the effects of the intervention immediately upon its completion and included surveying participants about their body image or attitudes toward food and comparing responses to preintervention data. Finally, the outcome evaluation assessed whether the intervention achieved its overall goal of improving diet content and reducing body weight. This was performed through surveys and anthropometric measures.

PATCH MODEL

PATCH, or the Planned Approach to Community Health model (Kreuter, Nelson, Stoddard, & Watkins, 1985), was developed by the CDC in the mid-1980s in response to a federal grant program called the Health Education-Risk Reduction Grants Program. PATCH was designed to improve the capabilities of state and local health departments and was largely based on the PRECEDE model. PATCH not only provides a model for program planning but also places a strong emphasis on community involvement and encourages communication among local, state, and national health organizations. The design of PATCH inspired the development of the PROCEED model (Green & Kreuter, 1992).

Phases of the PATCH Model

PATCH includes five phases: mobilizing the community, collecting and organizing data, choosing health priorities, developing an intervention plan, and evaluating PATCH. The first phase, mobilizing the community, involves gaining support from the target community. The target community is defined and participants are recruited. A demographic profile of the community is completed so that the individuals conducting PATCH can understand the community they are targeting. Partnerships are formed and the steering committee and working groups are formed in this phase. Also, the community is informed about the program to increase support.

The second phase of PATCH is collecting and organizing data. The working groups collect and analyze data regarding all facets of community health including mortality, morbidity, behaviors, and knowledge. The data are collected via varying methods including mining preexisting data, administering surveys, and conducting interviews, and are therefore both quantitative and qualitative. The data collected allow the PATCH participants to identify the leading health issues within the community and the behaviors contributing to the problem. In phase three, the community group ranks the health issues and analyzes all behavioral, social, economic, political, and environmental factors that influence the risk for poor health outcomes. It then selects the priority issues that will be addressed and establishes related objectives.

The fourth phase of PATCH includes developing and implementing a comprehensive intervention plan. The intervention components are selected based on the information collected during the previous three phases. The community group assesses prior programs, preexisting resources, and policies that may be applied to the intervention. The group develops an intervention plan based on its objectives that includes strategies, a timeline, and procedures for data collection, publicity, and evaluation. Once the plan is set, the intervention is implemented.

PATCH is formally evaluated in the fifth phase of the model, although the evaluation process is ongoing throughout the intervention. The evaluation assesses the successes or shortcomings of the intervention as it is being implemented and allows for appropriate adjustments to be made. A "successful" intervention must meet criteria set by the community. Following the completion of the intervention, the overall program is evaluated. The results are presented to the community to promote participation in future efforts.

APEX-PH MODEL

The Assessment Protocol for Excellence in Public Health, or APEX-PH model, was released by the National Association of County & City Health Officials (NACCHO) and the CDC in 1991 as a self-assessment tool for local health departments to "improve organizational capacity and strengthen their leadership role in their communities" (NACCHO, 1991, 2007).

APEX-PH is designed to be completed voluntarily by public health departments as a means of evaluating and improving effectiveness. It is a flexible and adaptable tool in that it can be altered to suit the unique resources available to any organization that uses the model and can also be combined with other planning tools. Originally available as a workbook, the tool can now also be utilized as an interactive online program available for purchase.

Completing APEX-PH can greatly benefit a health department in several ways. During the self-assessment process, the department is able to identify its strengths and weaknesses, enhance the community's involvement, increase public understanding of current health issues, and establish leadership within the community. The final result leads to the development of an appropriate plan of action for the future of the department. Although the benefits of the process are considerable, the process is ongoing and requires diligence and commitment to follow through. Prior to embarking on the APEX-PH process, the department director or management team must fully assess if the resources and time necessary to complete the APEX-PH process and to act on the results are available. For example, if through the APEX-PH process it is discovered that a new employee training program must be developed, the planners must try to anticipate whether it will be possible to accomplish this.

Phases of the APEX-PH Model

APEX-PH is a three-part process; it includes organizational capacity assessment, community process, and completing the cycle. The organizational capacity assessment is an internal assessment of the department's capabilities. During this phase, the department identifies and analyzes its strengths, weaknesses, and resources, then prioritizes the identified problems. The department develops an action plan for the next phases and prepares for data collection and analysis.

The community process is the data collection component of APEX-PH. During this second phase, both health data and community opinion data are collected. Health data will usually come from preexisting databases such as department or state records. Key community members are often surveyed or interviewed to determine the community's perceptions of its health problems. The health department is then able to identify its role in addressing the health problems. Health issues are prioritized by order of importance and changeability.

The third phase is completing the cycle. This phase is the culmination of all the research and data collection in the previous phases. The department uses the information it has collected to develop policies or interventions to improve health problems. Along with designing the next steps, the department also creates a plan for carrying them out. This requires ensuring that appropriate resources and partnerships are available to implement the plans and to evaluate their ongoing success.

The APEX-PH Model in Action

Since its publication, the APEX-PH model has been successfully applied within local health departments across the country. In fact, during its development in the late 1980s, the model was pilot tested in multiple rounds in more than 20 departments in the United States and revised based on the feedback received. Numerous state and local health departments utilized APEX-PH throughout the 1990s, such as Northern Kentucky Independent County (Kalos, Kent, & Gates, 2005; www .nkyhealth.org). Currently, the APEX-PH has been largely overtaken by more recent models; however, the key features of the model have been incorporated into several other models including IPLAN, PACE-EH, and MAPP.

MAPP MODEL

Mobilizing for Action through Planning and Partnerships (MAPP) is a strategic planning tool developed by NACHHO and the CDC and was first published in 2001 (NACCHO, 2001). MAPP was designed to provide communities with a framework for improving health and the overall quality of life throughout the entire community by identifying its resources and needs and establishing partnerships for strategic action. Several principles are critical to the implementation of MAPP, including using traditional strategic planning concepts, using systems thinking to emphasize the relationships among all units in the public health system, developing a shared vision, using data at each step, developing partnerships, using dialogue to represent all segments of the community, and celebrating success.

Communities that use MAPP can expect to experience many positive outcomes (NACCHO, 2001). Implementing MAPP strengthens partnerships within the local health organizations, allowing for more efficient use of resources and improved communication. Furthermore, by including the community throughout the process, local public health systems gain community support and bring attention to public health. Once the residents are aware of the health issues within their community, they may take ownership and strive to actively engage in the process for solving future issues. By bolstering public support for public health, the local organizations can continue to develop and implement successful programs. The cumulative effect of these benefits is an improved quality of life within the community, which is the ultimate goal of MAPP.

Phases of the MAPP Model

The MAPP process consists of six phases. The first phase, organizing for success and developing partnerships, aims to outline the planning process and identify who will be involved. Several steps are followed during this phase. First, the lead organizations should determine if and why the MAPP process is needed in their community and what they expect to get out of the process. Once it is determined that the plan is necessary, participants are identified and recruited. Ideally, participants will come from diverse organizations within the community and will also include community residents. Participants should include individuals who provide public health services. Participants are organized and subcommittees are formed by assessing their availability and expectations. The participants design the planning process by asking and answering certain questions like, "What steps need to be taken?" "How long will they take?" and "What results do we expect?" Once the plan is in place, participants assess the resource needs, such as meeting space and data collection costs, and secure commitment from the participating organizations that can provide the resources. The information gathered to this point forms a clear view of how prepared the community is to embark on the MAPP process, and a readiness assessment is performed to make certain all elements are ready. To complete the first phase of MAPP, participants plan how the rest of the process will be managed to ensure its success.

visioning is a process of structured brainstorming by program stakeholders that culminates in a statement of vision and values for a program.

The second phase in MAPP is **visioning**. Visioning is a process of structured brainstorming that culminates in a statement of vision and values. A vision statement should describe the capabilities the community and/or program hope to have in the future (i.e., "A community with an established system of preventive services that is available to all community members"). A value statement should explicitly state the priorities of the community and/or program (i.e., "This community is dedicated to providing equal access to preventive services"). Visioning takes place after an appropriate facilitator is selected and past visioning efforts in the community are identified. Visioning can be performed either as a community activity during which up to 100 residents convene, as a smaller meeting of key leadership figures, or at a large meeting with both residents and leadership figures. The larger, broader community meetings can begin the process of mobilizing the community but may require a large amount of resources to implement. The facilitator-led meetings identify common values and a shared vision of the future of the community, 5 to 10 years into the future. The vision and value statements become the constant driving force of the MAPP effort.

Four key assessments are conducted in the third phase of the MAPP process. The assessments are considered to be the strength and unique feature of the MAPP model and form the foundation of the process (NACCHO, 2001). The cumulative results of the four assessments show the gap between the community's current circumstances and their shared vision for the future. The first assessment, the Community Themes and Strengths Assessment (CTSA), is a qualitative appraisal of the community's opinions on what issues are most important. The CTSA can be scheduled to coincide with preestablished meetings such as PTA or town hall meetings or can be done through focus groups or one-on-one interviews. The second assessment is the Local Public Health System Assessment (LPHSA), which focuses on units in a community that contribute to public health services, or the local public health system. The LPHSA uses the 10 Essential Public Health Services (CDC, 2013) as a guide for assessing the local public health system. The third assessment, the Community Health Status Assessment (CHSA), identifies and prioritizes the current health issues faced by the community. The data collected during the CHSA allow the MAPP committee to compare the community's status and issues with peer communities and even national statistics. The fourth and final assessment in this phase is the Forces of Change Assessment (FCA). The FCA pinpoints the forces that are currently affecting or could in the future affect the community's health and quality of life. Examples of such forces include legislation, migration, or environmental changes. The information acquired during the assessments phase becomes a resource when identifying the strategic issues in the next phase of the model.

The fourth phase of MAPP is to identify strategic issues, or the "fundamental policy choices or critical challenges that must be addressed for a community to achieve its vision" (NACCHO, 2001). Identifying strategic issues is a precise process. MAPP participants must first come up with a list of all potential strategic issues identified during the assessment phase. Then they must discuss each issue and come to an understanding about why it is strategic. To prioritize the potential strategic issues, the group must discuss what the possible consequences are of leaving it unaddressed. Once the list is complete, overlapping issues can be consolidated and then arranged in order of importance. The MAPP team now has a prioritized list of strategic issues to focus on.

Goal statements pertaining to each strategic issue and broad strategies for achieving the goals are developed in the fifth phase of the MAPP model. Goals answer the question, "What do we want to achieve?" and strategies answer the question, "How do we want to achieve it?" (NACCHO, 2001). During this phase, the participants should consider the barriers they may encounter during implementation and develop back-up strategies. They also begin to consider the implementation of each strategy. The sixth phase of the MAPP model is the action cycle, which includes the planning, implementation, and evaluation of the program. Planning includes the development of specific program objectives and action plans. Implementation puts the plan in action. Evaluation of the project will determine its success and areas for improvement. This final MAPP phase culminates with recognizing the hard work that was done and celebrating the successes.

The MAPP Model in Action

The MAPP model is widely used across the United States. Numerous state and local health departments are currently implementing the MAPP process and have published their plans and progress on health department websites as a means of keeping the community informed and involved. For instance, Arlington, Virginia, has begun a program using the MAPP process called Destination 2017: Envisioning Public Health for the Future (http://www.arlingtonva.us/). The Arlington Human Services website provides the public with an overview of the

MAPP model and publishes the results of each phase as it is completed. This type of publicity is not unique to Arlington and demonstrates the success of MAPP in fostering community awareness and involvement.

CDCYNERGY MODEL

CDCynergy is a health communication model grounded in social marketing (CDC, 2003; 2010). CDCynergy is an interactive CD-ROM and web-based tool. CDCynergy was initially designed for use as a general planning model for health communication programs within the CDC but has since been modified and released for public use in numerous editions addressing specific health problems. In addition to the basic edition, other currently available editions include the cardiovascular edition, micronutrients edition, diabetes edition, tobacco prevention and control edition, American Indian/Alaskan Native diabetes edition, emergency risk communication edition, social marketing edition, and STD prevention edition.

Phases of the CDCynergy Model

The design of CDCynergy was based on a marketing model that had been successful for designing, implementing, and evaluating health communications programs. The model contains six phases, each with numerous steps. The first phase describes the problem. Although it sounds simple, the description must be thoroughly researched and precise. The problem statement can be very brief (i.e., "Unprotected sex causes serious public health issues, including sexually transmitted infections and unplanned pregnancies"), or it can be very detailed to include specific rates and population demographics. Program planners first write a concise problem statement, assess its relevance to the particular program, and research what the problem is and the groups affected by it. Based on the groups identified, planners develop a problem statement for each subgroup they plan to target and continue to gather information on the problem. At this time, planners also assess what issues may affect the project's progress, including strengths, weaknesses, opportunities, and threats (SWOT; CDC, 2003).

The second phase of CDCynergy is analyzing the problem identified in phase one. Planners determine both the direct and indirect causes of each problem, prioritize and choose subproblems for the intervention, and study theories pertinent to the possible interventions. After considering the SWOT and ethics of each option, interventions are selected for each subproblem. Planners identify resources and partners from whom they can obtain funding and with whom they can form partnerships.

The intervention planning takes place during the third phase and is when communication planning begins. For each problem, planners must determine whether communication will be a dominant intervention or used as support for other interventions and write communication goals for all subgroups of the audience that will be targeted. Establishing the subgroups is done through audience segmentation, in which a large group is segmented based on common traits such as age. Once initial communication goals are established, planners engage in formative research to define each audience segment and identify the best practices for health communication within the targeted segments. The planners then rewrite the communication goals as measurable objectives that describe what the audience segments should gain. Along with the communication objectives, planners write a creative brief that summarizes key findings and the intended methods of reaching the audience. The objectives and creative brief are presented to stakeholders who must approve the plans.

Phase four is the intervention development. Using the creative brief and objectives as a guide, planners work with partners to select and test the creative concepts, messages, and materials that will make up the intervention. A draft budget and timetable are also developed. The intervention settings, communication activities, and materials are developed, pretested, and produced. Planners finalize the communication plan and present it to stakeholders to obtain their support.

The fifth phase is the evaluation planning, which uses the CDC's *Framework for Program Evaluation in Public Health* (CDC, 1999). The first step in this phase is for planners to identify and meet with stakeholders to determine what information they need and when they need it. They then write a detailed description of the program and write intervention standards for each component of the intervention so that the particular component can be evaluated according to the stakeholders' expectations. Next, the sources and methods of data collection most appropriate for the intervention are selected, such as key informant interviews or secondary data sources. Finally, planners develop an evaluation design that will address the stakeholders' expectations and questions. A plan for data analysis and reporting results to the stakeholders is also developed, as well as an internal and external plan for communicating within and among all units involved. Finally, the evaluation plan is presented to all staff members and stakeholders.

During the sixth phase of the CDCynergy model, the plan is implemented. The sixth phase includes both the intervention and evaluation. During the implementation process, program members document all feedback received from stakeholders and the lessons learned throughout the process. Based on the feedback, the program can be modified as it is being implemented. At the conclusion of the intervention and evaluation, the findings from the evaluation are presented to the stakeholders.

Although it contains steps that overlap with other program planning models, CDCynergy offers some unique features. CDCynergy includes extensive research of and interaction with the priority population and stakeholders. CDCynergy users are guided through a stringent segmentation process and repeatedly engage stakeholders. When successful, CDCynergy programs offer a solid, research-based health communication plan that can greatly impact community health.

LOGIC MODELS

Logic models are widely used tools in public health programs. A logic model is a visual model depicting the associations between what goes into a program or intervention and what results are expected. Popular in part because of their brevity, logic models are not exactly program planning models but instead provide a broader program overview or evaluation model. However, while logic models may be simpler to use than other planning models, they can lack detail about the rationale behind the strategies selected and so are often used in conjunction with more specific program planning models such as PRECEDE-PROCEED.

Key Components of Logic Models

The particulars of a logic model can vary, but the basic structure always includes several key components: inputs, activities, outputs, outcomes, and the program goal (CDC, n.d.) The program goal states the overall purpose of the program. The model should clearly indicate how each component relates to the program goal. The inputs, activities, and outputs are referred to as the process components of a logic model, and the outcomes are referred to as the outcome components. The inputs of a logic model are the resources that are put into the program or intervention. Inputs include staff, time, funding, partnerships, and equipment. The activities are what the program is doing. Activities are anything from instructional sessions to a communication campaign. Outputs are the results of the activities. For example, if the activity is a class to teach elementary school parent volunteers how to tutor students in math, the output is the number of people who attended the class.

The outcome components are the intended results of the program and can be short term, intermediate, or long term. The short-term outcomes are the immediate effects of the program. Short-term outcomes usually reflect changes in knowledge, attitudes, and skills. Using the previous example of parent volunteer tutoring classes, the immediate outcome is the parents' new tutoring knowledge and skills. The intermediate outcomes take longer to change and include behaviors or policies. In our example, intermediate outcomes are the school requiring students with certain math grades to be tutored. Long-term outcomes are achieved years after the program has begun and represent the overall goals of the program—for instance, increased math scores on standardized tests within the school.

Other components that are often incorporated in a logic model are impacts, assumptions, and external factors (CDC, n.d.; U.S. Department of Justice, 2011). Impacts go a step beyond long-term outcomes by addressing the ultimate effects of the program. Going back to our example, the impact of the program could be increased funding to the school or higher college acceptance rates among the students. Assumptions are the planners' ideas about how the program will work. Specifically, assumptions include how one thinks the program will function, how participants will receive the information, what effect it will have on participants, or how long the funding will last. Although assumptions are based on research and prior experiences, they can be faulty and often are the reason programs are unsuccessful. External factors, also referred to as contextual factors, describe the larger environment in which the program operates. External factors can impact the success of the program and should be accounted for. These factors include the state of the economy, the cultural beliefs of the population, policies, and many others. While it may not be possible to alter external factors, it is important to document them so that planners can bear in mind the effects they may have on program implementation and success.

One problem that planners frequently encounter when using logic models is that the connection between the program components and the desired outcomes is unclear. A common method for creating a cohesive logic model in which the relationship between the activities and outcomes is clear is using "if-then" statements (CDC, 2010; U.S. Department of Justice, 2011). In an if-then statement, the "if" refers to the program activity and the "then" refers to the outcome. For example, "*if* we teach parents how to tutor math students *then* the students will earn higher grades" and "*if* the students earn higher grades *then* more students may be accepted into college."

Logic Models in Action

Figure 2-4 shows a sample logic model for a program with the goal of reducing incidence of melanoma among student athletes who participate in water sports. As the model shows, it follows this pattern: "*if* the students attend an educational session about the dangers of UV exposure *then* they will be more knowledgeable about skin cancer" and "*if* the students are provided with sunscreen at the pool *then* they will wear sunscreen." The assumptions are: funding will allow sunscreen to be provided to the students free of charge, the students will be receptive to the information, and they will use the sunscreen. The external factors are the social norms regarding sunscreen use and the media's reaction to the program. The impact of the program is reduced incidence of melanoma in the community.

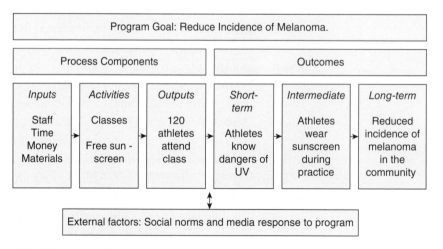

FIGURE 2–4 Sample logic model.

Summary

This chapter provided information on several program planning models. A general planning model was introduced, as well as six other popular models. The key message in this chapter is that program development is a meticulous process involving many steps that is vital to the success of a public health program; it includes identifying stakeholders, setting program goals and objectives, and establishing a system of evaluation to assess whether the program worked.

Review Questions

1. True or False: Planners set program goals and objectives prior to conducting the needs assessment.

2. Which program planning model is based on the principles of social marketing?
   a. CDCynergy
   b. MAPP
   c. APEX-PH
   d. PRECEDE-PROCEED

3. What is the unique feature of the MAPP model?

4. Which program planning model is used to build the capacity of health departments?
   a. Logic model
   b. MAPP
   c. PATCH
   d. APEX-PH

5. Which of the following is NOT a type of program objective?
   a. Evaluation
   b. Process
   c. Outcome
   d. Impact

6. During which phase of the PRECEDE-PROCEED model is the health status of the priority population defined?

    a. Phase I
    b. Phase II
    c. Phase III
    d. Phase IV

7. Priorities are set based on what criteria:

    a. Changeability
    b. Cost effectiveness
    c. Importance
    d. A and B
    e. A and C

8. True or False: Stakeholders only need to be included in the evaluation portion of a program.

9. Which of the following assesses how well a program was delivered compared to how it was designed?

    a. Impact evaluation
    b. Process evaluation
    c. Outcome evaluation
    d. None of the above

10. What does SMART stand for and why is it used in program planning?

11. Why it is important for planners to collect a combination of primary and secondary data when secondary data are often available at no cost?

12. Why do program planners need to involve stakeholders in all steps of program planning? What could happen if planners did not include stakeholders?

Web Resources

Visit the following websites to learn more about some of the topics presented in this chapter.

Centers for Disease Control and Prevention: www.cdc.gov

Centers for Disease Control and Prevention's National Center for Health Statistics: www.cdc.gov/nchs

Healthy People 2020: www.healthypeople.gov

CDCynergy program site: www.cdc.gov/healthcommunication/CDCynergy/

Authors of the PRECEDE-PROCEED Model: www.lgreen.net/precede.htm

National Association of County & City Health Officials' MAPP site: www.naccho.org/topics/infrastructure /MAPP/index.cfm

References

Bickman, L., & Rog, D. J. (1998). *Handbook of applied social research methods.* Thousand Oaks, CA: Sage Publications.

Centers for Disease Control and Prevention (CDC). (1999). Framework for planning evaluation in public health. *Morbidity and Mortality Weekly Report, 48* (RR-11), 1-40.

Centers for Disease Control and Prevention (CDC), United States Department of Health and Human Services. (2003). *CDCynergy 3.0: Your guide to effective health communication* (CD-ROM version 3.0). Atlanta, GA: Author.

Centers for Disease Control and Prevention. (2013). National Public Health Performance Standards Program (NPHPSP). 10 Essential public health services. Available at http://www.cdc.gov/nphpsp /essentialservices.html Accessed August 20, 2014.

Centers for Disease Control and Prevention (2014a). Behavioral Risk Factor Surveillance System Survey Data. Atlanta, Georgia: U.S. Department of Health and Human Services, Centers for Disease Control and Prevention.

Centers for Disease Control and Prevention. (2014a). National Center for Health Statistics (NCHS). National Health and Nutrition Examination Survey Data. Hyattsville, MD: U.S. Department of Health and Human Services, Centers for Disease Control and Prevention.

Center for Disease Control and Prevention (CDC). (n.d.). *State heart disease and stroke prevention program evaluation guide: Developing and using a logic model.* Atlanta, GA: U.S. Department of Health and Human Services, Department of Health and Human Services. Available at http://www.cdc.gov/dhdsp /programs/nhdsp_program/evaluation_guides/docs/logic_model.pdf. Accessed August 19, 2014.

Centers for Disease Control and Prevention (CDC). (2010). *CDCynergy: The Editions.* Available at http://www.cdc.gov/healthcommunication/cdcynergy/editions.html. Accessed August 20, 2014.

Cole, R. E., & Horacek, T. (2009). Applying PRECEDE-PROCEED to develop an intuitive eating nondieting approach to weight management pilot program. *Journal of Nutrition Education and Behavior, 41* (2), 120–126.

Cole, R. E., & Horacek, T. (2010). Effectiveness of the "My Body Knows When" intuitive-eating pilot program. *American Journal of Health Behavior, 34* (3), 286–297.

D'Onofrio, C. N. (2001). "Pooling information about prior interventions: A new program planning tool." In S. Sussman (Ed.), *Handbook of program development for health behavior research and practice* (pp. 158–204). Thousand Oaks, CA: Sage.

Erwin, P. C., Hamilton, C. B., & Welch, S. (2005). Students in the community: MAPP as a framework for academic-public health practice linkages. *Journal of Public Health Management and Practice, 11* (5), 437–441.

Frasure-Smith, N., Lesperance, F., Gravel, G., Masson, A., Juneau, M., Talajic, M., & Bourassa, M. (2000). Social support, depression, and mortality during the first year after myocardial infarction. *Circulation, 101*, 1919–1924.

Glanz, K., Rimer, B. K., & Viswanath, K. (2008). *Health behavior and health education: Theory, research, and practice.* San Francisco, CA: John Wiley & Sons, Inc.

Green, L. W. (1973). *Planning for patient educators: Considerations and implications.* Proceedings of the Maryland Conference on Patient Programming. Rockville, MD: Health Care Facilities Service, Health Resources Administration, DHEW Publication No. (HRA) 74-002.

Green, L. W. (1974). Toward cost-benefit evaluations of health education: Some concepts, methods, and examples. *Health Education Monographs, 2* (S1), 34–64.

Green, L. W., & Kreuter, M. W. (1991). *Health promotion planning: An educational and environmental approach* (2nd ed.). Mountain View, CA: Mayfield Publishing Company.

Green, L. W., & Kreuter, M. W. (1992). CDC's planned approach to community health as an application of PRECEDE and an inspiration for PROCEED. *Journal of Health Education, 23*, 140–147.

Green, L. W., & Kreuter, M. W. (1999). *Health promotion planning: An educational and ecological approach* (3rd ed.). Mountain View, CA: Mayfield Publishing Company.

Green, L. W., & Kreuter, M. W. (2005). *Health program planning: An educational and ecological approach* (4th ed.). New York, NY: McGraw-Hill.

Green, L. W., Kreuter, M. W., Deeds, S. G., & Partridge, K. B. (1980). *Health education planning: A diagnostic approach.* Mountain View, CA: Mayfield Publishing Company.

Howard-Graham, L., & Snetro, G. (2003). *How to mobilize communities for health and social change.* Baltimore, MD: Health Communication Partnership/USAID.

Kalos, A., Kent, L., & Gates, D. (2005). Integrating MAPP, APEXPH, PACE-EH, and other planning initiatives in Northern Kentucky. *Journal of Public Health Management and Practice, 11* (5), 401–406.

Kendall, W. E. (1984). The tools of industrial psychology, in C. Heyel & H. W. Nance (Eds.), *The foreman/ supervisor's handbook* (pp. 364–382). New York: Van Nostrand Reinhold Company Inc.

Kreuter, M. W. (1992). PATCH: Its origin, basic concepts, and links to contemporary public health policy. *Journal of Health Education, 23* (3), 135–139.

Kreuter, M. W., Nelson, C. F., Stoddard, R. P., & Watkins, N. B. (1985). *Planned approach to community health.* Atlanta, GA: Centers for Disease Control.

Leutzinger, J. (2005). *Building Your Wellness Budget.* WELCOA's *Absolute Advantage Magazine, 4*, 2–5.

National Association of County & City Health Officials (NACCHO). (1991). *APEX PH Assessment protocol for excellence in public health.* Washington, DC: Author.

National Association of County & City Health Officials (NACCHO). (2001). *Mobilizing for action through planning and partnerships (MAPP).* Washington, DC: Author.

National Association of County & City Health Officials (NACCHO). (2007, November). APEX*PH*, PACE EH, and MAPP: Local public health planning and assessment at a glance. Available at http://www .naccho.org/topics/infrastructure/mapp/upload/MappPaceApex.pdf. Accessed August 20, 2014.

National Cancer Institute (NCI). (1989). *Making health communications work.* Pub. No. NIH 89-1493. Washington, DC: U.S. Department of Health and Human Services.

Neiger, B. L., Thackeray, R., & Fagan, M. C. (2011). Basic priority rating model 2.0: Current applications for priority setting in health promotion practice. *Health Promotion Practice, 12,* 166–171.

Pickett, G. & Hanlon, J. (1984). *Public health: Administration and practice* (19th ed.). St. Louis, MO: Times Mirror/Mosby College Publishing.

Simons-Morton, B. G., Greene, W. H., & Gottlieb, N. H. (1995). *Introduction to health education and health promotion* (2nd ed.). Prospect Heights, IL: Waveland Press.

Thoits, P. (1995). Stress, coping, and social support processes: Where are we? What next? *J Health Soc Behavior,* Special Issue, 53–79.

Unchino, B. (2004). *Social support and physical health: Understanding the health consequences of relationships.* New Haven, CT: Yale University Press.

U.S. Census Bureau. (2011). *State & county quickfacts.* Available at http://quickfacts.census.gov. Accessed August 19, 2014.

U.S. Department of Health and Human Services (USDHHS). (2012). *Linking between program planning and budget development.* Available at http://eclkc.ohs.acf.hhs.gov/hslc/tta-system/operations/mgmt -admin/planning/planning/manage_pub_00512a_100405.html. Accessed August 19, 2014.

U.S. Department of Health and Human Services (USDHHS). (2014a). *Healthy people 2020: About the data.* Available at http://healthypeople.gov/2020/about/aboutdata.aspx Accessed August 19, 2014.

U.S. Department of Health and Human Services (USDHHS). (2014b). *Healthy people 2020: Physical activity.* Available at http://www.healthypeople.gov/2020/topicsobjectives2020/objectiveslist .aspx?topicId=33 Accessed August 19, 2014.

U.S. Department of Health and Human Services (USDHHS). (2014c). *Healthy people 2020: About healthy people.* Available at http://healthypeople.gov/2020/about/default.aspx Accessed August 19, 2014.

U.S. Department of Justice. (2006). *Guide to program evaluation.* Available at https://www.bja.gov /evaluation/guide/index.htm. Accessed August 19, 2014.

Chapter 3

Kyle Gutzmer, MA, Guadalupe X. Ayala, PhD, MPH, and Elva M. Arredondo, PhD

THEORY IN HEALTH PROMOTION

Key Terms

action
appraisal support
attitude
audience segmentation
behavior
behavioral capability
behavioral intentions
clinical information
  systems
community resources
  and policies
compatibility
complexity
conceptual models
consciousness raising
constructs
contemplation
contingency
  management
counterconditioning
cues to action
decision support
decisional balance

delivery system design
dramatic relief
early adopters
early majority
emotional arousal
  management
emotional support
environmental
  reevaluation
equivalence
exchange
framework
generalization
health care
  organization
helping relationships
informational support
innovators
instrumental support
laggards
late majority
maintenance
marketing mix

messages
model
observability
observational learning
outcome expectancies
outcome expectations
perceived barriers
perceived behavioral
  control
perceived benefits
perceived severity
perceived susceptibility
physical structures
precontemplation
preparation
reciprocal determinism
reinforcement
relative advantage
self-efficacy
self-liberation
self-management
  support
self-reevaluation

social liberation

social proximity

social structures

stimulus control

structural cohesion

subjective norms

termination

trialability

Learning Objectives

Upon completion of this chapter, the reader should be able to:

1. Define the terms "theory," "construct," "model," and "framework."
2. Identify the relevance of theory to public health promotion.
3. Describe what a conceptual model is.
4. Differentiate between theories at four levels of the Social Ecological Framework (individual, interpersonal, organizational, and community).
5. Demonstrate a basic understanding of the key concepts of each theory.
6. Analyze the use of theory in public health research.
7. Recognize limitations of each theory.

Chapter Outline

Theoretical Foundations of Health Promotion
   Importance of Theory to Health Promotion
   Conceptual Models in Health Promotion
Social Ecological Framework
   Application of the Social Ecological Framework
Individual-Level Theories
   The Health Belief Model
   The Transtheoretical Model
   The Theory of Reasoned Action
   The Theory of Planned Behavior
   Behavior Analysis
Interpersonal-Level Theories
   Social Cognitive Theory
   Social Support
   Social Influence
Organizational-Level Theories
   Chronic Care Model
   Diffusion of Innovations
Community-Level Theories
   Information Processing Paradigm
   Social Marketing
   Structural Model of Health Behavior
Special Considerations
   Resources

INTRODUCTION

Being asked to learn theory can seem daunting, even to those with a more inquisitive mind. For some, even the mention of theory elicits images of confusing terminology, complex models, and abstract relationships. Yes, there is some of that; but theory is also a way to put together a set of ideas that helps us understand *how*, *why*, and *what might happen next*. Kerlinger (1973) defined theory more broadly as "a set of interrelated constructs (concepts), definitions, and propositions that presents a systematic view of phenomena by specifying relations among variables or constructs, with the purpose of explaining and predicting phenomena" (p. 9). This definition highlights three important aspects of a theory. (1) A theory must *describe* the current relationships among concepts. (2) A theory must *explain* how these concepts work together to influence behavior. And, (3) a theory must use this explanation to *predict* future behavior. Not all theories provide descriptions, explanations, and predictions. However, theories that do not provide all three are limited rather than complete theories.

THEORETICAL FOUNDATIONS OF HEALTH PROMOTION

constructs are the main concepts of a theory.

A **model** presents and explains relationships between constructs.

framework provides a way of viewing the behavior but does not explain relationships between constructs.

Several terms are important to understand when discussing theories. These include "construct," "model," and "framework." **Constructs** are the main concepts of a theory (National Cancer Institute, 2005). They are the elements of the theory used to describe, explain, and predict behavior. For example, the constructs of the Health Belief Model include perceived susceptibility, perceived severity, perceived benefits, perceived barriers, cues to action, and self-efficacy. A **model** presents and explains relationships between constructs. For example, the Health Belief Model explains how attitudes and beliefs influence behavior. In contrast, a **framework** provides a way of viewing the behavior but does not explain relationships between constructs. For example, the Social Ecological Framework (SEF) describes different levels that influence behavior but does not necessarily explain the specific constructs and how these interact.

When distinguishing among theory, model, and framework, it is helpful to think of the term "theory" as the most all-encompassing of the three. Models and frameworks can exist within theories, the former by outlining a specific set of constructs and how they are related to a behavior, while the latter by providing a general idea of what influences behavior. Despite differences in the terms "theory," "model," and "framework," authors often use them interchangeably.

The next section provides a rationale for using theory in health promotion efforts and then a general orientation to conceptual models.

Importance of Theory to Health Promotion

Previous research indicates that interventions that apply theoretical principles and associated constructs to their design are more effective than those that do not (Glanz & Bishop, 2010). This provides a powerful argument for the importance of theory in practice. One reason for the greater effectiveness of interventions based on theoretical principles and associated constructs may be that theories help us understand behaviors and the process by which behavior change may occur (National Cancer Institute, 2005). For example, the Theory of Reasoned Action postulates that attitudes and beliefs influence intentions and that positive intentions influence behaviors. Theories describe and explain how and why attitudes, beliefs, and social influences such as friends, family, and the media, as well as the environment, influence our health behaviors and ultimately our health. This information is used to create models that predict future health behaviors and thus are relevant to health promotion efforts in that they identify potential targets of change. Theories differ in the extent to which they specify direct influences on health behavior and, as such, differ in their usefulness for informing health promotion interventions. For example, the Transtheoretical Model provides a specific set of processes

Model for Understanding
Application of Theory to Health Promotion

You are tasked with using theory to plan a health promotion intervention to increase physical activity among preteen girls. You ask yourself, "How do I know which theory to use? The list is enormous!" Start by thinking about what is influencing these girls' physical activity and how this might be changed. When making a decision about which theory is most appropriate to use, you need to consider what factors are most influential to increasing (or in some cases, decreasing, e.g., smoking, watching television) the behavior you are interested in and then identify those factors that are modifiable. For example, targeting preteen girls' attitudes and beliefs about physical activity, although modifiable, may be less effective at promoting physical activity than changing their environment, because preteens may be more constrained by their environment (such as limited access to physical activity opportunities) than adults. Also, because increasing physical activity is a long-term change, creating an environment that fosters physical activity may have a more lasting impact than targeting individual attitudes and beliefs.

When examining the application of theory, one should also consider aspects of the target population (i.e., their age, gender, cultural factors) and the target behavior (e.g., is it easy or difficult to perform?; National Cancer Institute, 2005). The theory needs to fit the sociocultural characteristics of the target population and be consistent with the behavior in question. Regarding the former, many theories are based on Western ideals of individualism, which may not be consistent with those of your target population. For example, in our research, we acknowledge the importance of the immediate family and extended family and friends when promoting Latino health; thus, individualistically oriented concepts such as self-efficacy are not always relevant in the communities in which we work (Elder et al., 2009). Regarding the latter, the application of a theory that supports a decrease in smoking should not be automatically applied to increasing physical activity without sufficient evaluation that the pathways are relevant.

to target in an intervention, whereas the Health Belief Model only specifies a relationship. Nevertheless, the use of theory serves as a guide for where to focus health promotion efforts (see the Model for Understanding feature "Application of Theory to Health Promotion").

Theories also allow us to join the academic conversation. One can study which theories past researchers have used with a similar population and health behavior currently being examined. Current findings build upon the work of others, changing, specifying, and updating the theories used. In this way, modern health promotion is influenced by theory, and, in turn, influences and changes theory. This process of theory building, destroying, and reconstruction forms the foundation of scientific progress and disseminates knowledge for future generations.

Conceptual Models in Health Promotion

conceptual models are physical depictions of causal relationships between constructs.

Conceptual models are a physical depiction of causal relationships between constructs (Earp & Ennett, 1991). Conceptual models can be used to depict a theory, to depict several theories, or to illustrate findings. Conceptual models, however, are not "theories" in their own right; they do not specify a common set of constructs that ultimately predict a behavior or other outcome. However, similar to theories, researchers use conceptual models to guide the design of health promotion interventions, and conceptual models are commonly used to succinctly explain how variables are related to each other in a potentially causal pathway.

Figure 3-1 presents an example of a simple conceptual model depicting three factors that may influence a college football player's use of chewing tobacco.

Figure 3-1 represents constructs in boxes and illustrates the relationships between constructs using arrows. This conceptual model, like most conceptual models, is read from left to right. The left side indicates the influences and the right side indicates the outcome of interest. In this model, teammates' use of chewing tobacco and knowledge of the health risk associated with chewing tobacco influence one's use of chewing tobacco. Additionally, the relationship of teammate use of chewing tobacco to one's use of chewing tobacco is further influenced by the importance of teammates to one's self-concept. This

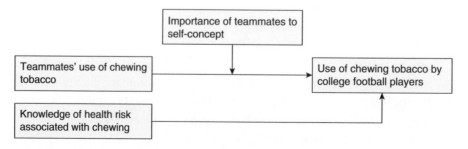

FIGURE 3-1 Conceptual model depicting factors that may influence a college player's use of chewing tobacco.

relationship is referred to as moderation. In this case, the importance the player places on his teammates for his self-concept will determine how much influence his teammates' behaviors will have over his own behaviors. This conceptual model depicts one health problem (chewing tobacco) and one target population (college football players). Thus it is distinguished from theoretical models, like the Health Belief Model, in that it specifies a limited set of factors that may influence the behavior.

In the next section, the SEF is presented to help guide the subsequent presentation of theories at each level of influence specified in the SEF. The SEF has guided much of health promotion research over the last 30 years given that it considers multiple levels of influence on health behaviors, making it one of the most relevant frameworks in the field of health promotion.

THE SOCIAL ECOLOGICAL FRAMEWORK

Think about the diverse factors influencing whether you are physically active. Why do you exercise the way you do (or neglect to exercise)? The SEF argues that factors ranging from one's personal beliefs to the way neighborhoods are designed will influence physical activity. The SEF explores the impact of multiple levels of influence on behavior (Stokols, 1992), including individual-, interpersonal-, organizational-, and community-level factors. These levels exert a direct influence on behaviors as well as interact with each other to influence behaviors.

Individual-level factors include personal opinions, beliefs, and attitudes that influence behavior. An example of an individual-level factor would be a person's enjoyment of physical activity. If an individual does not enjoy physical activity and instead believes that exercise is monotonous, then she is less likely to be physically active. Theories that consider individual-level influences are Classical and Operant Conditioning, the Health Belief Model, the Transtheoretical Model, the Theory of Reasoned Action, and the Theory of Planned Behavior.

Interpersonal-level factors are influences that derive from interactions with others. These include not only how family, friends, and peers think about a behavior but whether they engage in the behavior as well. An example of an interpersonal-level factor would be how often a friend goes to exercise class with you. If you have the support of your friend, whether in the form of encouragement or driving you to the gym, you may be more likely to attend the exercise class. Theories that consider interpersonal-level factors include Social Cognitive Theory, Social Support, and Social Influence.

Organizational-level factors are the values, policies, and routines of particular institutions and groups. An example of an organizational-level factor would be physicians at a certain hospital being required to refer obese patients to a free exercise program. In this case, an organizational policy may increase physicians' referrals to the exercise program and thus increase the physical activity of the physicians' patients. Theories that consider organizational-level factors include the Chronic Care Model and Diffusion of Innovations.

Community-level factors have the broadest scope and examine population-level factors. An example of a community-level factor for exercise would be how many parks have adequate lighting and are safe for people of all ages. Some studies show that parks with better lighting are more likely to be used by community members for exercise (Kaczynski, Potwarka, & Saelens, 2008). Theories that consider community-level factors include several communication theories such as Information Processing Paradigm and Social Marketing and the Structural Model of Health Behavior.

Authors differ on the labels and categories used for the different levels of the SEF. For example, some authors examine intrapersonal factors, social environments, physical environments, and policies. However, the essence of the SEF is that examining multiple levels of influence facilitates our understanding of where health promotion efforts are more urgently needed for sustained behavior change.

Application of the Social Ecological Framework

Sallis and colleagues (2006) illustrated use of the SEF to foster an active lifestyle. An active lifestyle involves physical activity not only as a leisure-time activity but also in the form of household chores, use of active transportation, and activity during work. Sallis used the SEF to visually depict these four types of physical activity and the various factors at multiple levels of influence that facilitate or create barriers for engaging in physical activity: intrapersonal, interpersonal, social environment, physical environment, and policy levels.

Intrapersonal factors include psychological, biological, and demographic variables. Interpersonal factors include family, friend, and peer influences such as the provision of social support and what these individuals role model in their daily lives. Social environmental factors include factors like social norms that are held by a particular community; for example, in some racial/ethnic communities, doing exercise for fun is not part of the culture. Perceived environment, an aspect of physical environment, incorporates factors such as perceived safety and attractiveness of the environment (e.g., is your neighborhood known for its gang activity and thus not conducive for walking?). Behavior settings, also an aspect of the physical environment, include factors such as the design and layout of the neighborhood and school environments (e.g., are you exposed to graffiti or do you see trees when you walk from home to school?). Lastly, the policy environment includes factors such as health care policy, zoning codes, and park policies. Sallis and colleagues argue that the best way to encourage an active lifestyle is to target as many levels of influence as possible by adopting a multilevel, multidisciplinary approach to promoting physical activity. Unfortunately, such efforts require a long time frame, significant funding, and extensive collaborations that are not always possible to foster with available resources.

The remaining sections will present theories that address factors at each level of the SEF, along with a conclusion section presenting limitations of this research and where health promotion theory needs to go next.

INDIVIDUAL-LEVEL THEORIES

How do your thoughts, feelings, and attitudes influence your health behaviors? For example, what thoughts, feelings, and attitudes influence what you eat? Do you drink soda because you believe it will provide the energy you need to pay attention in class regardless of what it will do to your waistline? Most individual-level theories focus on a person's thoughts, feelings, and attitudes toward the health behavior. These theories include the Health Belief Model, the Transtheoretical Model, and the Theory of Reasoned Action/Theory of Planned Behavior. One theory, Behavior Analysis, focuses less on these cognitive processes and instead on skill and performance deficits and the factors that reinforce or inhibit engagement of these behaviors.

The Health Belief Model

According to the Health Belief Model (HBM), beliefs and knowledge about a health behavior and its consequences affect whether the behavior is enacted. The HBM explores the influence of these beliefs and knowledge on a variety of health behaviors and health outcomes. The first version of this model emerged in the 1950s in Hochbaum and Rosenstock's work to examine prevention behaviors. Rosenstock, Janz Becker, and others further refined the theory to its current form (Janz, Champion, & Strecher, 2002). The Health Belief Model is a value expectancy theory. It is based on the assumption that if a person values an outcome (i.e., losing weight) and believes that a particular behavior (i.e., running daily) will help him achieve that outcome, then he is more likely to adopt that behavior.

The first models included the constructs of perceived susceptibility, perceived benefits, perceived barriers, and cues to action (Hochbaum, 1958). Later models added self-efficacy (Rosenstock, Strecher, & Becker, 1988). Researchers can assess participants' attitudes and beliefs by measuring the following constructs with questionnaires or interviews and then tailor their feedback based on these attitudes and beliefs. To understand how we can apply the concepts in an intervention, let us imagine we are assessing cigarette smoking in adolescent males. We are interested in factors influencing their decision to quit smoking. We plan to measure these concepts with a questionnaire. We could use the following constructs to craft our questions. The following concepts were defined by Rosenstock (1974).

- **Perceived susceptibility** is the belief that one is likely to contract a particular disease, condition, or negative health outcome. Perceived susceptibility is a person's *subjective* belief about risk rather than an objective measure. For example: In your opinion, how likely are you to develop lung cancer from cigarette smoking?

- **Perceived severity** is a person's belief in the negative consequences of contracting the disease, condition, or negative health outcome. It can include both negative health outcomes and negative personal or social outcomes as a result

perceived susceptibility is the belief that one is likely to contract a particular disease, condition, or negative health outcome.

perceived severity is a person's belief in the extent of negative consequences of contracting the disease, condition, or negative health outcome.

of contracting the disease. For example: How would your social life suffer if you developed lung cancer?

- **Perceived benefits** of taking action interact with perceived susceptibility and perceived severity. Specifically, if a person views a particular action as reducing susceptibility or severity, the individual will view the action as beneficial. The more a health behavior reduces perceived susceptibility and severity, the more beneficial. For example: How much will quitting smoking (taking action) reduce your chances of developing lung cancer? Will taking action add quality of life?

- **Perceived barriers** are obstacles to performing the recommended health behavior. Some individuals weigh the perceived benefits with the perceived barriers to determine if the action is worthwhile (Janz & Becker, 1984). For example: Do most of your close friends smoke, making it more difficult for you to quit?

- **Cues to action** are "triggers" for the proposed health behavior. Health promotion interventions informed by the HBM often consider this construct in their design. For example, a poster promoting smoking cessation in a bar's bathroom could function as a cue to not smoke despite the many temptations that might be present in this environment. Cues to action function as the prompting event. Interventionists using HBM focus on creating the ideal cues to prompt engagement in the behavior. They can be internal or external cues, the latter of which can take the form of billboards, public broadcasting commercials, and a myriad of other approaches. One group of researchers (Richard, Kosatsky, & Renouf, 2011) explored cues to air conditioning use during extreme ambient heat among chronically ill middle-aged and older adults. They examined both internal and external cues. Internal cues included how sensitive the person was to heat, and external cues included whether the person had heard an extreme heat warning or had been informed by a physician or nurse about how his or her chronic health condition influences heat sensitivity.

- **Self-efficacy,** within the context of health behavior, is one's perceived confidence in performing a specific health behavior (Rosenstock et al., 1988). Early versions of the HBM did not include self-efficacy, in part because the health behaviors upon which it was founded were relatively simple (i.e., vaccinations), and perceived confidence was not identified as an important construct to consider. In contrast, behaviors requiring habitual change, like diet and exercise, were perceived as more challenging to change and maintain. Thus Rosenstock and colleagues (1988) added self-efficacy to the model. Self-efficacy has been identified as an important construct to consider in the behavior-change process. As one might expect, higher levels of self-efficacy are associated with a greater likelihood of engaging in the behavior. For example, individuals who hold stronger beliefs that they can quit smoking are more likely to resist the temptation to smoke despite possible cues to do otherwise.

One critique of the HBM is that it does not present specific guidelines for health promotion interventions. Rather, the constructs are loosely applied. Another critique is that the HBM highlights the cognitive decision-making process and assumes that "people decide what to do based on the extent to which they expect their choices will produce results they value" (Jeffery, 2004, p. 4). However,

Model for Understanding

Using HBM to Design a Hypertension Intervention for the U.S. Hmong Community

One study described the use of the HBM to design health promotion campaigns to address hypertension in the U.S. Hmong community (Thalacker, 2011). Hmong people are from Laos, a small country near Thailand. The construct of perceived susceptibility was especially important to consider with this community because the Hmong view disease as a *felt* condition. Given that hypertension is not a physically painful condition, many Hmong do not view themselves as susceptible and, as a result, do not seek diagnosis or treatment of hypertension. In terms of perceived benefit, many Hmong are reluctant to accept Western disease treatment and instead turn to shamans and herbal medicines. As a result, behaving as prescribed by Western health care providers may not be perceived as a benefit. Perceived barriers include factors such as health care costs, accessibility to care, and community resources. These barriers would need to be considered in any intervention. Finally, cues to action could take the form of a group leader promoting diagnosis and treatment of hypertension, as this is consistent with the Hmong culture and community.

behavior is not always based on a rational decision-making process. A model emphasizing cognitive decision making neglects substantial evidence that behavior change can occur without rational decision making. The HBM also assumes that individuals understand their health condition and have the ability to make rational decisions based on their understanding. This is not always the case, particularly among less educated populations. Additionally, the HBM takes for granted that individuals view their health as important and have the ability to address health needs (Crosby, Kegler, & DiClemente, 2002). Individuals with fewer resources often have to prioritize other needs, for example, a roof over their head, before they can attend to physical ailments. Finally, the HBM, like the other individual-level theories, does not take into account relevant social and environmental factors (Brewer & Rimer, 2008).

The Transtheoretical Model

The Transtheoretical Model (TTM) frames health behavior as progressing through a series of stages and offers direction on how to promote behavior change in these various stages. In his research, Prochaska (1979) identified several processes of change that can be applied to a variety of behaviors. Prochaska later clarified his theory to include 10 processes of change in five stages (Prochaska & DiClemente, 1983). Some processes of change are more relevant than others at the various stages. For example, consciousness raising, which involves becoming aware of the problem, is more relevant at the earlier stages and less relevant at the later stages of change. Thus, motivating people to action involves understanding both their stage of change and the processes of change most applicable to them.

Stages of Change

The stages of change as defined by Prochaska, Redding, and Evers (2002) are pre-contemplation, contemplation, preparation, action, maintenance, and relapse. The stages represent an individual's stage at a particular time.

In the **precontemplation** stage, the person is not considering making a change. A person may occupy this stage for several reasons. At this stage. one is more apt to see the downsides of performing the change. One is unlikely to seek information about change because one sees no reason for change. A person may have attempted a change in the past and have now given up because of previous failure. In the **contemplation** stage, the person is intending to change in the near future (usually defined as 6 months). The person is often weighing the pros and cons of perform-ing the action. She may occupy this stage for a prolonged time before moving to preparation. In the **preparation** stage, the person is intending to change in the near future (usually defined as 1 month) and has done small actions to get ready for change. For example, at the preparation stage, a person could purchase a gym membership to prepare to get more physical activity. This stage can also include planning how the change will occur or consulting with experts. In the **action** stage, the person is either performing the desired behavior or not performing the unde-sired behavior. In the **maintenance** stage, the person has incorporated the change into daily life (usually for at least 6 months). Nonetheless, because the change is new, there is still a chance of relapse. A classic example of this stage is a smoker who has given up smoking but still desires to smoke. Although the person is no longer smoking, the temptation remains. In the **termination** stage, she has incorporated the change and is not tempted to relapse. For many behaviors, this stage is not relevant.

Decisional Balance. Decisional balance is the perception of the relative benefits and disadvantages of performing the behavior (Prochaska et al., 2002). Decisional balance is important in moving from one stage to another. For ex-ample, if a woman is in the preparation stage and has purchased a gym mem-bership to prepare for exercise, she has already realized many of the benefits of exercise. These benefits may have motivated her to consider exercising and pre-pare for exercising. The more benefits to exercising identified, the more likely she is to move from the preparation stage to the action stage. In contrast, the more she perceives the disadvantages to changing, the less progress she is likely to make through the stages.

Self-efficacy. Self-efficacy is how confident one feels in successfully making and maintaining a change. The construct of self-efficacy in the TTM is similar to the construct of self-efficacy in the HBM.

Processes of Change

Processes of change were identified by Prochaska (1979) in his comparative analy-sis of the various forms of therapy. These processes function as "the overt activi-ties that people use to progress through stages" (Prochaska et al., 2002, p. 103). The 10 processes include consciousness raising, dramatic relief, self-reevaluation,

precontemplation stage is when the person is not consider-ing making a change.

contemplation is a stage in which the person is intending to change in the near future (usually defined as 6 months). The person is often weighing the pros and cons of performing the action.

preparation stage is when the person is intending to change in the near future (usually defined as 1 month) and has done small actions to get ready for change.

action stage is when the person is performing the desired behavior or not performing the undesirable behavior for at least 30 days.

maintenance is the stage in which the person has incorpo-rated the change into daily life (usually for at least 6 months).

termination is the stage when a person has incorporated the change and is not tempted to relapse.

decisional balance is the perception of the relative benefits and disadvantages of performing the behavior.

environmental reevaluation, social liberation, helping relationships, counterconditioning, contingency management, stimulus control, and self-liberation. The first five are considered experiential and the latter five are considered behavioral. Interventionists can use these processes to motivate change in their target population. Certain processes of change are more beneficial at certain stages than others (Prochaska & DiClemente, 1983). For example, experiential (cognitive and emotional) processes (i.e., dramatic relief) are more relevant at earlier stages of change than are behavioral processes. Behavioral processes (i.e., contingency management), on the other hand, are more relevant at later stages of change. Each process functions to move individuals from one stage to another (Prochaska et al., 2002). In fact, one of the main contributions of the TTM is its discussion of how particular behavior-change strategies, or processes, are more effective for particular stages than others. This is critical information for those interested in promoting health behavior change.

Let us imagine that you are designing an intervention to reduce chewing tobacco use in male college football players. You could use the processes of change, defined by Prochaska and colleagues (2002), as follows.

Consciousness Raising. **Consciousness raising** is using new information to become more aware of a problem. Information can come from diverse sources. For example, college football players could become more aware of the negative health effects of chewing tobacco from an ad campaign, a physician's explanation, a segment on the news, or a school textbook.

> **consciousness raising** is using new information to become more aware of a problem.

Dramatic Relief. **Dramatic relief** is an emotional reaction to the problem behavior. Taking action to improve the behavior reduces the negative emotions. For example, personal testimonies, emotional media campaigns, and role playing could serve to encourage college football players to quit chewing tobacco. Anything that causes an individual to have an emotional response to the problem behavior is an example of the application of dramatic relief to the behavior change process.

> **dramatic relief** is an emotional reaction to the problem behavior. Taking action to improve the behavior reduces the negative emotions.

Self-Reevaluation. **Self-reevaluation** is conceptualizing the self with the problem behavior and without the problem behavior and then differentiating between these two possible identities to make a decision about which type of person to be. For example, self-reevaluation could include a football player picturing himself regularly chewing tobacco or not and what these two identities mean for that player.

> **self-reevaluation** is conceptualizing the self with the problem behavior and without the problem behavior and then differentiating between these two possible identities to make a decision about which type of person to be.

> **environmental reevaluation** is assessing how the behavior impacts others and society and can include both mental and emotional strategies.

Environmental Reevaluation. **Environmental reevaluation** is assessing how the behavior impacts others and society. This can include both mental and emotional strategies. For example, through empathy training or testimonies, the college football player could determine the effects of his behavior on younger players. This evaluation could be cognitive (e.g., a rational assessment of his behavior's impact), affective (e.g., "I don't want to harm my teammates"), or both.

> **social liberation** refers to changing social norms to promote healthy behaviors.

Social Liberation. **Social liberation** refers to changing social norms to promote healthy behaviors. For example, rather than spending time with teammates who frequently chew tobacco, the football player could find an alternative group that does not chew tobacco. Social liberation can also include advocacy for change at a societal level, which in turn can result in changes in social norms. An excellent example of this is changes in smoking policies in restaurants and bars, which have resulted in a more negative view of smoking.

Helping Relationships. **Helping relationships** emphasizes the role of trusting, nurturing relationships in promoting change. For example, teammates who have quit chewing tobacco could help those who are interested in quitting.

Counterconditioning. **Counterconditioning** involves replacement. Rather than changing a behavior by eliminating it and leaving a void, one replaces the unhealthy behavior with a healthy behavior. An example is replacing chewing tobacco with sunflower seeds.

Contingency Management. **Contingency management** is a type of behavioral conditioning. It frames behavior change as motivated through reinforcements for healthy behavior. For example, rewarding oneself with a dollar of spending money for each tobacco-free day is a type of contingency management. This process can also include social rewards in the form of group recognition after reaching a goal.

Stimulus Control. **Stimulus control** refers to the use of cues or prompts to promote healthy behaviors and counter engagement in unhealthy behaviors. For example, if a football player typically stops at a convenience store to pick up chewing tobacco on his way home from practice, he could control this stimulus by taking a different route home, thus removing the cue (the convenience store) for the unhealthy behavior.

Self-Liberation. **Self-liberation** is the belief that change is possible and the person has a personal commitment to follow through with the change. For example, a football player could hold the belief that he can successfully quit chewing tobacco and therefore be motivated to sign a personal commitment to quit.

helping relationships emphasizes the role of trusting, nurturing relationships in promoting change.

counterconditioning involves replacing one behavior with another. Rather than changing a behavior by eliminating it and leaving a void, one replaces the unhealthy behavior with a healthy behavior.

contingency management is a type of behavioral conditioning that frames behavior change as motivated through reinforcements for healthy behavior.

stimulus control refers to the removal of factors associated with unhealthy behaviors.

self-liberation is the belief that change is possible and the person has a personal commitment to follow through with the change.

Model for Understanding
Smoking Intention in Dire Dawna Town, Ethiopia

Girma, Assefa, and Deribew (2010) applied the TTM to a study of intentions to quit smoking in Dire Dawna Town, Ethiopia. The researchers were interested in the earlier stages of the TTM—precontemplation, contemplation, and preparation. They examined how the processes of change influenced the stages of change and intentions to quit smoking. They categorized participants into stages. Precontemplators were regular smokers who were not considering quitting smoking in the next 6 months. Contemplators were smokers who were thinking about quitting in the next 6 months but had not made any attempt to do so in the past year.

Those in the preparation stage were considering quitting in the next 30 days and had tried to quit in the past year. The researchers next explored the processes of change relevant for these earlier stages. These processes included consciousness raising, dramatic relief, self-revaluation, environmental reevaluation, and social liberation. Smoking self-efficacy and decisional balance were also included and measured for each participant. The researchers found that the processes of change corresponded as predicted with specific stages of change, thereby confirming the application of the theory to this health behavior within this population.

Application of the Transtheoretical Model

One critique of the TTM is that it is not suited to complex behaviors like exercise because an individual may be simultaneously at different stages, which is not accounted for by the model (Adams & White, 2005; Littell & Girvin, 2002). Some authors argue that the TTM oversimplifies complex behavior by artificially forcing it into stages (Littell & Girvin, 2002). Despite these critiques, other researchers argue that TTM "may still hold some promise" (Brug et al., 2005), because TTM helps researchers and practitioners to tailor their strategies to particular stages, making the process of change more relevant to the individual engaged in the behavior-change process.

The Theory of Reasoned Action

Like the HBM, the Theory of Reasoned Action (TRA) postulates that attitudes and beliefs are related to health behavior. However, unlike the HBM, the TRA also includes the concept of subjective norms, which is defined next. The TRA marks a shift from the exclusive focus on attitudes and beliefs and examines these constructs in a broader social context. Fishbein introduced this theory in 1967, and Ajzen and Fishbein further clarified it in 1975 (Montaño & Kasprzyk, 2002). The TRA includes the constructs of attitudes, subjective norms, and intentions. Attitudes and subjective norms determine intentions, which, in turn, influence behavior (Ajzen & Fishbein, 1980).

To understand how the TRA can be used, imagine you are designing an intervention to increase sun-protection behavior in teenagers, specifically sunscreen use.

behavior refers to performing the desired action.

Behavior refers to performing the desired action. A fundamental component of the TRA is the link between behavioral intentions and behavior. The TRA assumes that individuals can decide their own behavior, and what they intend to do predicts what they will do (Ajzen & Fishbein, 1980). Thus, a decision to act precedes action. For example, a teenager's decision to use sunscreen eventually results in her using sunscreen.

behavioral intentions represent a person's likelihood to engage in the behavior.

Behavioral intentions represent a person's likelihood to engage in the behavior (Montaño & Kasprzyk, 2002). How much weight you give to your attitude toward the behavior and your subjective norms (described further in what follows) determine how much these factors influence your intentions to act (Ajzen & Fishbein, 1980). Let us assume the teenager has a positive attitude toward use of sunscreen, yet her friends are pressuring her to get a tan instead and not use sunscreen. If she assigns higher weight to her own attitude and lower weight to her friends' attitudes, she will intend to use sunscreen. However, if the teenager assigns lower weight to her own attitude and higher weight to her friends' attitudes, she will not intend to use sunscreen. How much weight the teenager assigns to her own attitude versus those of her peers will affect her intention to perform the behavior of sunscreen use.

attitude toward the behavior is one's belief about the target behavior.

Attitude toward the behavior is one's belief about the target behavior. Attitudes are determined by behavioral beliefs (Ajzen & Fishbein, 1980). These include beliefs about the consequences of a behavior and an evaluation of the consequences.

For example, if a teenager is considering using sunscreen, her attitude toward use of sunscreen is determined by (a) her beliefs about the perceived probability of an outcome (i.e., not using sunscreen will lead to skin cancer) and (b) her evaluation of that outcome (i.e., getting skin cancer would be a "bad" thing).

subjective norms are the pressure one feels from others to engage in the behavior.

Subjective norms are the pressure one feels from others to engage in the behavior (Ajzen & Fishbein, 1980). Like attitudes, subjective norms are also influenced by beliefs, in this case, normative beliefs. This includes both the belief and the motivation to comply with that belief. For example, in the case of sunscreen use, the teenager's subjective norms about using sunscreen could include how her friends view sunscreen use and if she values their views.

The Theory of Planned Behavior

Although the TRA explains volitional influences on behaviors, it neglects to account for influences not under complete volitional control (Ajzen, 1988). Although the TRA and the Theory of Planned Behavior (TPB) both depict attitudes, subjective norms, and intention as influencing behavior, the TPB includes the construct of perceived behavioral control (PBC).

perceived behavioral control is one's belief regarding how much power one has over the enactment of the behavior.

Perceived behavioral control is one's belief regarding how much power one has over the enactment of the behavior (Ajzen, 2002). Control beliefs and perceived power influence PBC. Control beliefs are facilitators and barriers to engaging in the behavior. Perceived power is how much one believes these facilitators and barriers impact the behavior. Perceived behavioral control was included as part of TPB because a person's belief about his or her control over a behavior influences a person's intention to perform the behavior (Ajzen, 2002). For example, if you decided to increase your physical activity by attending aerobic classes three times a week, perceived behavioral control would help you determine how much control you think you have over attending the classes. If you share a car with your brother, there is a chance that attending classes three times a week may not be possible because you are not fully in control of your transportation. High perceived behavioral control leads to high intention and impacts behavior both directly and indirectly (Ajzen, 2002). Specifically, perceived behavioral control together with attitudes and subjective norms influences intentions. Additionally, perceived behavioral control and intentions directly influence behavior (Ajzen, 1991).

Like the other individual-level theories, the TRA and TPB are criticized for specifying cognitive predictors of behavior, like attitudes and beliefs, and therefore assuming that people are rational. Relatedly, researchers who apply TRA and TPB in their work often use behavioral intentions as a primary outcome. Data show that intentions are inconsistently linked with behaviors (Brewer & Rimer, 2008). In terms of application, past researchers using the TPB have tailored the original constructs to their specific study, making it difficult to compare studies or assess the effectiveness of the theory as a whole (White et al., 2010). A final limitation is that the TRA and TPB have mostly been tested in White populations. As a result, little is known about how this theory would function in non-White populations.

Model for Understanding
Sun-Safety Intervention for Adolescents

White, Hyde, O'Connor, Naumann, and Hawkes (2010) applied the TPB to test an intervention promoting sun safety for adolescents. They measured adolescents' behavioral beliefs (attitude), normative beliefs (subjective norms), control beliefs (perceived behavioral control), intentions, and behavior. Behavioral beliefs included beliefs in the advantages or disadvantages of performing sun-protective behavior. These behaviors included finding shade at times of peak sun exposure, using protective clothing, and applying sunscreen. Normative beliefs were how friends or family viewed the behavior. Control beliefs were factors that aided or inhibited performance of sun-protection behaviors. Intentions referred to the adolescents' intentions to perform the sun-protective behaviors. Behavior was how often the adolescent performed the sun-protective behaviors in the past week.

The study integrated an in-class intervention with three 1-hour sessions over the course of 3 weeks. The sessions targeted behavioral beliefs, normative beliefs, and control beliefs about sun protection. Specifically, session one targeted behavioral beliefs by discussing the advantages and disadvantages of sun protection. Session two targeted normative beliefs by encouraging sun-protection support. Session three targeted control beliefs by improving participants' views of their own ability to engage in sun-protective behaviors. The study found that intention significantly increased across time in the intervention group. Reported behavior also increased across time in the intervention group, although not significantly. In general, TPB provided a useful conceptual framework for designing the intervention for this health topic (sun protection) and for this age group (adolescents).

Behavior Analysis

According to the branch of learning theory known as behavior analysis or contingency management (Baer, Wolf, & Risley, 1968; Bandura, 1969; Miller, 1980), behaviors may or may not occur as a function of either performance or skill deficits. Performance deficits refer to the person knowing how to perform a given behavior and having the skills to do it but choosing not to because (a) there are too many aversive (or "punishing") consequences for doing so; (b) there are limited, if any, positive consequences for doing so; and/or (c) he is receiving positive reinforcement for performing a competing behavior (e.g., acceptance by peers for drinking heavily rather than for being physically active). In the case of dietary change, for example, a mother may receive complaints about the taste of commonly prepared family dishes when she uses a lower-fat preparation technique. Alternatively, her lower-fat food preparation efforts may go unnoticed and unpraised, while praise is given for the preparation of an unhealthy dessert, thereby reinforcing a competing behavior. A skill deficit implies that a person might like to perform a given behavior but is limited from the opportunity for doing so by a lack of ability. This is a common complaint heard from participants in dietary focus group research; men and women report not knowing how to prepare healthy dishes (Ayala et al., 2001), including those needed to manage a chronic disease like diabetes (Cherrington et al., 2011). Health promotion efforts are very different for these two types of deficits. Performance deficits imply a need to implement "environmental engineering" by way of altering behavior–consequence relationships in such a way as to strengthen healthy behaviors and weaken unhealthy behaviors. Skills training, in contrast, would be invoked to address specific skill deficits.

> **generalization** refers to whether a behavior will occur in a new physical or social context.

Principles of shaping and **generalization** are central to applied behavioral analysis. Shaping is the gradual development of a behavior through reinforcement of successive approximations (e.g., reinforcing a novice exerciser for walking 20 minutes three times weekly and then gradually proceeding to longer, more vigorous, and more frequent activity). Generalization takes three forms: stimulus (or situational, in a different location), response (from one behavior to another), or interpersonal (between people).

Behavior analysts give relatively more credence to quantifiable observable behaviors and their environmental determinants and question the scientific relevance of cognitive processes such as thoughts, feelings, and attitudes. In the "triple-term contingency," antecedent stimuli set the stage for the behavior, which, in turn, is strengthened or weakened by the reinforcing or punishing consequences.

INTERPERSONAL-LEVEL THEORIES

Think about the relationships in your life. How have your friends, parents, grandparents, siblings, and so on influenced your health behaviors like what you eat and how much television you watch? Interpersonal-level theories describe how the relationships between people influence health behaviors. The following interpersonal theories discussed include Social Cognitive Theory, Social Support, and Social Influence. Each theory uniquely addresses the convergence of relationships and health.

Social Cognitive Theory

Social Cognitive Theory (SCT) frames health behavior as a dynamic relationship among the person, the behavior, and the environment. First espoused by Bandura in 1962 as social learning theory, SCT highlights observational learning as a primary process in behavioral adoption (Baranowski, Perry, & Parcel, 1997). The theory underwent major changes for more than a decade. In 1977 and 1986, Bandura further refined the theory to include the current concepts. These current concepts are defined by Baranowski and colleagues (1997) as follows:

> **reciprocal determinism** refers to the dynamic relationship among the self, behaviors, and the environment, both social and physical.

- *Reciprocal Determinism.* **Reciprocal determinism** refers to the dynamic relationship among the self, behaviors, and the environment, both social and physical. Specifically, all three factors influence and are influenced by each other. For example, how you view your athletic ability (self) might influence how often you ride your bike (behavior). How often you ride your bike (behavior) might influence how often your group of friends rides their bikes (social environment). Conversely, how often your friends ride their bikes (social environment) could influence how often you ride your bike (behavior). How often you ride your bike (behavior) could influence how you view your athletic ability (self). Thus, there is no specific direction of causality, but rather they all continually influence each other.

- *Environment.* Environment is any factor outside the self. This can be a *physical environment*, like parks, or *social environment*, like a walking group. In the previous example on bike riding, the focus was on the social environment. However, whether one rides a bike is also influenced by the availability of safe streets (e.g., bike lanes).

- *Situation.* Situation is how you *perceive* the environment. The distinction between environment and situation acknowledges that a person's perception of the environment may differ from reality. There is substantial evidence that one's perceived environment affects health behaviors; for an example on how situational factors, like the neighborhood environment, affect physical activity among Latinos in the United States, see Martinez and colleagues (2012).

observational learning maintains that a person often learns by seeing others model the behavior and receiving a positive consequence as a result of its enactment.

- *Observational Learning.* **Observational learning** maintains that you often learn by seeing others model the behavior and receiving a positive consequence as a result of its enactment. For example, seeing someone feel good about their physical strength (positive consequence) after taking up bicycling (behavior) is likely to motivate you to take up bicycling.

behavioral capability is a person's *knowledge* and *skill* to enact the desired behavior.

- *Behavioral Capability.* **Behavioral capability** is your *knowledge* and *skill* to enact the desired behavior. Knowledge refers to knowing what is needed to engage in the behavior, and skill refers to understanding how to enact the behavior. SCT frames knowledge and skill as preceding behavior.

reinforcement originates from operant conditioning and includes positive reinforcement (i.e., rewards following the enactment of a behavior) and negative reinforcement (i.e., removal of unpleasant stimulus following the enactment of the behavior).

- *Reinforcement.* **Reinforcement** originates from operant conditioning. Positive reinforcement refers to rewards (e.g., praise, prize, etc.) following enactment of a behavior; receipt of a reinforcer leads to engagement and maintenance of the behavior. For example, if a family member praises you for choosing a healthy dessert at a restaurant, you are being reinforced for making that choice and are thus more likely to make a similar choice in the future. Negative reinforcement refers to the removal of an unpleasant stimulus following enactment of a behavior. One example of negative reinforcement is decreased muscle pain as a result of regularly biking.

outcome expectations are what a person thinks will happen as a result of enacting the behavior.

- *Outcome Expectations.* **Outcome expectations** are what you think will happen as a result of enacting the behavior. An example of outcome expectations is expecting to feel rejuvenated after riding your bike in the afternoon.

outcome expectancies are how much a person values the particular outcome.

- *Outcome Expectancies.* **Outcome expectancies** are how much you value the particular outcome. For example, outcome expectancies are how much you value feeling rejuvenated after riding your bike in the afternoon.

- *Self-Efficacy.* Self-efficacy is how much you believe you are able to perform the behavior. Bandura argued that self-efficacy was the most important concept in predicting behavior.

- *Self-Control.* Self-control is how much you are able to modify your own behavior to achieve the desired goal. Self-control is an important aspect of SCT because SCT frames the individual as a crucial component in the reciprocal relationship of self, behavior, and environment.

> **emotional arousal management** refers to how a person addresses and copes with the negative or positive emotions surrounding the performance of a behavior.

- *Emotional Arousal Management.* **Emotional arousal management** refers to how you address and cope with the negative or positive emotions surrounding the performance of a behavior. In fact, Bandura argued that emotional responses, like fear, stifle one's ability to learn.

Some critics have questioned the widespread application of SCT, as it is among the most frequently cited theories in public health intervention research. In addition, some have argued that the construct of self-efficacy, a central construct of SCT, is not strongly related to behavior (Jeffery, 2004) and is not well measured (Marzillier & Eastman, 1984). Thus, in applying SCT, one uses a theory with a controversial central construct. Additionally, because of the many constructs contained within SCT, it is rarely implemented as a whole. Rather, only parts of it are used in behavioral interventions (Munro, Lewin, Swart, & Volmink, 2007).

Social Support

The influence of human relationships on health behaviors is important and largely understudied. The study of relationships and health explicates how the "the degree to which an individual is interconnected and embedded in community is vital to an individual's health and well-being as well as to the health and vitality of entire populations" (Berkman & Glass, 2000, p. 137). Social support examines this intersection between relationships and health.

Social support considers the positive role of relationships in health outcomes. House (1981) delineated social support into four types of behaviors. These include

Model for Understanding
Sun-Protection Behavior of Preschoolers

Gritz and colleagues (2007) launched a 2-year intervention, Sun Protection Is Fun (SPF), to improve sun-protection behaviors in preschool staff of 20 schools. The intervention included three components: training sessions, a sun safety newsletter, and a curriculum and teacher's guide. Free sunscreen was also available during the 2-year intervention. The SPF intervention was founded on SCT, including skills training and modeling, which are part of the SCT constructs of behavioral capability and observational learning, respectively (Baranowski et al., 1997).

The researchers measured several SCT constructs including sunscreen self-efficacy, sun-avoidance self-efficacy, sunscreen use expectancies, and tanning expectancies. At follow-up, the researchers found that the effects of the SPF intervention on the behavioral and psychosocial constructs were in the hypothesized direction.

emotional support, appraisal support, informational support, and instrumental support.

emotional support is showing love, compassion, and care and incorporates behaviors like listening and physical affection. It refers to the amount of sympathy, care, and understanding provided by others.

appraisal support is facilitating social comparison, providing personal evaluation, and giving honest feedback.

informational support is providing helpful, relevant facts and information.

instrumental support is offering tangible help like money for a gym membership or a ride to the physician's office.

- *Emotional Support.* **Emotional support** is showing love, compassion, and care. It incorporates behaviors like listening and physical affection. Emotional support is the most fundamental type of social support, and most of the other supportive behaviors contain aspects of emotional support.

- *Appraisal Support.* **Appraisal support** is facilitating social comparison, providing personal evaluation, and giving honest feedback. An example is a mother evaluating her daughter's unhealthy eating habits and providing her daughter with feedback about these habits.

- *Informational Support.* **Informational support** is providing helpful, relevant facts. An example is a cancer survivor informing a cancer patient about the best radiologists.

- *Instrumental Support.* **Instrumental support** is offering tangible help like money for a gym membership or a ride to the physician's office.

Notably, these supportive behaviors are not always easy to delineate. Sometimes if you perform one type of supportive behavior, you also inadvertently provide additional types of support. For example, if a friend offered to drive another friend to the gym every week (instrumental support), this would also likely impart a type of emotional support because it would communicate caring and love.

SPOTLIGHT

Health promotion researchers often employ community members to deliver interventions to other community members. These types of interventions are often called community health worker (or lay health advisor, or promotor) models (Ayala et al., 2010, Cherrington et al., 2008). They are based on the assumption that the person who can provide the best type of support to someone learning to manage a chronic disease such as diabetes or helping to prevent one like obesity is someone who is like the individual and thus can relate to the challenges that the person might face. Community health workers are often naturally supportive individuals who are then trained to provide a specific type of support.

Social Influence

Social influence, like social support, explores the role of relationships in health behavior. However, unlike social support, social influence can be positive or negative; in other words, social influences can promote or hinder both healthy and unhealthy behaviors. Knowing who these influential people are and how they influence behaviors can be used to design more effective interventions. Three constructs important to social influence theory are social proximity, structural cohesion, and equivalence (Marsden & Friedkin, 1994).

social proximity is how close you are to someone else in your network.

structural cohesion frames social proximity in "terms of the number, length, and strength of the paths that connect actors in networks" (Marsden & Friedkin, 1994, p. 7).

- *Social Proximity.* **Social proximity** is how close you are to someone else in your network. Social proximity is one of the most important concepts in social influence theory. Notably, the closer two people are in a network, the more influence they have over each other.

- *Structural Cohesion.* **Structural cohesion** frames social proximity in "terms of the number, length, and strength of the paths that connect actors in networks" (Marsden & Friedkin, 1994, p. 7). For example, a best friend of 15 years would likely have more paths of influence of a longer duration with more strength per path than an acquaintance from college. Based on these aspects of structural cohesion, the best friend would be more socially proximate than the college acquaintance. By implication, the best friend would also have more influence on the attitudes and behaviors of the actor than the college acquaintance.

equivalence frames social proximity as similarity. Specifically, two people are equivalent if their social networks are similar.

- *Equivalence.* **Equivalence** frames social proximity as similarity. Specifically, two people are equivalent if their social networks are similar. In its most narrow sense, equivalence would mean two people having the same friends, acquaintances, and family. Thus, the more social connections two people share, the more equivalent they are. For example, brothers sharing the same group of friends would have more influence over each other than brothers who do not share the same group of friends. In a less narrow sense, equivalence can mean that two people have a similar social standing, regardless of whether they share the same social circle. For example, if two people are both regional bank managers at different banks, they have more social equivalence than a regional bank manager and a clerk. In both the restrictive and non-restrictive sense, the more social equivalence you have with someone else in the social network, the more socially proximate you are, and the more likely you are to influence each other. This is an important factor when designing interventions because more social equivalence provides more influence. For example, an intervention could engage group members who are more socially equivalent to the target audience to encourage healthy behavior.

Model for Understanding
Parents as Sources of Social Influence in Children's Risk for Obesity

Parents are an important source of social influence for their children. Given their proximity, cohesion, and equivalence, they are among the most influential people in children's adoption of healthy and unhealthy lifestyle behaviors. Previous research demonstrates that parents who role model healthy eating are more likely to have children who eat healthfully (Eisenberg et al., 2012).

One possible limitation of current social support research is that operationalizations of social support differ from study to study. This makes it difficult to compare between studies. One of the main critiques of studies using social influence theory is that because social influence is determined, in part, by one's social networks, interventions using this theory need to consider the individual, given that social networks and the influence of these networks greatly vary from person to person (Heaney & Israel, 2002).

ORGANIZATIONAL-LEVEL THEORIES

Organizational-level theories examine how the physical and social structures of organizations (e.g., systems) influence health behaviors and how these structures can be modified to promote health and well-being. Here we present two theories: the Chronic Care Model and the Diffusion of Innovation theory.

Chronic Care Model

The Chronic Care Model (CCM) emerged out of a need to provide a better quality of health care for patients with a chronic health condition such as diabetes, hypertension, and congestive heart failure. First developed by Edward H. Wagner, CCM is a comprehensive approach to chronic care management. It outlines significant changes in the way health care is organized and delivered to improve management of chronic diseases (Wagner, 1998). Bodenheimer, Wagner, and Grumbach (2002) argued that the health care system neglects the management of chronic diseases because the acute conditions of patients take priority. They provided the example of a patient with diabetes who visits his physician. Because the physician has limited time, they only discuss the patient's reason for the visit, which is his painful knee and gastroesophageal reflux disease. No time is left to educate the patient about how to manage his diabetes. The CCM was created to inform systems of care that include educating patients on how to manage their own chronic health conditions with the help of a team of medical professionals. This is achieved in part by improving communication between patients and their health care providers (Bodenheimer et al., 2002). To accomplish this, the CCM outlines three major spheres important to chronic care management: (1) the community, (2) the health care system, and (3) provider organizations (Bodenheimer et al., 2002). Within these overlapping spheres, there are six essential elements: community resources and policies, the health care organization, self-management support, delivery systems design, decision support, and clinical information systems. The six elements are mutually supportive; improving one element improves additional elements.

community resources and policies are linkages between the community and the health care organization.

- *Community Resources and Policies.* **Community resources and policies** are the first "essential element" in the CCM. These are linkages between the community and the health care organization. Specifically, the CCM emphasizes the importance of connecting patients with community resources. Let us imagine you were planning an intervention to improve diabetes management by incorporating the CCM. You could improve this element by meeting with community members, finding relevant community opportunities, and linking patients with diabetes to these opportunities. These could include opportunities like local cooking classes for people with diabetes, restaurants that offer meals suitable for people with diabetes, and community support groups.

health care organization
includes the organization's values, policies, training, and orientation toward patients.

self-management support
involves teaching patients with a chronic disease how to care for themselves.

delivery system design
refers to creating an ideal division of labor. This includes defining where specific medical staff (i.e., physicians vs. nurses) are needed and dividing the tasks accordingly.

- *Health Care Organization.* The **health care organization** includes the organization's values, policies, training, and orientation toward patients. Other potential factors are the organization's payment policies and relationships with insurance. The health care organization's support of the CCM is crucial to facilitation.

- *Self-Management Support.* **Self-management support** involves teaching patients with a chronic disease how to care for themselves. This includes teaching patients how to eat healthfully, exercise, use their medications, self-monitor symptoms, and other skills necessary for disease management (i.e., managing stress). It also includes providing routine support for patients by regularly evaluating their self-management and addressing any potential problems.

- *Delivery System Design.* **Delivery system design** refers to creating an ideal division of labor. This includes defining where specific medical staff (i.e., physicians vs. nurses) are needed and dividing the tasks accordingly. A well-designed delivery system improves medical care by defining the jobs of medical staff and lessening the burden of the physicians. This frees up time for the physicians to discuss chronic health issues with patients when needed (Carlini, Schauer, Zbikowski, & Thompson, 2010).

decision support means having a set of clear practice guidelines for the treatment and management of chronic diseases.

clinical information systems refer to the organization of patient medical records and other information sources within a health care setting.

- *Decision Support.* **Decision support** means having a set of clear practice guidelines for the treatment and management of chronic diseases. This includes providing practice team members regular reminders of these guidelines and educational programs for implementing these guidelines. The CCM argues that this will decrease reliance on specialist referrals.

- *Clinical Information Systems.* **Clinical information systems** refer to the organization of patient medical records. Efficient clinical information systems improve care by providing organized, easy access to patient medical information. This information can be used by the practice team to best treat the patient (Carlini et al., 2010). These systems include computerized registries, reminder systems, and physician feedback.

One of the main critiques of the application of the CCM is that it is complex to implement because it requires system-wide changes. A second critique is that it can be expensive to implement given this need for system-wide change. Additionally, it can be difficult to assess because the various components of the CCM can differ by context. Thus, the analysis is nuanced. To date, little is known about the "underlying mechanism" by which CCM as a whole improves patient outcomes. However, recent research has shown that although the CCM is expensive up front, it might be cost effective in the long run (Kuo et al., 2011).

Model for Understanding
Thrombosis Clinics in the Netherlands

A group of researchers from the Netherlands (Drewes et al., 2011) conducted a cross-sectional study assessing the impact of five elements of the CCM on patient outcomes (they did not include community resources). Their population included patients using oral anticoagulant therapy to prevent thrombosis, a disease affecting blood circulation. Improper dosage can lead to severe health consequences such as hemorrhaging. Within this context, quality chronic care is paramount. The researchers compared how different regions applied the CCM and if this affected patient outcomes. They operationalized the five elements of the CCM in the following way: health care organization =

quality of manager; self-management support = web-based support for patients; delivery system design = greater involvement of nurses; decision support = dosage advice information; and clinical information system = availability of the results of blood tests for specific patients. Patient outcomes included whether the therapy was in the "optimal target range." The researchers found that only patient orientation (health care organization) and specialized nurses versus physicians (delivery system design) resulted in statistically significant differences in patient outcomes. However, there was a positive association between application of the CCM as a whole and patient outcomes.

Diffusion of Innovations

The Diffusion of Innovation (DOI) theory, first introduced by Edward Rogers in 1962, defined innovation as any "idea perceived as new by the individual" and diffusion as "the process by which the innovation spreads" (Rogers, 1962, p. 13). In essence, DOI examines how new ideas spread in a social system. These concepts were ultimately applied to inform organizational change processes, including how systems change in response to the introduction of an innovation. Whether a system changes in response to an innovation is determined, in part, by characteristics of the innovation.

The characteristics of the innovation are the facets surrounding engagement of the desired behavior. These include the following five elements:

relative advantage is how much the new idea, or innovation, is superior to the current idea.

compatibility is the consistency between the innovation and current processes.

complexity is how difficult the innovation is to understand or accomplish.

- *Relative Advantage.* **Relative advantage** is how much the new idea, or innovation, is superior to the current idea. For example, are the potential benefits of introducing more signage in the produce department of a food store worth the additional efforts that are needed on the part of store staff? Would placing a sign in the produce department touting the benefits of vitamin C contained within oranges influence the purchase of oranges and thereby increase store sales?

- *Compatibility.* **Compatibility** is the consistency between the innovation and current processes. For example, are store staff already using signage to promote sales and simply need to change the message?

- *Complexity.* **Complexity** is how difficult the innovation is to understand or accomplish. For example, is the addition of health messages on store signage too difficult for store employees to implement?

trialability is how much one can "experiment" with the innovation before fully adopting it.

observability is how much others can perceive the effects of the innovation.

- *Trialability.* **Trialability** is how much one can "experiment" with the innovation before fully adopting it. For example, can store employees install temporary signs in the produce section to promote purchasing healthy products before installing permanent structures?

- *Observability.* **Observability** is how much others can perceive the effects of the innovation (Rogers, 2002). For example, will store staff notice that customers are buying more oranges after the signs about vitamin C are posted? People are most likely to accept innovations high in relative advantage, compatibility, trialability, and observability and low in complexity.

The innovation decision process is how one progresses toward adoption of the innovation. The steps progress as follows: knowledge about the innovation leads to attitude change about the innovation. Attitudes about the innovation lead to an acceptance or rejection of the innovation. The decision to accept or reject the innovation leads to implementation (or not) of the innovation. Implementation of the innovation leads to confirmation or disconfirmation (Rogers, 2002).

Characteristics of the adopter inform a categorization system of potential innovation adopters based on their level of acceptance of the innovation. These categories include innovators, early adopters, early majority, late majority, and laggards. Rogers delineates these categories by how early on the group adopts the innovation. **Innovators** are the first individuals to adopt the new idea. Rogers defines these individuals as the first 2.5% of the social system's population to accept the innovation. The subsequent 13.5% of the population to accept the innovation are the **early adopters**. This group is more socially integrated than the innovators. The next 34% of the population to accept the innovation are the **early majority**, and the subsequent 34% after that are the **late majority**. The final 16% of the social system's population to accept the innovation are the **laggards** (Rogers, 2002).

innovators are the first individuals to adopt the new idea.

early adopters are the 13.5% of the population, after the innovators, to accept the innovation and are more socially integrated than the innovators.

early majority are the 34% of the population, after the early adopters, to accept the innovation.

late majority are the 34% of the population that accepts the innovation after the early majority and before the laggards.

laggards are the final 16% of the social system's population to accept the innovation.

A criticism of the Diffusion of Innovation theory is the notion that once a scientifically validated approach is identified (e.g., a worksite wellness program reduces work absenteeism), it simply needs to be integrated into the system, and the system should, in turn, accommodate it. Green and colleagues argue that in order for organizational or policy changes to occur, five principles need to be considered that recognize the needs of the individual and the context (Green, Ottoson, García, & Hiat, 2009). Similar to Social Cognitive Theory, the importance of the person and the environment is critical for change, whether change is at the individual, interpersonal, or organizational level.

COMMUNITY-LEVEL THEORIES

Community-level theories include both communication and structural theories. These theories provide the broadest lens for examining behavior and ultimately how to change it. Rather than targeting specific individuals or organizations, these theories seek to inform change in the surrounding social and physical environments.

Communication theories in health behavior explore how mass media messages lead to behavior change. These include the Information Processing Paradigm and Social Marketing. They are included in the community-level section because these theories explore how mass media messages can be used to change societal norms and ultimately individual behavior. These are distinguished from interpersonal communication theories, which focus more on one-to-one interactions.

Information Processing Paradigm

The Information Processing Paradigm, also known as the Communication/Persuasion Matrix, delineates how certain factors impact persuasion (McGuire, 1985). Particular inputs (i.e., the source, message, channel, receiver, and target) influence the output steps (12-step journey toward behavioral adoption). McGuire framed the input factors as the independent variables and the output steps as the dependent variables. By improving the input factors, you can better persuade your audience to ultimately make a change. This is valuable when planning a health communication campaign.

Input variables include the source, message, channel, receiver, and target (McGuire, 1985). The source is who is saying the message. For example, in a public health commercial promoting fruit and vegetable consumption, the physician on the commercial is the source. The message is what the source is saying. In this example, the message is that the expectant mother should eat six to eight servings of fruits and vegetables a day. The channel is how the message is delivered. In the present example, the message is delivered via a television commercial. The receiver is to whom the message is directed. In the example, the message is directed at pregnant mothers watching the television channel. The target is the desired behavior, in this case, increased fruit and vegetable consumption by pregnant mothers. Public health researchers can manipulate these input variables to move their audience along the 12 output steps toward behavioral adoptions.

In order for behavior change to occur, the theory postulates that a person must progress through the various output steps: exposure, attention, liking, comprehension, generating related cognitions, skill acquisition, attitude change, memory storage, retrieval, decision, behaving in accord with decision, and consolidation (McGuire, 1985). *Exposure* is a necessary first step toward persuasion and involves contact with the message. For example, viewing a commercial about the importance of walking can represent exposure to the message. After being exposed to the message, it is important that you give the message your *attention*. *Liking* for the message causes you to continue to give the message your attention rather than disregarding it. You must also *comprehend* the message. Without understanding the information, the message will not move you toward persuasion. Understanding of the message should then lead to additional *related cognitions*, which are other thoughts and arguments supporting the message. For example, a television commercial encouraging you to walk may remind you that a friend of yours walked every day and lost 10 pounds. Many public health messages also require a level of *skill acquisition*. For example, a public health commercial could promote skill acquisition for increasing exercise by providing suggestions on *how* to increase exercise like taking your dog for a daily walk. After moving through these steps, you must next *accept* the message. This means that you agree with the message. If the researchers desire a long-term impact, the subsequent step is that you *retain* the message and are able to *retrieve* the message from memory. These are separate steps because one could

Model for Understanding
The Influence of Culture on Hispanic Women's Preference for Information

Oetzel, Devargas, Ginossar, and Sanchez (2007) explored the influence of culture on Hispanic women's source, message, and channel preference for breast health information. They elucidated three subjective cultural variables: self-construals, ethnic identity, and cultural health attributions. They posited that these variables might influence information preference. To test this assumption, they created questionnaires to measure the independent variables of subjective cultural factors and the dependent variables of sources, messages, and channels. They administered these questionnaires to 176 Hispanic women who were 35 years old or older. They found that source, message, and channel were influenced by cultural variables. Specifically, cultural variables accounted for 2 to 28% of the variance in source, message, and channel preference. For example, women with a bicultural identity preferred the message source to be family and the channel to be media. This implies that understanding what cultural variables are important to each subgroup will allow researchers to tailor their health communication campaigns appropriately. The study also underlines the importance of using the most relevant source, message, and channel for the population.

have the message in memory without actively remembering it. After retrieving the message from memory, you can use this information to make *decisions* ("I will take my dog for a walk") and then *behave* accordingly ("I take my dog for a walk"). After journeying through these 11 steps of persuasion, you end with *consolidation*. This means that the message is integrated into your belief system and you are now behaving according to your belief system.

A particular challenge of communication campaigns using the Information Processing Paradigm is that many of the audience members may not stay engaged enough to reach the final action stages. At each consecutive step in the 12-step process, more and more audience members lose interest. To account for this continual loss, exposure and awareness must be high (Huhman, Heitzler, & Wong, 2004). Also, progression through the 12 output steps may not occur in the linear sequence, as described in the theory. For example, one may comprehend the message (step 4) before liking it (step 3). In this way, the path to consolidation may be messier than the path outlined. Additionally, the theory frames human cognition similar to a computer processing information. However, humans are not computers and do not always behave logically (Corcoran, 2007).

Social Marketing

Social marketing uses the principles of commercial marketing to craft and guide behavior change programs (Grier & Bryant, 2005). Unlike commercial marketing, which usually promotes a particular company, social marketing promotes "social good" by encouraging health behavior change (Suarez-Amazor, 2011). Social marketing includes the central constructs of exchange, audience segmentation, competition, the marketing mix, consumer orientation, and continuous monitoring (Grier & Bryant, 2005). Researchers using a social marketing framework use these concepts to create and implement their program for a specific group of people, known as the target audience.

Exchange is the idea that self-interest, or the desire to maximize benefits and minimize costs, drives behavior. Unlike commercial marketing, social marketing is not promoting a consumer product; thus the rewards and costs in social marketing are often intangible. For example, the cost of increased physical activity may be less time relaxing at home after work. Social marketing researchers must take into account that their target audience wants the best deal. So they frame their programs to highlight the benefits of performing the desired behavior while acknowledging the costs (Grier & Bryant, 2005).

> **exchange** is the idea that self-interest, or the desire to maximize benefits and minimize costs, drives behavior.
>
> **audience segmentation** is dividing the target audience into groups based on certain characteristics, like behaviors, personal preferences, and values.

- *Audience Segmentation.* **Audience segmentation** is dividing the target audience into groups based on certain characteristics, like behaviors, personal preferences, and values. Audience segmentation assumes that people with similar characteristics will respond to the promotion in a similar way. By dividing the audience into groups based on certain characteristics, researchers can use the most appropriate strategies for each group. Social marketing researchers emphasize the importance of audience segmentation and spend a great deal of effort to divide the audience into meaningful groups. Unlike other types of public health research, social marketing researchers are less likely to use demographics to segment populations and are more likely to use behavior (Grier & Bryant, 2005). This allows researchers to tailor their messages to particular audiences based on behaviors (Suarez-Amazor, 2011). An example of audience segmentation for a health promotion program reducing fast food consumption would be dividing the target audience into separate groups based on how often they eat out at fast food restaurants.

- *Competition.* Competition has a distinct meaning in social marketing. In commercial marketing, competition is the company or product that may tempt consumers away from your company or product. In social marketing, competition is other behaviors that may tempt your target audience away from the desired behavior. For example, in a public health campaign that promotes increased walking, the competition would be sedentary behaviors like playing on the computer and watching television. Social marketing emphasizes the need to study and understand the competition and to ensure the desired behavior is more attractive to the target audience than the competing unhealthy behavior.

> **marketing mix,** or the "four Ps" (i.e., product, price, place, and promotion), is a foundational concept in commercial marketing and has been appropriated by social marketers to promote behavior change.

- *Marketing Mix.* **Marketing mix**, or the "four Ps," is a foundational concept in commercial marketing. The four Ps, which include product, price, place, and promotion, have been appropriated by social marketers to promote behavior change. Social marketing understands product as the benefits of performing the health behavior. For a program promoting walking, the product might be a trimmer figure and a healthier heart. In social marketing, price includes tangible and intangible costs of performing the desired behavior. For example, the cost of walking might be the loss of an evening watching television. Place is where the promotion occurs. It can also refer to where the target audience receives information or support. For example, place would be where the walking club meets. Promotion is how the social marketers communicate their message to the target audience. For example, the walking club is promoted using colorful fliers, radio-station announcements, and Facebook groups. Social marketers emphasize the need to integrate the four Ps in health promotion programs (Grier & Bryant, 2005). This means that the health program should include all four Ps and ensure that each element works well together. For example, if the walking program emphasizes the fun elements of walking, the product, place, and promotion should reflect this emphasis and the price should include any potential drawbacks.

- *Consumer Orientation.* Consumer orientation is thinking like the consumer. This means allotting significant time and money to discover how the consumer thinks and what the consumer wants. In social marketing, the consumer is the target audience of the health promotion. Social markets use formative research, like focus groups and interviews, to discover what the target audience needs and values, as well as the target audience's perceived benefits and barriers to performing the health behavior. For example, in a program promoting walking groups, the social marketers could first conduct a series of focus groups asking members of the target audience what barriers they face in joining a walking group. Social marketers also emphasize the need to change the program based on audience feedback.

- *Continuous Monitoring.* Continuous monitoring and revision includes evaluating the effectiveness of the promotion program at every stage. Although many public health programs include process evaluation at the end of the project, social marketers continuously assess and make relevant changes. This is a distinct attribute of the social marketing mindset.

Researchers using social marketing implement the central constructs in the following six steps. According to Grier and Bryant (2005), these steps include initial planning, formative research, developing a strategy, developing a program and pretesting, implementing, and monitoring/evaluating. For example, when planning a campaign to promote joining a walking group, researchers would first create a plan for what behavior they will target (initial planning). Next they would conduct focus groups and interviews to understand what the target population wants and needs and which strategies would be most effective (formative research). Based on the formative research, the researchers would design a plan for the campaign that includes development, implementation, and assessment as well as the project goals and target audience. The researchers also decide how they will incorporate the four Ps (strategy development). The researchers next develop the program and pretest the intervention and materials. They recruit several groups in the target population to read their promotional pamphlets, listen to their radio commercials, and provide feedback (developing a program and pretesting). They implement the program (implementation) and monitor and evaluate the progress at every stage (monitoring/evaluation).

Model for Understanding

Social Marketing to Promote Breastfeeding and Smoking Cessation

Lowry, Billett, Buchanan, and Whiston (2009) applied the social marketing framework to design and implement a campaign in northeast England to promote breastfeeding and smoking cessation in expectant mothers. The researchers demonstrated an understanding of exchange theory by clarifying the incentives of the program as health and self-esteem. The researchers used the four Ps to design their program. Specifically, their product was the promotion of breastfeeding and smoking cessation. They accounted for price by minimizing access cost and training professionals in effective communication skills. The places were maternity units, clinics, and community groups. The promotion included media advertising to promote awareness and skill building training for professionals working with the target audience. The researchers also conducted consumer research by utilizing focus groups and in-depth interviews to inform their program and adopt a consumer mindset. They included evaluating systems for continuous monitoring of breastfeeding and smoking cessation. The program was successful and resulted in increased breastfeeding and smoking cessation. The researchers attributed their success, in part, to social marketing.

One critique of social marketing is that it is mainly about advertising. Although social marketing can be used for this purpose, it also can be and has been used to design comprehensive public health campaigns (Grier & Bryant, 2005). Another critique of social marketing is that it does not account for the physical environment. In the example of social marketers promoting walking groups, the researchers communicate to community members rather than changing the environment by building more walking trails and offering tax benefits to walkers. A final challenge of social marketing is that it must compete within a "cluttered" environment with many opposing messages (Suarez-Amazor, 2011). Within this environment, the unhealthy messages of commercial marketing compete, and perhaps drown out, the health-promoting messages of social marketing.

Structural Model of Health Behavior

Consider again factors that influence your health behavior. Do you exercise regularly? If not, is it because you believe that exercise is painful and boring or because a gym membership is too expensive and there are no nearby parks where you can be physically active? Cohen, Scribner, and Farley (2000) explained that health interventions have two main targets. Either they target factors individuals can control (like attitudes or beliefs about exercise) or factors individuals cannot control (like park availability). They argue that most research has focused on factors individuals can control. Such research targets individuals at highest risk (i.e., teens who smoke, children who are already obese). As a result, a few high-risk individuals are targeted, but the community as a whole is not influenced and future risk is not prevented. To account for factors outside individual control, the researchers introduced the Structural Model of Health Behavior. They described four structural factors that can be used to promote population health: availability/accessibility of consumer products, physical structures, social structures and policies, and media and cultural messages (Cohen et al., 2000).

- *Availability.* Availability is how accessible products are that promote or inhibit health. For example, are fresh fruits and vegetables, healthy beverages, and clean water easily and cheaply available? Conversely, are cigarettes, alcohol, and high-fat foods accessible? Structural interventions can target availability by banning and taxing unhealthy products and subsidizing beneficial products.

- *Physical Structures.* **Physical structures** are the attributes of products, neighborhoods, and all other environmental objects that promote or inhibit healthy behavior. For example, the physical structure of a neighborhood would include its tangible attributes like walking paths, parks, lighting, and bike lanes. Researchers can target behavior by changing physical structures (e.g., improving a park) to encourage physical activity.

- *Social Structure.* **Social structures** are policies and laws that promote or inhibit healthy behavior. These can be formal (i.e., minimum-age drinking laws) or informal (i.e., a group of friends that take turns being designated drivers). Researchers can promote social structures that facilitate health either by advocating for government policy change or by encouraging community members to provide their own regulating groups.

- *Messages.* Media and cultural **messages** are communications from television, radio, Internet, and cultural groups that promote or inhibit healthy behavior. Although these messages may target individuals, they also change social norms. For example, television commercials that depict young, fit, and beautiful people enjoying soda reemphasize that drinking soda is normal and not harmful to health. Public health researchers can use media and cultural messages to create new norms for healthy behavior.

> **physical structures** are the attributes of products, neighborhoods, and all other environmental objects that promote or inhibit healthy behavior.
>
> **social structures** are policies and laws that promote or inhibit healthy behavior.

> **messages** both media and cultural, are communications from television, radio, Internet, and cultural groups that promote or inhibit healthy behavior.

These four structural elements can work together to promote health. For example, media commercials can promote joining a walking group. The neighborhood's physical structure (i.e., that there are many walking paths and trails) can facilitate this message. Meanwhile, social structures, in the form of a group of friends who agree to walk together several times a week, can further promote the healthy behavior. Finally, the availability of inexpensive walking shoes and workout clothes can further advance the goal. In this way, all four structural factors influence and encourage the same healthy behavior.

Structural interventions are ideal for achieving population-level changes. However, in a healthy population, a structural intervention may be less effective (Cohen et al., 2000). For example, in a community of people who are already physically active, changing government policy to budget for more walking paths may not be the best use of resources. An additional limitation to implementing structural interventions is that there is usually a disconnect between the researchers who desire the structural change (i.e., increased park budget) and the policy makers who enact the change (Katz, 2009). As a result, researchers are dependent on policy makers who may not see the need for structural changes. Collaboration between researchers and policy makers is essential for many types of structural interventions.

Model for Understanding
Park Improvement and Physical Activity

Veitch and colleagues (2012) tested the relationship between park improvement and park-based physical activity in Victoria, Australia. The local government planned to refurbish one of the local parks. This gave the researchers a unique opportunity to study park-based physical activity at this park pre- and post-renovations and to compare this park to another unrenovated park in the community. The researchers used behavioral observation (SOPARC) to note the total number of people in each park and the number of people being physically active. Researchers observed the intervention park (i.e., the park being renovated) and a control park (i.e., the park not being renovated) at baseline, after intervention park improvement, and 12 months after baseline. As expected, the researchers found that both park use and park-based physical activity increased in the intervention park after park renovations compared with the control park. Additionally, park use and park-based physical activity increased even more at the final time point, indicating that refurbished parks gain more and more visitors and promote more and more physical activity with time. This natural experiment highlights the importance of structural change in promoting healthy behavior.

SPECIAL CONSIDERATIONS

Public health researchers may need to take into account characteristics of the target population when considering a theory. For example, theories/models that take into account social influences (e.g., Social Cognitive Theory) may be more appropriate when considering adolescent populations, a period of time where the influence of peers is significant. Further, cognitive-focused theories/models (e.g., Health Belief Model) may not be appropriate for younger populations, as these theories/models assume that the individual's behavior is directly influenced by their attitudes without taking into account the important role of parental influence.

Resources

When considering which theories should inform health promotion research and practice, researchers and practitioners need to consider the types and amount of resources available to them, including organizational partners, as well as personnel and material resources. The application of some theories/frameworks may require more resources compared to others. For example, applying an organizational change theory requires changes within complex systems with implications for personnel and material resources. These partnerships and agreements are necessary to appropriately implement these types of health promotion interventions. In contrast, modifying an individual-level health behavior such as diet through the application of behavioral principles may require several visits with a dietician.

Summary

Theory is healthy. It links our study findings with previous and future research. It allows us to build upon the foundation of others to further the discipline. It also tells us how, why, and what we can expect in the future. It helps us improve our practices by guiding what we should do and what we should not do based on available evidence. Rather than being intimidating, theory can help us make decisions about how to design, implement, and evaluate our efforts to promote healthy behaviors.

To explore the various theories in health promotion, this chapter adopted the SEF. This framework depicts behaviors as influenced by multiple levels. These levels include individual, interpersonal, organizational, and community. Health behavior theories can be understood as examining factors on particular levels of the SEF.

The individual level includes the Health Belief Model, the Transtheoretical Model, the Theory of Reasoned Action, the Theory of Planned Behavior, and Behavior Analysis. These theories focus on how personal factors, like attitudes, beliefs, and intention, influence our behavior. The interpersonal level includes Social Cognitive Theory, Social Support, and Social Influence. These theories highlight the role of relationships on health. The organizational-level theories, the Chronic Care Model and Diffusion of Innovations, describe the role of institutions in constraining or enabling health and what is needed to improve these organizations. Finally, the community level includes Communication Theories (i.e., Information Processing Paradigm and Social Marketing) and the Structural Model of Health Behavior. These theories explore how messages, marketing, and the environment shape health.

Understanding and correctly applying theory is crucial to scientific progress and to informed practice. By incorporating and refining theory, future researchers and practitioners can build upon the findings of the past and create improved ways of understanding and ultimately promoting better health in the future.

Review Questions

1. True or False: One application of theory to our health promotion research and practice is to build scientific evidence.

2. True or False: An individual or intrapersonal factor within the Social Ecological Framework includes how our family treats us.

3. Which of the following is not a central construct in the Health Belief Model?

    a. Perceived benefits
    b. Perceived barriers
    c. Perceived outcomes
    d. Perceived severity
    e. Perceived susceptibility

4. What construct was added to the Theory of Reasoned Action when it was modified to the Theory of Planned Behavior?

    a. Perceived behavioral control
    b. Perceived environment
    c. Perceived attitude
    d. Perceived norms
    e. Perceived adoption

5. True or False: Social Cognitive Theory is a value expectancy theory.

6. Which of the following is not a type of social support?

    a. Informational support
    b. Emotional support
    c. Appraisal support
    d. Personal support
    e. Instrumental support

7. True or False: Structural cohesion refers to the number, length, and strength of relationships between people.

8. According to the Chronic Care Model, the three major spheres important for chronic care management are _____, _____, and _____ _____.

9. The Marketing Mix is represented by the four Ps. Which of the following is not one of the Ps?

    a. Price
    b. Product
    c. Place
    d. Promotion
    e. Position

10. True or False: The Structural Model of Health Behavior delineates factors outside the individual's control that may be modified to promote healthy behaviors.

Web Resources

Visit the following websites to learn more about some of the topics presented in this chapter.

National Cancer Institute: Theory at a Glance-A Guide for Health Promotion Practice: http://www.cancer .gov/cancertopics/cancerlibrary/theory.pdf

References

Adams, J., & White, M. (2005). Why don't stage-based activity promotion interventions work? *Health Education Research*, *20*(2), 237–243. doi:10.1093/her/cyg105

Ajzen, I. (1988). *Attitudes, personality, and behavior*. Chicago, IL: Dorsey Press.

Ajzen, I. (1991). The theory of planned behavior. *Organizational Behavior and Human Decision Processes*, *50*(2), 179–211. doi:10.1016/0749-5978(91)90020-T

Ajzen, I. (2002). Perceived behavioral control, self-efficacy, locus of control, and the theory of planned behavior. *Journal of Applied Social Psychology*, *32*(4), 665–683. Wiley Online Library. doi:10.1111/j.1559-1816.2002.tb00236.x

Ajzen, I., & Fishbein, M. (1980). *Understanding attitudes and predicting social behavior*. Englewood Cliffs, NJ: Prentice Hall.

Ayala, G. X., Elder, J. P., Campbell, N. R., Engelberg, M., Olson, S., Moreno, C., & Serrano, V. (2001). Nutrition communication for a Latino community: Formative research foundations. *Family and Community Health*, *24*(3), 72–87.

Ayala, G. X., Vaz, L., Earp, J. A., Elder, J. P., & Cherrington, A. (2010). Outcome effectiveness of the lay health advisor model among Latinos in the United States: An examination by role type. *Health Education Research*, *25*(5), 815–840.

Baer, D., Wolf, M., & Risley, T. (1968). Some current dimensions of applied behavior analysis. *Journal of Applied Behavior Analysis 1*, 91–97.

Bandura, A. (1969). *Principles of behavior modification*. New York, NY: Holt, Rinehart & Winston.

Baranowski, T., Perry, C. L., & Parcel, G. S. (1997). How individuals, environments, and health behavior interact: Social cognitive theory. In K. Glanz, F. M. Lewis, & B. K. Rimmer (Eds.), *Health behavior and health education: Theory, research, and practice* (pp. 165–184). San Francisco, CA: Jossey-Bass.

Berkman, L. F., & Glass, T. (2000). Social integration, social networks, social support, and health. In L. F. Berkman & I. Kawachi (Eds.), *Social Epidemiology* (pp. 137–173). New York, NY: Oxford University Press.

Bodenheimer, T., Wagner, E. H., & Grumbach, K. (2002). Improving primary care for patients with chronic illness. *JAMA: The Journal of the American Medical Association*, *288*(14), 1775–1779. Retrieved from http://www.ncbi.nlm.nih.gov/pubmed/12377092

Brewer, N. T., & Rimer, B. K. (2008). Perspectives on health behavior theories that focus on individuals. In K. Glanz, B. K. Rimer, & K. Viswanath (Eds.), *Health behavior and health education: Theory, research, and practice* (4th ed., pp. 1–13). San Francisco, CA: Jossey-Bass.

Brug, J., Conner, M., Harré, N., Kremers, S., McKellar, S., & Whitelaw, S. (2005). The Transtheoretical Model and stages of change: A critique: Observations by five commentators on the paper by Adams, J. and White, M. (2004) Why don't stage-based activity promotion interventions work? *Health Education Research, 20*(2), 244–258. doi:10.1093/her/cyh005

Carlini, B. H., Schauer, G., Zbikowski, S., & Thompson, J. (2010). Using the chronic care model to address tobacco in health care delivery organizations: A pilot experience in Washington state. *Health Promotion Practice, 11*(5), 685–693. doi:10.1177/1524839908328999

Cherrington, A., Ayala, G. X., Amick, H., Scarinci, I., Allison, J., & Corbie-Smith, G. (2008). Applying the community health worker model to diabetes management: Using mixed-methods to assess implementation and effectiveness. *Journal of Health Care for the Poor and Underserved, 19*(4), 1044–1059.

Cherrington, A., Ayala, G. X. Scarinci, I. Corbie-Smith, G. (2011). Developing a family-based diabetes program for Latino immigrants: Do men and women face the same barriers? *Family and Community Health, 34*(4), 280–290.

Cohen, D. A., Scribner, R. A., & Farley, T. A. (2000). A structural model of health behavior: A pragmatic approach to explain and influence health behaviors at the population level. *Preventive Medicine, 30* (2), 146–154. doi:10.1006/pmed.1999.0609

Corcoran, N. (2007). Theories and models in communicating health messages. In N. Corcoran (Ed.), *Communicating health: Strategies for health promotion* (pp. 5–31). Thousand Oaks, CA: Sage. Retrieved from http://www.corwin.com/upm-data/13975_Corcoran___Chapter_1.pdf

Crosby, R. A., Kegler, M. C., & DiClemente, R. J. (2002). Understanding and applying theory in health promotion practice and research. In R. J. DiClemente, R. A. Crosby, & M. Kegler (Eds.), *Emerging theories in health promotion practice and research: Strategies for improving public health* (pp. 1–15). San Francisco, CA: Jossey-Bass.

Drewes, H. W., Lambooij, M. S., Baan, C. A., Meijboom, B. R., Graafmans, W. C., & Westert, G. (2011). Differences in patient outcomes and chronic care management of oral anticoagulant therapy: An exploratory study. *BMC Health Services Research, 11*(18), 1–7.

Earp, J. A., & Ennett, S. T. (1991). Conceptual models for health education research and practice. *Health Education Research, 6*(2), 163–171. doi:10.1093/her/6.2.163

Eisenberg, C. M., Ayala, G. X., Crespo, N. C., Lopez, N. V., Zive, M. M., Corder, K., Wood, C., & Elder, J. P. (2012). Examining multiple parenting behaviors on young children's dietary fat consumption. *Journal of Nutrition Education and Behavior, 44*(4), 302–309.

Elder, J. P., Ayala, G. X., Parra-Medina, D., & Talavera, G. A. (2009). Health communication in the Latino community: Issues and approaches. *Annual Review of Public Health, 30*, 227–251.

Glanz, K., & Bishop, D. B. (2010). The role of behavioral science theory in development and implementation of public health interventions. *Annual Review of Public Health, 31*, 399–418.

Girma, E., Assefa, T., & Deribew, A. (2010). Cigarette smokers' intention to quit smoking in Dire Dawna Town, Ethiopia: An assessment using the Transtheoretical Model. *BMC Public Health, 10*, 320–326. doi:10.1186/1471-2458-10-320

Green, L. W., Ottoson, J. M., García, C., & Hiatt, R. A. (2009). Diffusion theory and knowledge dissemination, utilization, and integration in public health. *Annual Review of Public Health, 30*, 151–174.

Grier, S., & Bryant, C. A. (2005). Social marketing in public health. *Annual Review of Public Health, 26*(9), 319–339. doi:10.1146/annurev.publhealth.26.021304.144610

Gritz, E. R., Tripp, M. K., James, A. S., Harrist, R. B., Mueller, N. H., Chamberlain, R. M., & Parcel, G. S. (2007). Effects of a preschool staff intervention on children's sun protection: Outcomes of Sun Protection Is Fun! *Health Education and Behavior, 34*(4), 562–577. doi:10.1177/1090198105277850

Heaney, C. A., & Israel, B. A. (2002). Social networks and social support. In K. Glanz, B. K. Rimmer, & F. M. Lewis (Eds.), *Health behavior and health education: Theory, research, and practice* (3rd ed., pp. 185–209). San Francisco, CA: Jossey-Bass.

Hochbaum, G. M. (1958). *Public participation in medical screening programs: A socio-psychological study.* Washington DC: U.S. Government Printing Office.

House, J. S. (1981). *Work stress and social support.* Reading, MA: Addison-Wesley.

Huhman, M., Heitzler, C., & Wong, F. (2004). The VERB campaign logic model: A tool for planning and evaluation. *Preventing Chronic Disease, 1*(3), 1–6.

Janz, N. K., & Becker, M. H. (1984). The Health Belief Model: A decade later. *Health Education Quarterly, 11* (1), 1–47.

Janz, N. K., Champion, V. L., & Strecher, V. J. (2002). The Health Belief Model. In & K. Glanz, B. K. Rimmer, & F. M. Lewis (Eds.), *Health behavior and health education: Theory, research, and practice* (3rd ed., pp. 45–66). San Francisco, CA: Jossey-Bass.

Jeffery, R. W. (2004). How can health behavior theory be made more useful for intervention research? *International Journal of Behavioral Nutrition and Physical Activity, 1*(1), 1–10.

Kaczynski, A., Potwarka, L., & Saelens, B. (2008). Association of park size, distance, and features with physical activity in neighborhood parks. *American Journal of Public Health,98*(8),1451–1456.

Katz, M. H. (2009). Structural interventions for addressing chronic health problems. *Journal of the American Medical Association, 302,* 683–685.

Kerlinger, F. N. (1973). Foundations of behavioral research (2nd ed.). New York, NY: Holt, Rinehart and Winston.

Kuo, S., Bryce, C. L., Zgibor, J. C., Wolf, D. L., Roberts, M. S., & Smith, K. J. (2011). Cost-effectiveness of implementing the chronic care model for diabetes care in a military population. *Journal of Diabetes Science and Technology, 5*(3), 501–513. Retrieved from http://www.pubmedcentral.nih.gov/articlerender.fcgi?artid=3192617&tool=pmcentrez&rendertype=abstract

Littell, J. H., & Girvin, H. (2002). Stages of change: A critique. *Behavior Modification, 26* (2), 223–273. doi:10.1177/0145445502026002006

Lowry, R. J., Billett, A., Buchanan, C., & Whiston, S. (2009). Increasing breastfeeding and reducing smoking in pregnancy: A social marketing success improving life chances for children. *Perspectives in Public Health, 129*(6), 277–280. doi:10.1177/1757913908094812

Marsden, P. V., & Friedkin, N. E. (1994). Network studies of social influence. In S. Wasserman & J. Galaskiewicz (Eds.), *Advances in social network analysis: Research in the social and behavioral sciences* (pp. 3–26). Thousand Oaks, CA: Sage.

Martinez, S. M., Ayala, G. X. Patrick, K., Arredondo, E. M., Roesch, S., & Elder, J. P. (2012). Associated pathways between neighborhood environment, community resource factors, and leisure-time physical activity among Mexican-American adults in San Diego, CA. *American Journal of Health Promotion, 26*(5), 281–288.

Marzillier, J., & Eastman, C. (1984). Continuing problems with self-efficacy theory: A reply to Bandura. *Cognitive Therapy and Research, 8,* 257–262.

McGuire, W. J. (1985). Attitudes and attitude change. In G. Lindzey & E. Aronson (Eds.), *Handbook of social psychology* (3rd ed., pp. 233–346). New York, NY: Random House.

Miller, K. L. (1980). Principles of everyday behavior analysis (2nd ed.). Montgomery, CA: Brooks/Cole.

Montaño, D. E., & Kasprzyk, D. (2002). The Theory of reasoned action and the theory of planned behavior. In K. Glanz, B. Rimer, & F. M. Lewis (Eds.), *Health behavior and health education: Theory, research, and practice* (3rd ed., pp. 67–98). San Francisco, CA: Jossey-Bass.

Munro, S., Lewin, S., Swart, T., & Volmink, J. (2007). A review of health behavior theories: How useful are these theories for developing interventions to promote long-term medication adherence for TB and HIV/AIDS? *Biomedical Central Public Health, 7*, 104–119.

National Cancer Institute. (2005). *Theory at a glance: A guide to health promotion practice.* Retrieved from http://www.cancer.gov/cancertopics/cancerlibrary/theory.pdf.

Oetzel, J., Devargas, F., Ginossar, T., & Sanchez, C. (2007). Hispanic women's preferences for breast health information: Subjective cultural influences on source, message, and channel. *Health Communication, 21* (3), 223–233.

Prochaska, J. O. (1979). *Systems of psychotherapy: A transtheoretical analysis.* Pacific Grove, CA: Brooks-Cole.

Prochaska, J. O., & DiClemente, C. C. (1983). Stages and processes of self-change of smoking: Toward an integrative model of change. *Journal of Consulting and Clinical Psychology, 51* (3), 390–395. Retrieved from http://www.ncbi.nlm.nih.gov/pubmed/6863699

Prochaska, J. O., Redding, C. A., & Evers, K. E. (2002). The transtheoretical model and stages of change. In K. Glanz, B. Rimer, & F. M. Lewis (Eds.), *Health behavior and health education: Theory, research, and practice* (3rd ed., pp. 99–120). San Francisco, CA: Jossey-Bass.

Richard, L., Kosatsky, T., & Renouf, A. (2011). Correlates of hot day air-conditioning use among middle-aged and older adults with chronic heart and lung diseases: The role of health beliefs and cues to action. *Health Education Research, 26* (1), 77–88. doi:10.1093/her/cyq072

Rogers, E. M. (1962). *Diffusion of innovations.* New York: Free Press.

Rogers, E. M. (2002). Diffusion of preventive innovations. *Addictive Behaviors, 27*, 989–993.

Rosenstock, I. M. (1974). Historical origins of the Health Belief Model. *Health Education Monographs, 2*, 1–8.

Rosenstock, I. M., Strecher, V. J., & Becker, M. H. (1988). Social learning theory and the Health Belief Model. *Health Education Quarterly, 15* (2), 175–183.

Sallis, J. F., Cervero, R. B., Ascher, W., Henderson, K. A., Kraft, M. K., & Kerr, J. (2006). An ecological approach to creating active living communities. *Annual Review of Public Health, 27*, 297–322. doi:10.1146/annurev.publhealth.27.021405.102100

Stokols, D. (1992). Establishing and maintaining healthy environments: Toward a social ecology of health promotion. *American Psychologist, 47*(1), 6–22.

Suarez-Amazor, M. E. (2011). Changing health behaviors with social marketing. *Osteoporosis International, 22* (Suppl 3), S461–S463.

Thalacker, K. M. (2011). Hypertension and the Hmong community: Using the Health Belief Model for health promotion. *Health Promotion Practice, 12* (4), 538–543. doi:10.1177/1524839909353735

Veitch, J., Ball, K., Crawford, D., Abbot, G. R., Psych, G. D., & Salmon, J. (2012). Park improvements and park activity: A natural experiment. *American Journal of Preventive Medicine, 42* (6), 616–619.

Wagner, E. H. (1998). Chronic disease management : What will it take to improve care for chronic illness? *Effective Clinical Practice, 1*, 2–4.

White, K. M., Hyde, M. K., O'Connor, E. L., Naumann, L., & Hawkes, A. L. (2010). Testing a belief-based intervention encouraging sun safety among adolescents in a high-risk area. *Preventive Medicine, 51*, 325–328.

PART 2

HEALTH SPECIFIC PROMOTION

Chapter 4

Jennifer A. Emond, PhD and Guadalupe X. Ayala, PhD, MPH

NUTRITION

Key Terms

biomarker	dietary pattern	food security
community health workers	dose	market basket
competitive foods	energy-dense foods	nutritional epidemiology
dietary behaviors	environmental food audit	self-monitoring

Learning Objectives

Upon completion of this chapter, you should be able to:

1. Explain how the United States Department of Agriculture defines a healthy dietary pattern.
2. Differentiate between dietary intake and dietary behavior.
3. Give examples for when a food diary, a 24-hour dietary recall, or a food frequency questionnaire is an appropriate method to use when measuring dietary intake.
4. Design a scenario in which an individual's family has a positive influence on her own self-efficacy to adopt healthy dietary behaviors.
5. Provide recommendations to improve the dietary intake of students attending elementary and secondary schools in an organizational level intervention.
6. Develop methods to measure the physical and social environmental influences of employees' dietary behaviors within a workplace.

7. Select a tool to measure the community's access to fresh produce.
8. Describe how socioeconomic differences in health status across the U.S. may be partially explained by a lack of access to healthy foods.
9. Provide an example of a state or federal policy that was designed to promote healthy dietary behaviors of individuals.
10. Describe how a policy at the state or federal level based on taxing unhealthy foods could impact the dietary behaviors of individuals.

Chapter Outline

Nutrients in Food
    Basic Physiological Functioning
    Dietary Patterns
The Role of Healthy Eating Programs
Dietary Intake
Factors That Influence Dietary Behaviors
    Individual-Level Influences on Dietary Behaviors
    Interpersonal-Level Influences on Dietary Behaviors
    Organizational-Level Influences on Dietary Behaviors
    Community-Level Influences on Dietary Behaviors
    Policy-Level Influences on Dietary Behaviors
Summary

INTRODUCTION

A large component of health is based on the foods a person eats. Most adults are aware of certain dietary recommendations. For example, many people know that eating lots of fruits and vegetables is recommended for optimal health and that too much salt can harm health. Because most people eat a variety of foods, no one food or meal on a given day is going to have a dramatic impact on one's overall health. However, longer-term exposure to certain nutrients found in foods can influence health. Consider the timeframe of a month or even a year: most individuals will tend to choose from the same types of foods over this time. It is this general **dietary pattern** that health researchers want to optimize for good health and to prevent diseases such as heart disease, diabetes, and cancer.

Nutritional epidemiology studies have linked certain dietary patterns to an increased risk of certain diseases. For example, evidence from nutritional epidemiology studies support that diets high in sodium increase the risk of hypertension, diets low in calcium and vitamin D increase the risk of osteoporosis, and diets high in refined carbohydrates contribute to developing type 2 diabetes (Graudal, Hubeck-Graudal, Jurgens, 2011; IOM 2011; Willett, Manson, & Liu, 2002).

A **dietary pattern** describes an individual's usual dietary intake of foods and beverages.

nutritional epidemiology is the study of how dietary intake and nutritional status impact the distribution of disease and mortality among humans.

SPOTLIGHT

Nutritional epidemiology is the study of how dietary intake and nutritional status impact the distribution of disease and mortality among humans. Nutritional epidemiology often involves prospective cohort studies (e.g., studies that follow people over time) and case-control studies (e.g., studies that compare people with and without a disease). These studies determine the associations between individuals' reported dietary intake and the likelihood of developing a specific disease or health condition. Health promotion researchers often use the results from nutritional epidemiology studies when designing programs to promote a healthy diet. For an easy-to-read introduction to nutritional epidemiology, see *Nutritional Epidemiology—Past, Present, Future* (Michels, 2003).

What defines a healthy dietary pattern? Defining a healthy dietary pattern is not a simple task. Health promotion professionals need to consider the evidence linking the intake of specific food groups to health, the relative intake of specific food groups compared to one's overall dietary pattern, and even how specific food groups interact with each other. Much attention has been given to the Mediterranean diet, a dietary pattern that emphasizes healthy fats, whole grains, fish, fruits, and vegetables. The Mediterranean diet has been linked to decreased risks of heart disease, some cancers, and even Alzheimer's disease (Bosetti, Pelucchi, & La Vecchia, 2009; Kris-Etherton, Eckel, Howard, St. Jeor, & Bazzarre, 2001; Solfrizzi et al., 2011). Think about all the different foods that are part of a Mediterranean dietary pattern. How would health promotion professionals technically define what makes the Mediterranean dietary pattern "healthy"? Would it be appropriate to promote the increased consumption of individual food groups such as fish or whole grains to improve health, or would health promotion professionals need to promote the entire dietary pattern? What evidence would researchers need to answer such questions?

NUTRIENTS IN FOOD

Besides tasting good, food provides the nutrients needed for our bodies to function normally. Nutrients are needed to regulate normal physiological processes including cell growth, tissue repair, and hormone regulation. Because these processes are so varied, the human body needs many different nutrients to maintain normal, healthy functioning.

Basic Physiological Functioning

The human body needs various types of nutrients for basic physiological functioning. These types of nutrients are classified as essential versus nonessential and also as macronutrients, micronutrients, or other nutrients. Essential nutrients are those that are required for normal body functioning. The human body cannot generate these nutrients on its own, or the human body generates these nutrients in quantities too low for adequate functioning. Therefore, humans get these nutrients from food. Essential nutrients include some vitamins, minerals, fatty acids, and amino acids. Nonessential nutrients are those that improve health yet may not be required for basic functioning. Fiber is considered a nonessential nutrient. Macronutrients are nutrients that provide energy to the body. Macronutrients are needed in large amounts (macro = large scale), as they provide the material for many bodily functions. Essential macronutrients include carbohydrates, fats, and proteins; nonessential macronutrients include alcohol. Macronutrients are the main source of energy for the body and provide the building material needed for tissue growth and repair and even provide the material needed for hormone synthesis. Micronutrients are nutrients that are also needed for normal body functions, yet these nutrients are needed only in small quantities (micro = small scale). Micronutrients include vitamins and minerals. Micronutrient deficiencies can result in severe health consequences. For example, anemia can result from a deficiency of the micronutrient iron, and blindness can result from a deficiency of the micronutrient vitamin A. The human body also needs other nutrients for normal functioning. These other nutrients include water and electrolytes such as sodium chloride, potassium, and inorganic sulfate (USDA Dietary Guidelines, 2010).

Dietary Patterns

The United States Department of Agriculture (USDA) is charged with defining a healthy dietary pattern for residents of the United States. The USDA reviews the scientific literature every 5 years, and their final set of dietary recommendations is published as the USDA Dietary Guidelines for Americans. The goal of the dietary guidelines is to define a dietary pattern that provides all of the essential nutrients needed for adequate health. However, because people eat foods and not nutrients, dietary guidelines are based on food groups that share similar nutritional profiles. For example, the current USDA Dietary Guidelines are based on five distinct food groups: grains, fruits, vegetables, low-fat dairy, and protein. For the current dietary recommendations, visit the USDA's website, www.ChooseMyPlate.gov.

The USDA Dietary Guidelines are *evidence based*. An appointed committee reviews the scientific literature regarding diet and health and makes recommendations related to the intake of certain food groups based on their nutritional profiles. For the 2010 USDA Dietary Guidelines, more than 180 scientific questions were analyzed. Specific diseases reviewed included cardiovascular disease (CVD), hypertension, diabetes, cancer, and osteoporosis. Recommended intakes for specific food groups are based on levels found to be related to a reduced risk of chronic disease. Recommendations include limiting those foods or nutrients related to an increased risk of disease and increasing the intake of foods or nutrients related to a decreased risk of disease. Recommendations are relative to the average American diet at the time of the scientific review phase.

Model for Understanding
The USDA Dietary Guidelines

The USDA Dietary Guidelines for Americans are used to inform nutrition-related policies and public health promotion efforts. For example, the dietary guidelines inform national child nutrition programs such as the School Lunch Program and the Special Supplemental Nutrition Program for Women, Infants, and Children (WIC). The Dietary Guidelines also inform the nutrition-related objectives of the Healthy People program, a program sponsored by the U.S. Department of Health and Human Services (HHS) to improve the health of all Americans.

The USDA Dietary Guidelines for Americans are written for an intended audience of policy makers and health care or nutrition professionals; the dietary guidelines are not specifically written for the general public. The dietary guidelines are complex, and the USDA and the HHS work together to develop a communication program to explain and promote the guidelines to the public. The published version of the 2010 Dietary Guidelines is 112 pages long—imagine the difficulty of condensing that into a simple set of messages that the public can understand! Past communication programs have encouraged Americans to choose foods from the "basic four" food groups, from the Food Pyramid, or from an individually tailored program called My Pyramid. Each of these health communication programs has had its share of criticism. The current communication program is the Choose My Plate program (www.ChooseMyPlate.gov). For an interesting review of the history behind the development of the various communication models for the dietary recommendations, see the book *Food Politics* by Marion Nestle (Nestle, 2002).

THE ROLE OF HEALTHY EATING PROGRAMS

Most Americans fall short of following a health dietary pattern as defined in the USDA Dietary Guidelines. For example, most Americans still fail to meet the recommended servings of fruits and vegetables per day (Blanck, Gillespie, Kimmons, Seymour, & Serdula, 2008) and consume too much fat, often in the form of fast food (Briefel & Johnson, 2004).

To help address these deficiencies, the goals for Healthy People 2020 include seven specific nutrition and healthy eating–related objectives. Unfortunately, due to many regional, cultural, economic, and even biological differences, certain population groups are more affected by diet-related diseases than others. For example, in the United States, rates of hypertension are highest among African-American men (CDC, 2010a), and rates of type 2 diabetes are highest among Mexican-American adults (Flegal, Carroll, Kit, & Ogden, 2010). Obesity rates are also disproportionately distributed by racial and socioeconomic status in the United States: African Americans and Mexican Americans are more likely to be overweight or obese compared to White, non-Hispanic Americans, and those who live in lower-income communities are more likely to be overweight or obese than those who live in upper-income communities. Healthy eating programs are therefore important tools not only to help all Americans follow a healthy dietary pattern but also to help reduce disparities seen in diet-related diseases.

SPOTLIGHT

The USDA Dietary Guidelines Address Weight Management

One key recommendation of the USDA Dietary Guidelines for Americans is for individuals to balance their caloric intake and caloric expenditure to achieve and maintain a healthy weight. Overweight or obese status is usually defined in terms of body mass index (BMI), which is a ratio of weight in kilograms over height in meters squared. An individual is considered overweight with a BMI > 25 kg/m^2 and obese with a BMI > 30 kg/m^2. Most recent studies report that 33.6% of American adults are overweight and 34.9% are obese (Ogden, Carroll, Kit, & Flegal, 2014). Overweight and obese status leads to many health complications, including an increased risk of developing metabolic syndrome, type 2 diabetes, cardiovascular disease, and even some types of cancers (National Institutes of Health and National Heart, Lung and Blood Institute, 1998). Therefore, one important aspect of a healthy eating program is to promote a healthy dietary pattern that manages total caloric intake compared to caloric expenditure to promote weight loss when needed and to also maintain a healthy weight once a healthy weight is achieved.

SPOTLIGHT

Breastfeeding is an excellent way for a mother to provide her newborn with proper nutrition. Breast milk is free, contains all of the nutrients needed for proper growth, is easy for newborns to digest, and also provides newborns with antibodies from the mother to help fight off infections such as lower respiratory and ear infections. The American Academy of Pediatrics recommends that all newborns be fed only breast milk for the first 6 months of life and are fed breast milk and appropriate foods up to 1 year. The Academy encourages mothers to continue breastfeeding for as long as they desire. Compared to babies who are fed infant formula, breastfed babies have lower rates of gastrointestinal illnesses and ear infections and even have lower rates of obesity, type 2 diabetes, and asthma as they grow up. However, breastfeeding alone is not the full answer; racial/ethnic and socioeconomic inequities continue to drive many of the outcomes seen in children as recent evidence suggests.

Unfortunately, breastfeeding can be challenging for women. Many women lack appropriate information about the benefits of breastfeeding and lack the support needed from medical professionals and trained experts such as lactation nurses to help overcome the emotional, physical, and even time-management challenges often posed by breastfeeding. Many women may also be confused about breastfeeding in public (a women's right to breastfeed in public is protected under federal and many state laws). Visit the U.S. Department of Health and Human Services' Women's Health website for more information (http://www.womenshealth.gov/breastfeeding/index.html).

DIETARY INTAKE

dietary behaviors include food and beverage purchasing behaviors, meal, snack, and beverage preparation behaviors, and what people and situations cue the consumption of certain foods and beverages, which all ultimately influence what foods and beverages are consumed.

Dietary patterns reflect an individual's usual food intake; **dietary behaviors** are those actions that influence what people eat—for example, whether a family eats their dinner at the dinner table or in the living room in front of the television.

Subsequent sections focus on dietary behaviors, because intervention programs target individuals' dietary behaviors in an effort to improve their dietary intake. However, it is important to understand the ways in which dietary intake is measured and how dietary intake differs from dietary behaviors.

Dietary intake represents the ultimate behavior: what a person puts in her mouth. To determine whether a healthy eating intervention works, dietary intake is tracked for changes over time. In an ideal world, researchers could simply ask individuals what they ate yesterday, the last week, or the last year, free of concern about these individuals' ability to remember what they ate. Yet, measuring dietary intake is an imperfect science, and one source of variation is how well people remember what they ate yesterday, or even the past year. Methods for measuring dietary intake differ, and it is important to understand the limitations of their use.

Food diaries or dietary records are considered an imperfect "gold standard" of intake at the individual level. For these measures, individuals keep a log of all foods and beverages consumed over a set amount of time (e.g., 3 to 7 days). They must be trained on how to track intake as foods and beverages are consumed. Records can be paper based or completed using a computer or smart phone. For example, MyNetDiary (http://www.mynetdiary .com) is an application that users can download to any mobile device or computer. MyNetDiary offers a free basic service as well as more advanced pay-for-service options. Once registered, users track dietary intake. The user simply enters the foods consumed and the application tracks the total caloric intake and nutritional content using a database of more than 515,000 food items. MyNetDiary also tracks physical activity levels and any desired weight loss goals to consider total caloric intake and expenditure. For more examples, search popular stores for mobile and computer applications such as the Google Play store (https://play.google.com/store) or the Apple Store (http:// www.apple.com/iphone/from-the-app-store/). Food diaries or dietary records require participants to be literate and requires high levels of cooperation. Adults can use this method to track intake for children.

During a 24-hour dietary recall, individuals are asked to recall all foods and beverages they consumed in the prior 24 hours. Individuals can complete these assessments on their own using a computer or with a trained researcher in person or over the phone. A 24-hour dietary recall assessment may have a lower level of participant burden than dietary diaries, yet this type of assessment is still burdensome to the participant. Assessments require between 1 and 2 hours of a participant's time and require the participant to recall everything she ate in the previous 24 hours. Additionally, many studies use multiple 24-hour dietary recall assessments, further increasing the level of participant burden. Finally, 24-hour dietary recall assessments are expensive for researchers to conduct due to the need for trained personnel and software required to track participant response. The 24-hour dietary recall is the dietary assessment method used by the National Health and Nutrition Examination Survey (NHANES).

Food frequency questionnaires (FFQs) are questionnaires that include a checklist of foods and beverages consumed over a previous period of time, such as the past 30 days or past year. FFQs can be administered using paper forms or completed online. FFQs reflect usual intake and are not as precise as diet diaries or 24-hour recalls for measuring specific intake at the individual level, and FFQs are limited in the precision of specific nutrients consumed. The food items included on an FFQ can be tailored to be culturally appropriate. The Southwest FFQ is an example of an FFQ tailored to foods typically consumed in the American Southwest (Taren et al., 2000). Completing FFQs requires adequate literacy and cognitive skills. Data from FFQs are useful to describe the average intake of a group, and they can be used to rank individuals within a group.

A brief dietary assessment (BDA) is similar to an FFQ except that it is modified to focus on a smaller set of specific foods or beverages, typically with a focus on the intake of one or a few select nutrients. BDAs include a limited number of items (e.g., 15–30) that are chosen from those foods that are high in the micronutrient or macronutrient of interest. For example, a 20-item BDA has been designed to measure the usual dietary intake of foods containing soy among postmenopausal women (Frankenfeld et al., 2004).

Remember, measuring dietary intake is an imprecise science. Dietary intake methods that ask individuals about past intake are affected by recall bias; people may have difficulty remembering every food or beverage consumed and may not remember the actual serving size, for example. In addition to not remembering well, participants may underreport their total food and beverage intake and specifically underreport their intake of unhealthy foods. Similarly, participants may overreport their intakes of healthy foods. This source of bias is known as a social desirability bias or impression management. Such bias in self-reported intake is more common among certain subgroups such as those who are overweight. Additionally, measuring dietary intake can be time consuming and expensive. Trained counselors are needed to record intake based on 24-hour dietary recall, and calls may take 30 minutes to complete. FFQs can be lengthy, including as many as 125 individual items over multiple pages. For an in-depth review of methods for measuring dietary intake, including specific measures, their validity and reliability, and recommendations of which measures to use, see *Dietary Assessment Methodology* by Thompson and Subar (Thompson & Subar, 2008).

> A **biomarker** is a biological molecule sampled from an individual that reflects a specific metabolic process or biological state.

SPOTLIGHT

The Use of Biomarkers to Validate Dietary Intake

There are various **biomarkers** used to estimate the intake of certain foods. Biomarkers are biological molecules sampled from individuals that reflect a specific metabolic process or biological state (National Cancer Institute, 2012). Samples are obtained through the collection of blood, urine, saliva, hair, and so on. For example, carotenoids, obtained through the collection of blood (plasma), are pigments that give fruits and vegetables their red, yellow, and orange coloring, and plasma carotenoid concentrations can be measured as a proxy of fruits and vegetable intake. Other examples include plasma concentrations of isoflavones to reflect soy intake, urinary nitrogen concentrations to reflect protein intake, and hemoglobin A1C (HbA1C) values to estimate average blood glucose levels over the previous 3 months. It is important to remember that the concentration of any biomarker will differ based on many factors, including an individual's metabolism and food preparation methods. For example, tomatoes are high in lycopene (a carotenoid), and cooking tomatoes increases the bioavailability of lycopene. Also, lycopene is fat soluble, which means more lycopene will be absorbed when foods high in lycopene are consumed with fat. Just think, pizza is a great food for lycopene intake! Obtaining biomarkers as part of a health promotion study requires substantial resources to collect, store, and analyze the samples.

FACTORS THAT INFLUENCE DIETARY BEHAVIORS

There are many factors that influence dietary behaviors. When choosing a snack, an individual may choose to purchase the less expensive potato chips compared to the more expensive fresh fruit, providing an example of how individual characteristics (e.g., concerns related to cost) may influence dietary behaviors (e.g., purchasing the less expensive snack), which ultimately influences dietary intake (e.g., decreased fruit intake and increased high-fat, high-salt snack). Community-level differences in access to healthy foods may make it difficult to follow a healthy dietary pattern, particularly if there is an abundance of unhealthy food in the environment. Similarly, cultural differences in food preparation may impact other dietary behaviors that can greatly influence what is consumed. For example, deep-frying chicken, a popular method of preparation in the Southern United States, greatly increases the level of fat per serving compared to steaming or baking chicken. It is important for health promotion researchers to understand the factors that influence specific dietary behaviors to help individuals lead a healthier lifestyle.

Many federal organizations, such as the USDA, the HHS, and the Centers for Disease Control and Prevention (CDC), recognize the need to consider the multiple influences on dietary behaviors in order to design successful healthy eating efforts. These various influences can be explained as factors within the levels of the Social Ecological Framework (see Chapter 3 for more information on the Social Ecological Framework). The remainder of this chapter describes the key influences on following a healthy dietary pattern under each of the various levels of the Social Ecological Framework. Examples of important considerations for promoting healthy eating are provided.

Individual-Level Influences on Dietary Behaviors

Individual-level influences on dietary behaviors can be grouped into three main categories: *psychosocial*, *biological*, and *lifestyle* (adapted from Story, Neumark-Sztainner, & French, 2002). How much each of those influences what we ultimately consume varies with age, gender, race, ethnicity, and socioeconomic status. Healthy eating efforts need to consider these differences when working with specific populations.

Psychosocial Influences

Psychosocial influences include *knowledge*, the *value an individual places on her health* and her *perceived risk* of disease, and *self-efficacy*. Healthy eating efforts also need to be sensitive to additional psychosocial influences such as the *meaning of food* and *food preferences*.

Knowledge Knowing is an essential component of identifying and selecting healthy food options. A study in New York City showed that among urban Black men (African-American, Caribbean, or African), a greater level of knowledge of the recommend servings of fruits and vegetables was related to a higher intake of fruits and vegetables (Wolf et al., 2008). Knowing how to define an appropriate serving size is also a critical component of monitoring overall intake and total caloric intake of specific food groups. For example, the recommended serving size for meat is 3 ounces, which translates to about 215 kilocalories for one hamburger. Compare that to the 7 ounces per serving of hamburger the typical American eats (Nielsen & Popkin, 2003). That means the typical American eats twice the recommended serving of meat when choosing a hamburger as a meal! For an entertaining comparison of serving sizes and caloric intake 20 years ago compared to today, see the National Heart Lung and Blood Institute's (NHLBI) Portion Distortion quiz (http://www.nhlbi.nih.gov/health/educational/wecan/eat-right/portion-distortion.htm).

The Value of Health and Perceived Risk Some healthy eating programs use health or freedom from disease as a motivator for improving dietary intake. Some researchers argue that in order for individuals to make positive dietary change, they need to first believe they are at risk of developing any related diseases. For example, those who believe there is a strong relationship between diet and developing cancer are more likely to make positive dietary changes (Cohen, Clark, Lawson, Casucci,

& Flocke, 2011), and those with a recent diagnosis of cancer are likely to adopt healthy dietary patterns (Demark-Wahnefried, Aziz, Rowland, & Pinto, 2005). Novel interventions targeting dietary change are also focusing on physical appearance as a motivating factor for increasing fruit and vegetable intake (Whitehead, Ozakinci, Stephen, & Perrett, 2012). For example, the carotenoids found in fruits and vegetables add color to the skin tones of light-skinned individuals, such that those who eat more fruits and vegetables have a deeper yellow skin tone, which is rated as more attractive.

Self-Efficacy Self-efficacy for healthy eating refers to one's confidence to engage in healthy dietary behaviors. That can include one's perceived confidence to act on knowledge, such as purchasing a cereal with recommended levels of fiber by reading the nutrition facts label. Self-efficacy can also extend to confidence in avoiding temptations such as forgoing the dessert table at a family picnic. Individuals are more likely to follow a healthy dietary pattern when they are confident in their abilities to do so.

Biological Influences

Biological states drive hunger, and differences in age, gender, race, and ethnicity influence biological drive. Current physical fitness levels, weight status, level of fatigue, and disease state can also influence the biological drive of hunger. It is important to separate biological drives of hunger from psychosocial drives such as stress or emotional state.

Lifestyle Influences

Dietary behaviors are influenced by many lifestyle factors, including the *time* available to prepare and consume a meal or snack or the *price* of different food choices. The level of influence a lifestyle factor ultimately has on dietary behaviors can vary with individual characteristics. Among lower-income adults, price can be a barrier to purchasing quality fruits and vegetables (Kaufman, MacDonald, Lutz, & Smallwood, 1997), while price may not be a barrier among those with greater incomes. *Culture* is another lifestyle factor that influences dietary behaviors. The influence of culture on dietary behaviors can be seen among individuals and families who recently immigrate to the United States: as individuals begin to identify more with the American culture, dietary patterns change to reflect the typical Western dietary pattern marked by higher intakes of saturated fat, refined grains, and added sugar (Sofianou, Fung, & Tucker, 2011).

Many health promotion efforts target adolescents, and increasing levels of *autonomy* felt among adolescents can impact their dietary behaviors and food choices (Story, Neumark-Sztainer, & French, 2002). Adolescents who spend increasing amounts of time outside of their home with peers may choose to purchase snack foods and fast foods as a symbol of their growing autonomy. Therefore, healthy eating efforts that encourage adolescents to reduce their consumption of soda, snack foods, or fast foods may face resistance from adolescents if they see these messages as challenging their growing independence. More information on the influence of friends is found in the interpersonal section.

Measuring Individual-Level Influences on Dietary Behaviors

Questionnaires, knowledge scales, and quizzes can be used to measure an individual's knowledge of what defines a healthy dietary pattern. Knowledge assessments must consider that the cognitive abilities of individuals are influenced by factors such as age, literacy, and disease state. There are validated scales that measure self-efficacy for healthy eating. Questionnaires are also available to measure an individual's self-reported dietary behaviors related to various lifestyle factors. For example, the National Health and Nutrition Examination Survey (NHANES) study includes a dietary behavior questionnaire. This assessment includes questions such as the number of meals eaten away from home, the number of fast food meals, and even the number of frozen meals eaten in the past week. Other questions include how often a school-aged child eats meals at school and if the family receives any federal assistance from nutritional programs such as WIC. These subjective measures can help estimate how lifestyle factors may influence dietary choice.

Behavioral observation offers an objective technique to gauge an individual's dietary behaviors. Innovative studies have used eye-tracking sensors to measure the frequency and duration of nutritional label reading by customers (Graham & Jeffery, 2011). Not surprisingly, customers actually looked at a product's nutritional label much less frequently than they claimed to have when asked with a self-report instrument. Objective measures also include observing an individual preparing a meal to record foods used and cooking methods, observing an individual as she estimates portion sizes, and even weighing a plate of food before and after eating to measure the actual amount of food consumed.

Interventions Targeting Individual-Level Influences on Dietary Behaviors

Print material can provide tips on identifying healthier foods, identifying appropriate serving sizes, and tips for overcoming lifestyle barriers to healthier eating. Material developers must consider the target audience's educational level as well as their cultural differences to be most effective. There are a variety of print materials available from state and federal government agencies. For example, the USDA offers a series of tip sheets for healthy eating, including how to eat well on a budget. Often these materials are free to use in research studies, although there may be specific guidelines related to the use of the agency's logo. Materials available from the USDA, CDC, NHLBI, National Cancer Institute (NCI), and American Heart Association (AHA) include tip sheets for making positive dietary changes, self-monitoring worksheets, and recipe booklets. These agencies also provide promotional and program planning materials. One limitation to consider is that individuals rarely make dietary changes based on print material alone.

Counseling can effectively target individual-level influences on dietary behavior as a way to encourage dietary change. Counseling can target knowledge by including education about appropriate dietary recommendations, serving sizes, and healthier meal preparation techniques. However, beyond print material alone, counseling increases the likelihood of dietary change by helping individuals self-monitor their progress, by providing social support, and by building their confidence, their self-efficacy for making dietary changes.

In health behavior research, **self-monitoring** is a technique individuals often use to track behaviors in an effort to document patterns of behavior and to use those patterns to effect behavior change. For example, individuals may use collected data to identify barriers to behavior change (e.g., time of day, emotional state, physical location). Self-monitoring is also a method to empower individuals with a way to monitor progress toward a behavior-change goal.

For example, healthy eating counselors can train individuals on how to identify healthier food options in stores or restaurants, how to select appropriate serving sizes using food models, and even how to prepare healthier meals and snacks based on different cooking techniques. Health promoters can teach individuals healthier meal preparation techniques and then observe individuals practice those techniques with cooking demonstrations. Counseling programs can be delivered one-on-one in a clinic setting, at the participant's home, over the phone, or over the Internet. Instruction can also be delivered as part of a group or classroom setting. A limitation of counseling programs is that they often require large resources. Staff must be hired and trained. Counseling delivered over the phone or Internet can greatly reduce the cost of counseling programs compared to in-person meetings.

Finally, healthy eating efforts can even target certain biological influences of dietary behavior such as taste preferences. For example, school gardening programs have been shown to be an effective way to increase children's willingness to taste new vegetables, and taste ratings for vegetables are higher among children in these school garden programs compared to children not part of these programs (Jaenke et al., 2012). Chef and activist Alice Waters is often credited with starting the farm-to-school movement with the Edible Schoolyard Project, supported by the Chez Panisse Foundation in 1996 (http://edibleschoolyard.org/). That project provides students in primary and secondary public schools in urban areas with land for gardening and kitchen space to prepare foods.

Model for Understanding
Self-Monitoring of Dietary Intake

Many healthy eating programs that target dietary change include some aspect of self-monitoring. Self-monitoring of dietary intake increases the likelihood of long-term dietary change and is an effective tool when used in weight loss programs. Specifically, individuals are most successful in making positive dietary change when they set goals, self-monitor their progress toward meeting those goals, and review their progress with others (Michie, Abraham, Whittington, McAteer, & Gupta, 2009). Self-monitoring of dietary intake can involve keeping a food diary or using a worksheet or checklist to track dietary intake. Self-monitoring can be done with traditional paper logs or worksheets or electronically with smart phones, PDAs, or computers. Counselors can review an individual's dietary intake log and then help that individual identify and overcome barriers to adopting healthy dietary changes. One reason self-monitoring works is that it can serve as a feedback loop to individuals, making them more aware of what they are eating, where they are eating certain foods, and who they are around when they eat these foods. As will become evident in the next sections of this chapter, identifying these influential factors is important for sustained dietary change.

Targeting Individual-Level Influences

Benefits of targeting individual-level influences on dietary behaviors are that they are the most immediate precursors of dietary behavior. However, there are many influences on dietary behavior that are outside the control of an individual. Other people can influence dietary behaviors through role modeling, through peer pressure, or by setting social norms. Additionally, some groups, such as children and the elderly, have limited control over their diet if others prepare their meals. Also, the foods that are available in schools, at work, and in the community all influence an individual's ability to access healthy food options. These factors will be discussed next.

Interpersonal-Level Influences on Dietary Behaviors

As with other health behaviors, other people influence our dietary behaviors. These people include family members (immediate and extended), close friends, and even acquaintances. The ways in which they influence our dietary behaviors are extremely varied, as are the dietary behaviors that they influence, depending in part on the influential sources and the context of the behavior (at home versus at a restaurant). However, one important distinction to consider immediately is whether the influence is *direct* or *indirect*. For example, parents have a direct influence on the dietary intake of their young child by deciding what foods are purchased for the home and how accessible those foods are to young children in that home (e.g., chips in a bottom drawer or washed and precut vegetables in the fridge). Conversely, friends can have an indirect influence on dietary behaviors and intake by influencing what type of restaurant is chosen for lunch. Even a recommendation from a store employee can change what you buy at a grocery store. Healthy eating efforts are concerned with the impact that these interpersonal influences have on dietary behaviors. Health promotion researchers and practitioners are interested in how to change these interpersonal sources of influence so that they are health promoting.

Social Support

Social support is among the most important variables to consider when examining interpersonal levels of influence that occur naturally and that are changeable (i.e., can be improved). The interactions we have with others reflect the various forms of social support that promote healthy eating. There are four classifications of social support: instrumental, emotional, informational, and appraisal (see Table 4-1 for a description of each type of support). Each type of social support is unique and can be targeted in different ways and in synergy to promote healthy eating.

As with sources of influence, the provision of social support can be direct, such as a spouse preparing a special meal for a partner who was recently diagnosed with diabetes. Or it can be indirect, such as a father congratulating his son for eating the vegetables on his plate.

TABLE 4.1 The Four Types of Social Support

Type of Social Support	Description
Emotional	Empathy, love, caring
Informational	Advice, suggestions, information
Instrumental	Tangible aid and services
Appraisal	Feedback used for self-evaluation

SPOTLIGHT

Do Social Support and Social Influence Mean the Same Thing?

As the term suggests, social support is generally considered to reflect the positive support offered by others. Social support is a specific example of social influence, where social influence is the more general term used to describe the influences of others. Social influences can be positive or negative. Peers can be a source of positive influence if they are engaging in healthy lifestyle behaviors (e.g., suggesting bringing a brown-bag lunch instead of stopping to get fast food); however, peers can be a source of negative influence if peer pressure and social norms are directed at unhealthy eating behaviors (e.g., always choosing to go to the restaurant that does not have a vegetarian option).

Social Norms and Social Networks

A lesser-studied area of social influence relates to social norms. Social norms refer to the socially, culturally, and contextually relevant factors that guide what a society values and expects from its people. In some cultures, it may be disrespectful to refuse to eat what is served on one's plate even if it is twice as much as you might need to maintain energy balance. Social norms are driven, in part, by what is communicated through mass media. For example, it is not uncommon for young immigrant children to request certain foods from their parents based on what they see on television, and their parents to comply with these requests to ensure that their children are adapting to the perceived norms of their new community.

Social scientists also have examined the concept of social networks and their influence on eating and weight and, more generally, on health. Social networks can be considered in terms of their size (the number of people in the network), their homogeneity (how similar network members are to each other—for example, in terms of race/ethnicity, gender, and socioeconomic status), their density (how much they interact with each other), and their dispersion (how close in proximity they live to each other). Social networks may support or impede healthy eating behaviors.

The Influence of Family

Family members are the most influential persons in determining our dietary behaviors and our intake. This is evident as a direct influence in terms of sharing meals together. And it is evident as an indirect influence based on what is brought home from the grocery store or ordered over the phone for dinner. All family members likely have an influence on our dietary behaviors, though most of this research has focused on mothers. This is not surprising given that mothers, in most families, have the longest and most impactful influence on dietary behaviors. From how long she breastfeeds to what she buys at the grocery store, from how much oil she uses in the frying pan to the size of cereal portions served, mothers are influential in forming dietary behaviors. As a result, mothers are often the target of interventions to improve dietary behaviors within a family.

Model for Understanding
Are Families or Friends More Important?

Consistent with social development theories like those proposed by Eric Erikson, the dietary behaviors of children become more susceptible to the behaviors and norms of their peers as they age into preadolescence and adolescence. This is due in part to the fact that more time is spent eating outside the home, including with friends at child care and in school. However, the influence of friends is not limited to children. In an experimental study to examine sources of influence on how much we eat, women were randomly assigned to receive a larger portion versus a smaller portion and to eat with someone who ate a larger portion versus a smaller portion (think a 2 × 2 table). These researchers from the Netherlands found that women ate bigger portions of food when they were served the larger portion and when the person they were with ate the larger portion (Hermans et al., 2012). This shows the multiplicative effect of being served larger portions and someone modeling eating larger portions.

An observational study by Salvy and colleagues (2011) exemplifies the complex power of family versus friend influence on dietary behaviors. In that study, researchers examined the influence of mothers or same-sex friends on food selection among children (5–7 years old) and adolescents (age 13–15). Children consumed fewer unhealthy snacks in front of their mothers than with friends. In this case, it seems that children were aware of their mothers' expectations of limiting their intake of unhealthy snacks. Female adolescents, on the other hand, ate fewer unhealthy snacks and more healthy snacks when they were with their friends than when with their mothers. That pattern was not seen among the male adolescents. Thus, these results may reflect the growing sense of body image among teenage girls and the resultant social norms related to food that influence dietary intake.

Davison and Campbell (2005) created a model showing how the parents' dietary behaviors contributed to the development of their children's food preferences, dietary behaviors, and ultimately their risk for obesity. Specifically, parents who are overweight, who have problems controlling what they eat, or who are concerned about their child's intake will engage in controlling feeding behaviors, which in turn is associated with unhealthier dietary behaviors and greater risk for obesity.

Finally, family support is important for healthy eating. Researchers have consistently found a relationship between family support and healthy eating, with a potentially more pronounced relationship among men than among women. This may be because women still have the primary role for the food shopping and food preparation for the household. Family support is important for children's eating behaviors. Children who receive higher levels of family support for healthy eating consume fewer sugar-sweetened beverages.

Measuring Interpersonal-Level Influences on Dietary Behaviors

Similar to individual-level influences, interpersonal influences can be measured with questionnaires. Given that social support is among the most studied aspects of interpersonal influence, its many characteristics have been captured through self-report and using observational methods as described in what follows. For example, researchers have asked mothers to report on the amount of support they provide their children that promotes healthy eating, including instrumental support (e.g., "Provide your child with low-fat foods as a snack"), emotional support (e.g., "Encourage your child to eat lower-fat foods"), and informational support (e.g., "Share information about how to read the nutrition label"). A variety of family and friend support scales are available on on-line (e.g., http://sallis.ucsd.edu/).

Other self-reported measures of interpersonal influence include asking how often family members go to fast food restaurants during a typical week, how often family members share meals during a typical week, and how often the TV is on during those shared meals.

Researchers have also observed the direct and indirect behaviors of family members and how this might influence children's risk of being obese (McKenzie et al., 2008). Using an innovative method known as BEACHES (Behaviors of Eating and Activity for Child Health Evaluation System), trained research assistants went into the homes of Mexican-origin families and observed the types of prompting that parents were using to encourage eating, what foods were available in the home, and how both of these were related to what the child ate and his/her BMI. The variables that explained part of why the children were obese were having unhealthy foods available at home, including both sweet and salty snacks, as well as sugary beverages. Observed data are important to collect, as they are less subject to social desirability bias, particularly when asking parents about how they are supporting (or not) the health of their children.

> ## SPOTLIGHT
>
> Mealtime is not the only time when parents and children interact that ultimately influences children's dietary behaviors. Increasing evidence points to the importance of examining child influence in other contexts such as grocery stores. How many of us have seen a child throw a temper tantrum in a grocery store in order to get his or her parent to buy him or her a product? Any given food shopping trip provides many opportunities for food purchasing–related interactions between children and parents. Children begin to ask their parents to purchase particular products by 18 to 24 months of age (Valkenburg & Cantor, 2001). Previous research has shown that parents underestimate the influence that children have over their shopping decisions (Ebster, Wagner, & Neumueller, 2009). This is an innovative line of research that few people are examining that has the potential to change the way healthy eating efforts are designed for parents.

Interventions Targeting Interpersonal-Level Influences

Consistent with the Social Ecological Framework, researchers have identified numerous variables at the interpersonal level that could be targeted in health promotion efforts. Among the many strategies that have been used to promote healthy eating at the interpersonal level is targeting improvements in social support. Methods for intervening on social support include the provision of new sources of social support, as in community health worker programs (see "Spotlight" box). Alternatively, one could focus on building the capacity of existing social network members to engage in more supportive behaviors. For example, parents can be taught how to communicate more effectively with their teenagers to negotiate healthier dietary behaviors when out with friends. Spouses can be taught about how to negotiate dietary changes as a result of a diagnosed health condition in their significant other. There is strong and consistent evidence that efforts that reach the parents are most important for both parent and child dietary change; child and other family member involvement is desirable though not a necessary condition for change.

Interpersonal interventions are often delivered in a group format, though as with individual-level interventions, they can occur via print materials, telephone calls, Internet, and text messaging, among other methods. The group format capitalizes on the social aspect of change. Groups can occur with family members only, such as with a family-based intervention in which a coach comes to the family's home, or they can occur with other families such as in a skills development group or support group.

community health workers are members of the community they are trying to reach who are trained to provide various forms of support to promote health and reduce risk of illness.

SPOTLIGHT

Community health workers (CHWs) are individuals who are similar to the target community, sharing cultural and language preferences. They understand how country-of-origin factors influence dietary decisions and behaviors. CHWs engaged in dietary behavior change efforts most commonly share information about what it means to eat healthy, how to identify healthy foods in the grocery store and in restaurants, how best to estimate portion sizes, and how to create a healthy plate. CHWs have been trained to help women improve the dietary behaviors of themselves and of their families (Elder et al., 2006, 2009). Similarly, CHWs have been trained to conduct home visits with women and their children to engage in home-based strategies to promote healthy eating and physical activity (Duerksen et al., 2007). These efforts have resulted in improvements in parenting skills (Ayala, Elder, et al., 2010) and in children's health behaviors (Crespo et al., 2012). Introducing this source of support to the family system is an evidence-based approach for intervening on a number of health behaviors (Viswanathan et al., 2009) and specifically among Latinos (Ayala, Vaz, et al., 2010). An important factor to consider when examining CHW–led family based efforts is how much contact (or overall **dose**) is needed to achieve dietary behavior change. This is important given that each contact is associated with a certain cost, and communities in which such efforts are needed often lack the resources to implement them.

The **dose** of a health behavior intervention represents the level of exposure that individuals who are enrolled in the program have to the behavior change material and activities, such as the number of educational sessions or support groups attended. For programs implemented at the family level, dose could be counted as number of home visits completed.

How much dose is needed is one area of much-needed research. As part of the development of a family-based intervention, a dose of eight contacts was identified as the amount of contact needed for dietary behavior change. However, in a more recent look at the literature examining changes in childhood obesity and other measured indicators of child health, a dose of 16 contacts was identified as being closer to what is needed for sustained behavior change and improvements in measured health indicators.

Targeting Interpersonal Influences

Substantial evidence supports the importance of the interpersonal level of influence. The sources of influence are varied, as is the type of influence that they can exert, and on a varied number of dietary behaviors. Many of these influences are modifiable. However, targeting interpersonal influences has its challenges, including knowing who to target in your effort. For example, should a program encouraging school-aged children to eat more fruits and vegetables enroll the children, just the parents, or both? What about teachers? Finally, interpersonal sources of influence do not occur outside a larger context, among them the organizations in which dietary behaviors occur. This is the focus of the next section.

Organizational-Level Influences on Dietary Behaviors

The *physical* and *social environment* of an organization can influence an individual's dietary behaviors and ultimately their ability to maintain a healthy diet. *Physical environmental* influences include the food environment, such as access to healthy or unhealthy foods. The physical environment also includes appropriate areas for eating such as cafeterias and break rooms. For example, an office building with a designated kitchen area can help employees follow a healthy diet by providing an appropriate place to store and prepare foods. Conversely, a high school that allows outside vendors to sell fast foods such as pizza and hamburgers during lunchtime creates an environment with easy access to unhealthy food options. *Social environmental* influences refer to an organization's culture, and often this is reflected as social norms within the organization. Management often dictates the corporate culture of workplaces, and administrators often dictate the culture within schools. For example, a workplace that values productivity first and foremost may create a social environment in which employees choose not to take meal breaks, possibly encouraging an employee to choose less healthy yet more convenient meal options at lunch.

Examples of social environments that are supportive of following a healthy lifestyle include workplaces that implement wellness programs or provide incentives such as discounts on health insurance premiums when employees maintain a healthy lifestyle. Schools can develop a culture that is supportive of healthy dietary behaviors. Examples include encouraging student-led fundraisers to offer healthy food options instead of candy or requiring students to enroll in a course focused on healthy dietary habits. Shift workers, or employees with variable work schedules, are more likely to be overweight or obese than are day workers (Antunes, Levandovski, Dantas, Caumo, & Hidalgo, 2010). Organizations such as hospitals often take extra steps to create physical and social environments that can help shift workers maintain a healthy diet.

The Influence of Schools on Dietary Behaviors

By 2000, nearly one third of U.S. children and adolescents were overweight (age- and sex-adjusted BMI ≥ 85th percentile), and while obesity rates have slightly declined among preschoolers, this rate has remained relatively stable since 2003 (Ogden, Carroll, Kit, & Flegal, 2014). During this time, diseases previously seen only among adults such as type 2 diabetes and hypertension were being reported among children. It is no wonder that many healthy eating programs have focused on schools.

The School Nutrition and Dietary Assessment Study started in 1995 to measure the dietary intake of students. The goal of that survey was to measure the dietary quality of meals prepared in schools as part of the School Breakfast Program and the National School Lunch Program and to compare the dietary intake of students who participated in these school meal programs to that of students who did not. Data from this survey not only provide nationally representative estimates of the dietary quality of school meals but also provide estimates of the prevalence of **competitive foods** sold on school campuses.

competitive foods are foods and beverages including snacks, meals, and sodas sold on campus that are not funded under school-based meal programs. Competitive foods are also referred to as a la carte items and include foods sold by outside vendors such as fast food companies and also foods sold by school groups as part of fundraisers.

Public health researchers can use results from this survey to inform nutritional health programs focused on schools. For example, the most recent data showed that vending machines were available on 97% of high school campuses, and the most common competitive foods offered on campuses were energy-dense snacks such as candy, cookies, and sugar-sweetened beverages (Gordon et al., 2007). Studies have demonstrated that exposure to competitive foods influences the dietary patterns of students: students who attend schools where competitive foods such as soda and fast food meals are available have diets of lower nutritional quality than students in whose schools the availability of competitive foods is limited (Kubik, Lytle, Hannan, Perry, & Story, 2003). These lower-quality diets are marked by lower intakes of fruits and vegetables and greater intakes of added sugars and saturated fat. On the other hand, competitive foods can be a significant source of income for primary and secondary schools, often in the form of contract fees paid to the schools and as profit sharing from products sold. Schools also receive materials and supplies (e.g., football scoreboards) from food manufacturers. Those products often display the company's logo. One study among Oregon public schools (Pinson, 2005) in 2004 found that school districts received between $12 and $24 dollars per student based on contacts with soda companies, which lasted an average of 9 years. Revenues for the manufacturers were much greater. With many public schools in the United States struggling financially, it is easy to see how contracting with food manufacturers may be an attractive model for increasing revenue. Unfortunately, the current food and beverage offerings may put public school children's health at risk.

In 2011, the USDA updated the standards for breakfasts and lunches served in public schools in the United States. Nutritional standards increased the required amounts of fruits, vegetables, whole grains, and low-fat milk servings per meal. Standards also limited the amount of sodium and saturated fat offered per meal. Upper limits on the total calories per meal were also set, based on age and grade level of students. These guidelines were praised by public health organizations as one way to help improve dietary intakes of public school children while also helping children consume an appropriate amount of total calories (compared to previous meals that were often too high in total calories). Many school professionals and parents were concerned that children were not eating the updated meals and possibly not consuming enough calories. The USDA published a report to summarize comments to the 2011 school lunch and school breakfast nutritional standards along with the organization's response (USDA, 2012).

Daycare Centers More than 3 million children attend day-care Centers, where attitudes about eating and nutrition are often formed (Anzman-Frasca et al., 2012). Many day-care provide drinks, meals, and snacks to children and are therefore important outlets to providing proper nutrition to children. The USDA funds the Child and Adult Care Food Program (CACFP, http://www.fns.usda.gov/cacfp/child-and -adult-care-food-program) to help centers meet appropriate nutritional needs of children and adults in day-care facilities. The CACFP, established in 1968, provides financial and educational support to day-care centers. Meals and snacks provided must meet certain nutritional requirements for reimbursement. However, meals and snacks consumed at day-care centers may still not meet appropriate nutritional standards: meals and snacks are too often based on starchy carbohydrates with added sugars and fats, and children may not be consuming enough fruits and vegetables (Copeland, Neelon, Howland, & Wosje, 2013). Programs are needed to help support day-care centers in providing nutritionally appropriate meals and snacks (Robert Wood Johnson Foundation, 2007).

Measuring Organizational-Level Influences

Individual self-report by members of an organization can be used to gauge an organization's physical and social environment with respect to healthy eating. It is important to remember that the rating of an organization's environment depends on who is being surveyed. For example, employees may rate the food environment differently than their supervisors do, and students may have a different perspective than teachers within schools, in part because they may be interacting with different aspects of the food environment.

An **environmental food audit is** often done to assess the physical food environment of an organization. Audits of an organization's physical environment include checking for the presence of designated food storage areas, checking for eating areas such as break rooms or cafeterias, and counting the number of available competitive food options. Audits can be extended to assess the quality of food offered within organizations, such as the quality of school lunches or the quality of items offered in vending machines. Audits can also gauge the social environment of an organization. Counting the number of visible posters that encourage healthy eating habits is one method to gauge the social environment of an organization toward healthy eating; surveying an organization about any wellness programs that support healthy dietary behaviors is another. The National Cancer Institute (NCI) provides a listing of food environment audit instruments; this listing includes 5 instruments for work sites and 18 instruments for schools (see Web Resources section at end of chapter for more information).

Programs can also measure sales of healthy or unhealthy food options at an organization over a period of time. While this method cannot reflect an individual's intake, it can reflect an average intake at an organization and can be used to track changes in intake over time. Food waste measurements can be used to compare the food offered to students or employees during mealtimes; food is measured before and after mealtime, and any food left uneaten can gauge the overall intake of specific food items.

An **environmental food audit** is a precise measurement of physical or social aspects of that environment that can influence the quality, accessibility, and availability of various food items. Environmental food audits are typically completed with standardized forms; examples include audits that measure the physical environments of institutions, food retail outlets, workplace organizations, and even communities. Additional resources on environmental food audits can be found on the National Institutes of Health website for the NCCOR initiative.

Targeting Organizational-Level Influences

Organizations commonly targeted with healthy eating programs include schools, worksites, and hospitals. As mentioned earlier, organizations can encourage healthier dietary choices by altering the physical environment. Adequate food storage and eating areas can be designated, and healthier food can be offered in cafeterias or in vending machines. Healthier food options can also be priced lower than less-healthy options to encourage an individual to purchase these healthier choices. For example, one study found that a 50% price reduction on fresh fruit increased sales of fresh fruit by 400% (French, 2003).

Social norms that support healthy dietary choices can shape the social environment related to dietary behaviors. Promotional material encouraging a healthy dietary pattern such as posters can be made visible at the organization. The organization can sponsor wellness and nutrition programs for its members. Incentive programs can also tap into individual motivating factors to promote dietary change.

For example, a workplace wellness program could offer free nutritional counseling or provide medical insurance discounts for employees who maintain a healthy weight. Schools could encourage a healthy eating environment by limiting access to unhealthy, competitive foods and by supporting food service workers in preparing healthier meal options.

Implementing Change at the Organizational Level Students and employees spend a large portion of their day in schools and worksites, and patients in hospitals or long-term-care facilities are many times dependent on the physical food environment of the organization. Healthy eating efforts implemented at the organizational level have the potential to reach a large audience. Healthy eating efforts that modify the foods available at the organization, or their price, can have a direct impact on the foods individuals have access to in the organization. These approaches require no direct involvement of the individual. Offering healthier meals and snacks at the organizational level may provide other benefits in addition to better nutrition for members of the organization. Offering students, teachers, employees, and patients healthier food options can improve attention and focus and can even improve morale by offering individuals meals and snacks they desire. From the organization's perspective, offering less-processed, healthier food options may be more labor intensive and expensive than offering meals based on more-processed foods. However, the overall benefits to the organization must also be considered.

Limitations of targeting organizational influences include limited control over the foods individuals bring to the organization, such as premade lunches. Additionally, individuals in an organization are only exposed to the physical and social environments that support healthy eating while at the organization. However, incentive programs may carry over to time spent outside of the organization, and any positive social norms acquired while at the organization may carry over to behaviors outside of the organization. Also, the level of attentiveness to healthy eating promotional material may be dependent on the level of social integration an individual has with the organization. An employee who feels disgruntled about his employer may not be receptive to promotional material. Finally, the implementation of a healthy eating effort at an organization is dependent on the key decision makers of the organization. Many times, these decision makers need to also consider other factors such as financial cost. Finally, decision makers may change over time, which can impact the sustainability of a healthy eating initiative.

Community-Level Influences on Dietary Behaviors

In 2012, the American College of Sports Medicine named Minneapolis, MN, as the healthiest city in America. Minneapolis received the highest ranking on more than 25 indicators of health, including low rates of heart disease and diabetes and high access to farmers' markets. In comparison, Oklahoma City, OK, ranked last out of the 50 cities included in the survey (for all listings and study details, see the ACSM American Fitness Index website in the Web Resources section). As discussed in the physical activity chapter, access to public parks is just one important aspects of a city's ability to support the health of its residents; the availability and affordability of quality, healthy food is another component of how a community can influence the health of its residents. A community with a healthy food environment is one where residents have access to quality, affordable healthy foods, which supports residents in following a healthy dietary pattern.

Critical Thinking

The Centers for Disease Control and Prevention's Strategies for Healthy Food Environments

The Centers for Disease Control and Prevention (CDC) considers healthy food environments a key health topic related to community design. The CDC outlines nine strategies for the creation and maintenance of a healthy food environment. These strategies are (1) zoning, (2) land use planning and urban/peri-urban agriculture, (3) farmland protection, (4) food policy councils, (5) retail food stores, (6) community gardens, (7) farmers' markets, community-supported agriculture, and local food distribution, (8) transportation and food access, and (9) farm-to-institution and food services. Think about the various levels of the Social Ecological Framework each one of these strategies involves. Think about how each one of these strategies can support a healthy food environment. Who do you think would be the key players involved in creating and maintaining each of these strategies?

A healthy food environment is a vital component to individual health. For example, individuals who live in areas with limited access to healthy food options are at a disadvantage in their ability to follow a healthy dietary pattern. Grocery stores have been frequently used as a proxy for the availability of affordable, healthy foods in a community. Studies have shown that residents in communities with a greater density of grocery stores are less likely to be overweight (Morland, Diez Roux, & Wing, 2006) and are more likely to follow a healthy dietary pattern (Moore, Diez Roux, Nettleton, & Jacobs Jr., 2008). Conversely, communities with excess exposure to **energy-dense foods** such as fast food and snacks foods can support unhealthy dietary choices.

energy-dense foods are foods and beverages high in calories and low in nutritional value per serving. The high caloric content of these foods and beverages is often due to high levels of added sugar and fat. Energy-dense foods include candy and snack foods such as chips and cookies but can also include other foods consumed as meals, such as packaged sweetened breakfast cereals and frozen or prepared meals such as pizza.

Energy-dense snacks and meals are often less expensive per calorie than healthier alternatives. When these foods are freely available within a community, the ability of an individual to follow a healthy dietary pattern may be jeopardized by offering temptations of less healthy and less expensive food alternatives. Studies have found a positive correlation between the number of fast food restaurants in a community and residents' BMI (Li, Harmer, Cardinal, Bosworth, & Johnson-Shelton, 2009). In fact, students of secondary schools are more likely to be overweight and less likely to follow a healthy dietary pattern with a greater number of fast food restaurants near the school (Davis & Carpenter, 2009). Adolescents in communities with a greater density of convenience stores, a common outlet for energy-dense snacks, are more likely to be overweight (Powell, Auld, Chaloupka, O'Malley, & Johnston, 2007).

Measuring Community-Level Influences

There are many ways to measure the community food environment. One way to do this is to measure the presence of food outlets in an area. The idea here is that a greater presence of certain food outlets (e.g., fast food restaurants) will be associated with greater consumption of high-fat and high-sugar foods. As such, studies categorize food outlets by their type; for example, stores include super-centers, supermarkets, farmers' markets, and grocery, ethnic, convenience, and liquor stores. Among restaurants there are sit-down, buffet, and fast food. Food banks are another example of a community outlet to help those who are food insecure follow a healthy dietary pattern.

food security refers to the minimum level of socially acceptable access to food required to sustain normal functioning. Food security also includes access to healthy foods items required for proper nutrition.

SPOTLIGHT

Food Security

The World Food Summit of 1996 defined **food security** as "when all people at all times have access to sufficient, safe, nutritious food to maintain a healthy and active life" (World Health Organization, 2012). While food security includes access to healthy food items, this term is also used to define the minimum level of socially acceptable access to food required to sustain normal functioning. For example, in the American culture, accessing quality food at a food bank or shelter is less socially acceptable than purchasing those foods at a supermarket. The USDA defines households as having *low food security* when members have to modify their diet quality because of limited income or limited access. Such households may still be able to consume enough food to meet their energy needs; however, diet quality is compromised. An even more extreme situation exists for households with *very low food security*. These households have had to limit overall food intake at some point in the previous year. The most recent estimates show that 9.1% of U.S. households have low food security and 5.4% of U.S. households have very low food security (USDA & ERS, 2011).

One way to count the presence of different types of food outlets in a community is by integrating lists from different organizations. This process is called enumeration, and it may include cross-referencing state and local databases to collect current food retail licenses, followed by checks in the field to assess validity (i.e., how representative the list is of the true food environment). The presence and location of outlets can be measured using geographic information systems (GIS) technology. Those methods often require trained researchers to visit areas (e.g., field surveys) and record the location of specific food outlets using GIS software. The software is then able to summarize the locations visually and provide data related to density and proximity. For example, researchers in California used GIS technology to map the location of supermarkets, grocery stores, and other vendors providing fresh produce (in addition to many other outlets) in lower-income communities; authors recommended that the data be used to help inform community-level polices regarding access to healthy food options (Ghirardeli, Quinn, & Foerster, 2010). As described further in what follows, this can be followed by a detailed environmental audit to better understand what is specifically in the environment. Likewise, transportation opportunities are another critical feature of a community's food environment. Vehicle ownership, access to public transportation, and even walkability within a neighborhood can all impact residents' abilities to access outlets that provide affordable, healthy foods (Ver Ploeg et al., 2009).

There are many food environment measurement tools available. The CDC provides a series of measures and toolkits for assessing a community's food environment. These resources include the USDA's Community Food Security Assessment Toolkit, which has measures for food availability within a community while considering other barriers to food access such as a lack of transportation (Cohen, 2002).

Access and exposure can also be measured by the *presence of food items within food outlets* collected using a within-store environmental audit. The amount of shelf space devoted to fresh fruits and vegetables or the number of displays of snack foods and soda quantifies exposure to foods within stores. Within-store audits can also record the *availability*, *quality*, and *price* of various items. The food items included in a within-store audit tool can vary. Some audits focus on specific food types, while more general audits include a range of basic food items considered to make up a standard food **market basket**.

A **market basket** is defined by the USDA as the sum of a variety of food and beverage items that will allow an individual to follow the recommended dietary guidelines for 1 week. Market baskets can also be computed for households. The USDA creates a series of recommended market baskets based on four income levels to help individuals and households maintain a healthy diet while considering price (Carlson, Lino, Juan, Hanson, & Basiotis, 2007).

Some audits even focus on a few food items specific to managing certain chronic diseases. For example, researchers in New York conducted within-store audits to measure the availability of five foods that were recommended to manage type 2 diabetes: low-carbohydrate or high-fiber bread, low- or nonfat milk, fresh fruit, fresh green vegetables, and diet or club soda (Horowitz, Colson, Hebert, & Lancaster, 2004). The results of that study demonstrated that lower-income communities had limited access to these five recommended foods, especially when compared to upper-income communities.

The NCI provides a listing of food environment audit tools (see Web Resources). Audit tools focusing on the organizational level of the Social Ecological Framework were previously mentioned; however, this resource from NCI also lists measurement tools targeting community-level influences on dietary behaviors. Instruments for food stores, the home, public facilities, and restaurants are included. Research studies that have used each instrument are also cited. One popular within-store environmental audit tool is the Nutrition Environment Measures Survey for Stores (NEMS-S). This survey measures availability and price of various healthy food items and, when appropriate, any less-healthy alternatives. For example, the NEMS-S survey audits the availability and price of whole milk, low-fat milk, and skim milk, as well as 80% lean ground beef, 90% lean ground beef, and > 90% lean ground turkey. Results from the NEMS-S can be used to compare the availability and price of healthier options such as skim milk or extra-lean ground beef across stores. Results from the NEMS-S are one way to gauge the ability of a community to meet the needs of its residents who wish to maintain a healthy diet.

Disparities in Access to Healthy Food Items Unfortunately, the quality of a community's food environment varies greatly with different community characteristics. Within-store audits completed in various U.S. cities have shown that lower-fat milk and lower-fat meat options are less available in stores located in lower-income communities than in stores located in upper-income communities (Laska, Borradaile, Tester, Foster, & Gittelson, 2009). Often when these lower-fat options were available, they cost more than the fuller-fat, less-healthy options. This limited access and price barrier puts residents of these lower-income communities at a disadvantage in terms of acquiring these lower-fat food products. Evidence also supports that the quality of healthier foods may be compromised in lower-income communities. Studies comparing produce quality in lower- and upper-income communities of Chicago, IL, and also between Kansas City, KS, and Kansas City, MO, found lower-quality produce offered in stores in lower-income communities compared to upper-income communities (Block & Kouba, 2006; Lee et al., 2010). Finally, lower-income communities are often disproportionately exposed to unhealthy, energy-dense foods from convenience or corner stores, liquor stores, or fast food restaurants (Powell, Slater, Mirtcheva, Bao, & Chaloupka, 2007). The frequent exposure to these outlets, the ease of access to these outlets, and the often low price of items at these outlets can encourage residents to follow an unhealthy dietary pattern (Rose et al., 2009).

Targeting Community-Level Influences

Healthy eating programs at the community level can influence dietary change by altering the environment. Environmental changes studies can take advantage of "natural experiments" by comparing the dietary intake of residents in a community before and after the introduction of a new grocery store. Environmental change studies can also manipulate the availability of foods within food outlets. The Healthy Bodega Initiative is a program sponsored by the New York City Health Department to support New York City corner stores in stocking healthier food options such as low-fat milk, fresh produce, and healthier snack food options (New York City Department of Health and Mental Hygiene, 2012). Another ongoing innovative effort in Southern California is working with small to medium-sized Latino food store managers/owners to modify the food store, both physically (via structural changes) and socially (via employee training and a point-of-purchase campaign), to increase purchasing and consumption of healthy foods. Introducing farmers' markets or mobile food vendors into neighborhoods is another way to improve the healthy food environment of a community (for more information on similar efforts, please visit the Institute for Behavioral and Community Health website [www.ibachsd.org]).

Healthy eating programs can also be incorporated as part of larger community projects (Twiss et al., 2003). These community projects could be centered on food security, cultural integration of immigrant groups to the community, and even neighborhood beautification. Community garden projects and community food co-ops are just two examples of larger community projects that can easily incorporate healthy eating programs. Many community projects take a "bottom-up" or grassroots approach to community building by empowering community residents to organize and execute community projects with minimal outside interference. Financial support is available for such programs. For example, the USDA administers the

Community Food Projects Competitive Grant Program to fund community-based programs that target improvements to a community's food system.

Implementing Change at the Community Level Measuring the community food environment requires significant resources from the research team. Enumerating locations requires access to current databases of retail food outlets. Databases are often large, requiring trained data managers to handle them. Also, food outlet entries in these databases require trained research staff to verify that food outlets remain in business. Enumeration efforts that incorporate GPS data require additional technical expertise. Within-store audits also require significant resources. It is important to use instruments with good psychometric properties, and researchers should incorporate some verification of these properties such as measuring the interrater reliability. Auditors must be trained in the instrument's protocol to ensure that their observation match those of someone who is considered the gold standard; when it matches in all or most cases, this is referred to as high interrater reliability. Some within-store audit instruments may be lengthy, possibly taking up to 1 hour to complete. Finally, the availability and price of food items may change over time.

Community food environment interventions are intended to target the overall well-being of a community's residents. There is often no specific measurement of an individual's exposure to, purchase of, and consumption of specific foods. Programs at the community level cannot guarantee that all residents will be impacted by specific environmental changes. For example, some residents may choose to shop for groceries in other communities that are close to their work or school as opposed to their neighborhood food store that is participating in a healthy eating initiative.

As with organizational changes, changes at the community level require no direct input from an individual. However, there is always the risk that some residents of the community will object to an environmental change. It is also important to distinguish between community-*placed* healthy eating programs and simply community-*based* programs.

Community-placed programs are those that are implemented by researchers or organizers outside of the community. While these program planners may be able to bring in significant funding for a healthy eating initiative, there is always the risk that community residents may reject the outside involvement. Program planners who are not based in a specific community need to be sensitive to a community's social and political structure and should work to establish connections with key stakeholders in the community.

Conversely, a community-based program that takes more of a grassroots approach may have more direct insight into the immediate needs of the community. However, a community-based program may face many delays and hurdles when program planners are inexperienced in dealing with the intricate details of planning, funding, and implementing a community effort. Additionally, coordinating the time available to work on a community-based program may be difficult, especially when working with various community interest groups.

It is also possible to have a hybrid of these two models. In this case, an outside agency provides funding and organizational structure for a community project yet allows community members to direct and execute the project with periodic oversight.

SPOTLIGHT

Special Considerations When Trying to Change Dietary Behaviors

Context. Programs that teach and encourage individuals to adopt new dietary behaviors may be more successful at promoting sustained behavior change when programs are implemented in a setting where those dietary behaviors naturally occur. For example, if the goal is to change food-purchasing behavior, an intervention implemented at the grocery store or restaurant level may be more successful at promoting sustained behavior change than an intervention disseminated in a classroom setting.

Resources. Time, funding, and partners. Multilevel interventions are needed to effect long-term changes, but they are costly. Planners must select the intervention context and approach that will have the greatest potential to effect the needed change and then be sustained in that context

Stakeholder preference. Listening to and working with organizations and community members to identify where and how to intervene will strengthen implementation.

Policy-Level Influences on Dietary Behaviors

There are many ways that policies can support an individual's ability to maintain a healthy diet. Policies set at the federal level are consistent across states, while policies set at the local level can be tailored to the particular needs of any one state, county, or city. At the most macro level, federal policy sets the nutritional standards for many government programs based on the USDA Dietary Guidelines for Americans. The Supplemental Nutrition Assistance Program (SNAP) and the Special Supplemental Nutrition Program for Women, Infants and Children (WIC) program are two examples of federally funded programs to help low-income individuals purchase healthy food items. In 2011, the SNAP program helped 40 million individuals each month purchase healthy food, and the WIC program covered more than 9 million individuals. Many community-level organizations have outreach programs to enroll eligible individuals and families in federal- and state-run programs such as WIC and SNAP. For example, California funds the First Five program (http://www.ccfc.ca.gov/). First Five consists of community outreach and promotional programs to encourage families with children 0 to 5 years old to learn about federal- and state-level programs available to them, including nutrition assistance programs. The SNAP program in California, CalFresh, also runs many community enrollment clinics to encourage eligible individuals to apply for SNAP benefits; clinics are often held in lower-income communities at housing developments, at community centers, and at senior living centers. Clinics are often held in conjunction with food distribution events. For example, the San Diego Food Bank in San Diego County hosts many "occasional" and "emergency" food distribution events to provide food-insecure individuals with food. Foods are often donated by grocery stores and organizations in the community. For more information about the San Diego Food Bank outreach programs, including programs with CalFresh, visit their website (http://sandiegofoodbank.org/programs).

Policies can increase access to nutritious foods and encourage the consumption of healthy foods. Funding for the Community Food Projects Competitive Grant Program is set by legislation formally called the Food, Conservation, and Energy Act (informally referred to as the U.S. Farm Bill). Policies can also be designed to discourage the consumption of unhealthy foods. Two examples of policies intended to curb unhealthy eating are those that require fast-food restaurants to post the caloric content of menu items and policies that require taxes on sugary beverages.

Policies related to healthy eating efforts can begin with a bottom-up or grassroots approach. A grassroots approach includes community activism or lobbying to introduce a bill on local or state ballots. Advocacy groups such as the California Center for Public Health Advocacy have lobbied for the introduction of state bills requiring a tax on soda or a fee on fast-food meals that include toys for children. Policy change can also happen with momentum from scientific and consumer organizations. As part of the 2010 Affordable Care Act, restaurants are required to post the caloric content of foods and beverages they serve. Many advocacy groups including the American Cancer Society lobbied for that legislation (U.S. Food and Drug Administration, U.S. Department of Health & Human Services, 2011). Finally, policy could even be set with legislation as the result of a civil lawsuit. In California, a public-interest lawyer sought to ban the sale of Oreo cookies due to their trans-fat content; the case was dropped in 2009.

Measuring Policy-Level Influences

Measuring the effectiveness of policy implementation is a complex process. As a starting point, health promotion researchers studying healthy eating policies can turn to published guidelines used to measure the impact of general public health policies. For an example, see *Measuring the Impact of Public Health Policy* (Brownson, Seiler, & Eyler, 2010).

One method to measure the effectiveness of a healthy eating policy on behavior change is to take advantage of natural experiments. Specifically, an outcome related to healthy eating can be measured and compared before and after the implementation of a policy. Possible outcomes include self-reported dietary intake of healthy or unhealthy foods, rates of chronic disease including obesity, the availability of healthy food items within a community, or even the availability and price of healthy food items within food outlets. It is important to remember that the chosen outcome must reflect a direct consequence of the policy change. For example, policies that limit the availability of competitive foods during lunchtime within schools in an attempt to improve the diets of students could measure fruit and vegetable intake (e.g., components of a healthy diet) among students before and after the policy change; it would be wasteful to measure dietary intake of all community residents since not all residents would be affected by such a policy.

Finally, it is important to remember the rule of unintended consequences with any policy change. Specifically, a policy change may inadvertently shift the targeted behavior to another undesirable behavior. For example, if a school implemented a policy to limit the availability of competitive foods at school, perhaps students would adapt by bringing in their own unhealthy snacks and lunches. In fact, it is not uncommon to hear about "black markets" for candy and snack foods at secondary schools!

Another method to measure the effectiveness of a healthy eating policy is to compare a relevant outcome between communities with and without the policy. It is important that communities being compared are similar in demographics when taking this approach. As an example, in July 2008, New York City became the first U.S. city to require certain fast-food restaurants to post the caloric content of menu items. A study was conducted soon after the implementation of this policy to gauge its effectiveness on changing customer behavior. That study compared the food purchases of customers in fast food restaurants in New York City to customers of the same fast food restaurant in nearby Newark, New Jersey, where menu labeling was not required. Results showed that posting the caloric content on menus in these fast food restaurants had no influence on the items consumers purchased (Vadiveloo, Dixon, & Elbel, 2011).

Targeting Policy-Level Influences

Policies by their nature are interventions. This section expands on three ways policies can be constructed to support healthy eating.

SPOTLIGHT

Farm-to-What?

Farm-to-school, farm-to-hospital, and farm-to-work programs are examples of programs that connect organizations with local farms that provide fresh food to the organization. Farm-to-organization programs connect local farmers (e.g., farms within a 100-mile radius) to a local distribution center to sort and store foods. Program administrators organize the various food items and work with organizations to meet meal requirements. By working with local farmers, programs are often able to save on operating costs by reducing costs related to distribution and loss related to food spoilage due to long-distance travel. In that way, programs can offer fresh produce to local organizations. Programs also benefit the communities they are located in by supporting local business. The National Farm-to-School Network provides information on programs and events at the state level (http://www.farmtoschool.org/). The USDA also provides information on current farm-to-school programs and their details in becoming established. For example, the USDA helped the Boston Public School District in Massachusetts set up a farm-to-school program with the aid of local nonprofit organizations. A coordinator was hired by the school district to help with program details, and a 1-year pilot program was established to phase in local foods as part of special programs such as Local Lunch Thursdays. Local nonprofits such as Food Corps (a program of AmeriCorps) continued to help with program administration after the 1-year pilot period.

Reducing Barriers to Purchasing Healthy Foods SNAP and the WIC program were mentioned as two examples of federally funded programs to help low-income individuals purchase healthy food items. These programs are designed to reduce the barrier of price in purchasing healthier food items. Policies that require nutritional information to be provided on food packages target the barrier of limited knowledge in determining if a food can be considered a healthy option. Policies that provide funding for farm-to-school or farm-to-hospital programs can help increase access to healthy foods within organizations. Policies that provide funding for farmers' markets help reduce the barrier of access to fresh fruits and vegetables in the community. Policies can also help target disparities in access to healthy foods in communities by encouraging the development of grocery stores by providing tax incentives or subsidies. Even policies that determine the scheduling and cost of public transportation routes can reduce the lack of transportation as a barrier to healthy eating.

Increasing Barriers to Purchasing Unhealthy Foods Previous sections discussed policies to implement taxes on sugary beverages and fees on fast food meals that include a toy for children. These policies are intended to decrease the likelihood of purchasing these products by introducing an additional barrier based on price. At the most macro level, federal policies impact the subsidies provided to U.S. farmers when growing commodity crops such as corn, soy, and wheat. Since these crops are major ingredients of energy-dense meals, snacks, and drinks, many food companies are able to offer these energy-dense foods at prices that are much lower than those of healthier food or beverage options. Change in these policies that might limit the subsidies provided for these crops may therefore increase the cost of many energy-dense foods, thus increasing the barrier of price in purchasing these foods.

Decreasing Demand for Unhealthy Foods Policies that require restaurants to post the caloric content of menu items are intended to reduce the demand for unhealthy foods. Customers may be surprised to learn how many calories (and possibly grams of fat or salt) a meal has. Posting this information is also intended to help customers make healthier food choices by comparing different items. Policies that limit the marketing of energy-dense meals, snacks, or drinks to children are another way to decrease the demand for these products among a vulnerable group. Many food industries specifically promote products to children to increase "pester power": the likelihood that parents will break down and purchase a product for their children after continued pestering. Marketing can include television advertisements to children, sponsorships and promotions aimed at children, even product placement within video games or movies. Policies can be implemented that limit the marketing of unhealthy food items to children, much in the way that polices limited the way tobacco companies could market to children.

Many food industries promote self-regulation with respect to healthy eating as an alternative to federal or state policy changes. Health promotion experts have rated industry efforts as mixed. For example, the Smart Choice program was an industry-led effort to promote certain snacks and beverages as healthy options. These products were identified with a green check mark on the front of the package. However, many of the products given Smart Choice labels did not meet standard nutritional requirements as defined by a nonindustry health group (Roberto et al., 2012).

The program was highly criticized and was discontinued after only a few months (Neuman, 2009). For detailed information on nutritional health policy in the United States, visit the Yale Rudd Center for Food Policy & Obesity website (http://www.yaleruddcenter.org).

Implementing Change at the Policy Level

An advantage of healthy eating policies is that a large group of individuals is influenced, with no direct involvement from the individual. Unfortunately, those who disagree with a policy may divert their behavior to another unhealthy option. Bans on competitive foods in secondary schools may result in a black market for snack foods, for example. A policy may also have unintended consequences. If a tax on sugary beverages was implemented in California and not in neighboring states, residents near the state border might divert their business outside of California.

Policies that impact organizations such as schools also have to consider unintended consequences. Soft-drink companies often provide large financial incentives to secondary schools for exclusive contracts with that school. A policy banning competitive foods sold in schools would jeopardize that additional funding.

Policy change can be a slow process. Time is needed to build support for the health issue being targeted and to draft legislation. For a policy to be effective, the policy needs to be properly implemented and enforced. These actions require state, federal, or organizational resources. Penalties for noncompliance also need to be defined and enforced.

Summary

This chapter provided a comprehensive examination of diet, how to measure it, and how to promote a healthy diet across the Social Ecological Framework, with case examples provided at all levels of influence.

4-1   CASE STUDY

Nutritional Education and Dietary Behaviors of WIC Enrollees

The Special Supplemental Nutrition Program for Women, Infants and Children (WIC) is a federally funded program to help low-income individuals purchase healthy food items. Those eligible include women who are pregnant, breastfeeding, or recently gave birth and children under the age of 5. The WIC program provides enrollees with money to purchase food; the food purchased must be from a list of specific items called the WIC food package. In October 2009, the WIC food package underwent a major revision. For the first time, the food package included fresh fruits and vegetables, whole grains, and lower-fat milk. These changes were made so that the WIC food package better agreed with the USDA Dietary Guidelines for Americans.

Women who receive WIC benefits and caregivers of children who receive WIC benefits must participate in nutrition education counseling. The state of California required that a new nutrition curriculum be developed for WIC enrollees before the introduction of the new WIC food package in October 2009. The new education curriculum, called Healthy Habits Every Day, would provide education related to increasing the intake of fruits and vegetables, whole grains, and lower-fat milk. The new curriculum was designed to include three sessions delivered over a 6-month period and was tailored to consider the large proportion of Latino enrollees in California. Nutrition education counselors were trained in administering the new curriculum, and all 82 WIC sites in California began using the new curriculum in April 2009. Since the new WIC package was set to be introduced in October 2009, this provided a unique opportunity for researchers to measure the impact of a targeted, nutrition education program on the dietary intake of WIC enrollees before changes in the WIC food package.

This study is an example of a *natural experiment*. To determine whether the curriculum was effective, the researchers conducted two separate cross-sectional surveys at two time points: before the implementation of the new curriculum in April 2009 (preexposure) and after implementation of the new curriculum in September 2009 (postexposure). Surveys asked enrollees about their dietary intake of fruits, vegetables, whole grains, and lower-fat milk. The survey was informed by the Transtheoretical Model (TTM), and enrollees were asked a series of questions to classify them based on their readiness to change, a condensed version of the TTM's stages of change, in adopting the healthier dietary behaviors. For each food group, enrollees were classified as not thinking about eating these foods (precontemplation stage), intending to eat these foods (planning stage), or already eating these foods (action stage).

At each time point, two random samples of 3,000 WIC participants were surveyed, and more than 90% of those surveyed agreed to participate. It is important to note that two separate groups were surveyed at each time point. The goal of the study was to determine if exposure to the new curriculum increased awareness and consumption of fruits, vegetables, whole grains, and lower-fat milk for participants and their families. Therefore, the main outcomes of the study were awareness of nutritional messages, movement in readiness to change to the new dietary behaviors, and self-reported dietary intake for the participant and participant's household. These outcomes were measured for each of the three food groups targeted and were measured pre- and postexposure to the new curriculum to determine if any changes occurred after implementation of the new curriculum.

The results were mixed. For all food groups, awareness of nutritional messages promoting each food group increased from pre- to postexposure to the new curriculum, supporting the prediction that WIC enrollees were aware of the new educational messages. However, self-reported intake of fruits and vegetables was not different between the two time points. Nevertheless, a slightly greater number of participants who were surveyed postexposure reported eating whole grains compared to participants surveyed preexposure, and an even larger number of participants who were surveyed postexposure reported consuming lower-fat milk compared to participants surveyed preexposure. Lower-fat milk intake was also greater for the entire family among the group surveyed postexposure. In agreement with the self-reported dietary intake data, the percentage of participants in each stage-of-readiness-to-change category was similar pre- and postexposure for fruits and vegetables, yet at postexposure to the new curriculum, a greater number of participants reported being in the planning and action stages for increasing intake of whole grains and lower-fat milk.

There are several aspects of this study worth highlighting. First, the study was a natural experiment. Researchers took advantage of a state-mandated change to the WIC nutrition education curriculum to measure the effectiveness of a nutrition education curriculum on changing dietary behaviors. The WIC program is an established program with a developed infrastructure in place, which allowed for a relatively easy way to incorporate the study measures. One limitation is that the curriculum was already designed, and researchers could not modify any of the curriculum components.

This study did not include *repeated measures* on the same participants. If the researchers did design a repeated-measures study, the study would have followed the same participants pre- and postexposure to the new curriculum. Instead, two large, random, cross-sectional samples of enrollees were collected at both time points. Each sample had a high participation rate, and the sample characteristics such as age, race, ethnicity, and WIC specific enrollment criteria were similar between the two samples. Also, this study was not a randomized trial. All WIC sites in California were required to use the new curriculum in April 2009, meaning that there were no *comparison* WIC sites (i.e., those that did not use the new curriculum) to compare the findings to.

Source: Ritchie, Whaley, Spector, Gomez, & Crawford (2010)

Thought Questions

1. What levels of the Social Ecological Framework are represented in this study?

2. This study was designed using the Transtheoretical Model, and participants were classified based on a condensed version of TTM's stages of change. However, the nutrition education curriculum primarily targeted knowledge: identification of these foods and the health benefits related to eating these foods. After reading this chapter, think about ways the curriculum could have been enhanced to address dietary behaviors instead of simply knowledge.

3. The nutrition education curriculum was found to be most effective in increasing awareness of health messages for lower-fat milk and for increasing reported intake of lower-fat milk. Why might this program be most effective in changing dietary behaviors for milk compared to the other food groups included?

4. At the time this study was completed (April and September 2009), the WIC food package did not include fresh fruits and vegetables. The new WIC food package, introduced in October 2009, did include subsidies for fresh fruits and vegetables. Consider how the allowable WIC food package may impact the dietary intake of enrollees and their families. How you do think the results of this study may have differed if the WIC package included fresh fruits and vegetables at the time this study was completed?

Family Meal Decision-Making Styles and Dietary Behaviors Among Hispanic Families in Southern California

In the United States, women in households that value traditional, patriarchal values typically are the sole planners and preparers of meals and snacks for their partners and families. When women take on these traditional roles, meals are primarily prepared with the taste preferences of their husbands or partners in mind. Typically, these meals tend to be low in fruits, vegetables, and whole grains and high in saturated fat. As decision making within the household becomes more shared, women gain more support in preparing meals that are higher in fruits and vegetables and lower in saturated fat.

Most previous research on meal decision-making styles has focused on non-Hispanic, White families; little research had been conducted with Hispanic families, particularly families from Mexico or whose parents were from Mexico. Traditional Mexican culture values a patriarchal household structure, and the female head of household traditionally prepares all meals and snacks. Further, when Mexican families immigrate to the United States, members become acculturated to a "U.S." lifestyle, in part because of the need for women to work outside the home, and thus traditional family roles give way to a more egalitarian, shared decision-making process. Researchers of this study were interested in understanding how dietary behaviors change with changes in meal decision-making patterns as reported by Mexican-origin families in the United States.

Researchers recruited 357 Mexican-origin women and their families living in central and southern San Diego County, California (southern San Diego County shares a border with Mexico). Most women were born in Mexico (95%), and most women were married (79%). Women were asked to keep a dietary intake diary for 3 days, and at the end of 3 days, trained researchers visited the women in their homes to input their dietary data into a computer program (see 24-hour recalls for more information on this methodology). The intake data were entered into the Nutrition Data System managed by the University of Minnesota to compute the average daily intake of various food groups and nutrients (e.g., calories consumed per day).

Women were asked about their meal decision-making process in the home for breakfast, lunch, and snacks, and responses were categorized as traditional (women plan or prepare meals alone) or shared (women plan or prepare meals with their partner and/or children). Women were also asked about their *expectations* (an individual psychosocial variable) related to healthy eating. Women were asked to rate their responses to 10 statements such as "Eating more fruits and vegetables will make me healthier" and "Eating high-fat foods now increases my chance of getting cancer later in life." Finally, women were asked to similarly rate their response to a series of 19 items related to *barriers* to eating fruits and vegetables and to eating low-fat foods (an individual psychosocial variable). Barriers included "Fresh fruits and vegetables will spoil before my family and I can eat them" and "High-fat foods are more convenient than low-fat foods."

As expected, results from this study showed that women who practiced shared meal decision making were more likely to be employed and more likely to be acculturated to the American culture than were women in traditional decision making households. However, in contrast to previous studies, this study showed that Mexican women who practiced shared meal decision making followed less healthy diets. Specifically, women with shared meal decision making had a greater intake of saturated fat than did women with traditional meal decision-making roles. Women with shared meal decision making reported more barriers to preparing low-fat snacks for themselves and their households compared to women with traditional meal decision-making roles, and women with shared meal decision making employed fewer *behavioral strategies* for eating more fruits and vegetables. Finally, women with shared meal decision making were more likely to eat outside of the home (e.g., at fast-food restaurants) than women in households with traditional meal decision-making styles. In short, it seems that women who work outside the home and adopt a more American way of life are more likely to use shared decision-making strategies when it comes to meal preparation; however, unlike what was hypothesized, they are also likely to engage in behaviors that result in less healthy eating.

The results of this study demonstrate the importance of understanding cultural differences when working with different races and ethnicities. While previous studies that enrolled non-Hispanic, White women showed a better in diet quality with shared meal decision making, results from this study showed the opposite: women with shared meal decision making in Hispanic families tended to have a less healthy diet marked by higher intakes of saturated fat, and these women used fewer behavioral strategies to add more fruits and vegetables to household meals. Interestingly, the ratings of *expectations* of healthy eating did not differ by meal decision-making style, and with the exception of increased barriers to eating low-fat snacks, women in shared meal decision-making households did not report any fewer or more *barriers* to increasing fruit and vegetable intake overall or for reducing saturated fat intake at meal time. Again, these results were in contrast to previous studies among non-Hispanic, White women that suggested women in traditional meal decision-making households face greater barriers to preparing healthier meals. The researchers concluded that dietary intervention programs targeting Hispanic families may be best served by focusing on the entire household or family. Programs should also incorporate negotiation and communication strategies for meal preparation among Hispanic women, in contrast to simply supporting Hispanic women in their efforts to overcome barriers in preparing healthier meals.

Source: Arredondo, Elder, Ayala, Slymen, & Campbell, (2006)

Thought Questions

1. What levels of the Social Ecological Framework are represented in this study?

2. Research in theories of social support have identified several types of support that family and friends can provide. For example, family members can provide *emotional support* by giving a relative a pep talk before caving into serving a second helping of potato salad. What other types of social support are represented in the case study?

3. If you were put in charge of designing a program to promote healthy eating in the family, what strategy might work in this case study?

4. Change in dietary behaviors following the immigration process has been identified as an important area of study given that these changes are often unhealthy and lead to negative health consequences for these immigrants. What can communities do to prevent dietary changes from happening?

Review Questions

1. Describe how the USDA's Dietary Guidelines for Americans influence the dietary intake of children in the United States.

2. The most appropriate data collection method for a researcher to use when trying to understand the usual dietary intakes of a group of participants over the previous year would be:

    a. 24-hour dietary recall
    b. Food diary
    c. Objective measurement
    d. Food frequency questionnaire

3. Maria has had a long day at work as the CEO of a Fortune 500 company, and as a result, she is very tired on her way home. She has two young children at home, and she still needs to prepare dinner for her family. Instead of preparing a meal from foods at home, she decides to stop at the drive-through window of a fast-food restaurant near her office to pick up dinner. Provide examples of factors at the individual, interpersonal, organizational, community, and policy levels that may have impacted Maria's decision to purchase fast food for dinner.

4. Fill in the blank: Once Maria arrives at home, she serves the fast food to her children. Maria is _____ influencing her children's dietary intake.

    a. Directly
    b. Indirectly

5. David works at a company that values employee health. His office offers fresh fruit for employees in the morning and offers an employee discount at a local farmers' market. His company also encourages employees to submit their favorite healthy recipes to a workplace cookbook each summer. In this example, how is David's company hoping to influence the dietary behaviors of its employees?

6. Meals and snacks sold on school campuses that are not part of school-based meal programs are referred to as:

    a. Energy-dense foods
    b. Competitive foods
    c. SNAP benefits
    d. WIC benefits

7. A researcher counted all of the convenience stores and other outlets known to sell energy-dense snack foods that were within a 1-mile radius of 10 elementary schools. She also collected dietary intake data on a sample of students at each of those 10 schools. In her study, she found a positive correlation between the amount of energy-dense snack foods consumed by students and the number of outlets that sold energy-dense snack foods near the school. Provide an example of how her study results could be used to inform a public health program that targets individual-, interpersonal-, organizational-, community-, and policy-level influences of dietary behavior.

8. True or False: In the United States, differences in community-level influences on dietary behaviors contribute to diet-related health disparities observed between different racial and ethnic subgroups.

9. A state representative has proposed a bill that will ban all mobile food vendors within a 1-mile radius of every elementary school in her state. For example, no food trucks or ice cream carts would be allowed within this 1-mile radius of each school. What type of dietary behavior influence does this action represent?

   a. Interpersonal
   b. Organizational
   c. Community
   d. Policy

10. Describe how a policy to implement a 25-cent state tax per 12 ounces on sugar-sweetened beverages could be used to increase barriers to purchasing unhealthy food items. For whom would that type of policy be most effective?

Web Resources

Visit the following websites to learn more about some of the topics presented in this chapter.

The Centers for Disease Control and Prevention's Strategies for Creating and Maintaining a Healthy Food Environment: http://www.cdc.gov/healthyplaces/healthtopics/healthyfood_environment.htm

The Centers for Disease Control and Prevention's Community Food Assessment resources: http://www.cdc.gov/healthyplaces/healthtopics/healthyfood/community_assessment.htm

The Centers for Disease Control and Prevention's National Health and Nutrition Examination Survey (NHANES): http://www.cdc.gov/nchs/nhanes.htm

New York City's Healthy Bodega Initiative: http://www.nyc.gov/html/doh/downloads/pdf/cdp/healthy-bodegas-rpt2010.pdf

The Nutrition Environment Measures Survey (NEMS): http://www.med.upenn.edu/nems/

The U.S. Department of Agriculture, Food and Nutrition Service's School Nutrition Dietary Assessment Study (SNDA): http://www.fns.usda.gov/school-nutrition-dietary-assessment-study-iv

The U.S. Department of Agriculture, Economic Research Service's briefing of food security in the United States: http://www.ers.usda.gov/topics/food-nutrition-assistance/food-security-in-the-us.aspx

The U.S. Department of Agriculture and U.S. Department of Health and Human Service's Dietary Guidelines for Americans: http://www.cnpp.usda.gov/dietaryguidelines.htm

References

Antunes, L. C., Levandovski, R., Dantas, G., Caumo, W., & Hidalgo, M. P. (2010). Obesity and shift work: Chronobiological aspects. *Nutrition Research Reviews, 23*, 155–168.

Anzman-Frasca, S., Savage, J. S., Marini, M. E., Fisher, J. O., & Birch, L. L. (2012). Repeated exposure and associative conditioning promote preschool children's liking of vegetables. *Appetite, 58*(2), 543–553.

Arredondo, E. M., Elder, J. P., Ayala, G. X., Slymen, D., & Campbell, N. R. (2006). Association of a traditional vs. shared meal decision-making and preparation style with eating behavior of Hispanic women in San Diego County. *Journal of the American Dietetic Association, 106*(1), 38–45.

Ayala, G. X., Elder, J. P., Campbell, N. R., Arredondo, E., Baquero, B., Crespo, N., & Slymen, D. J. (2010). Longitudinal intervention effects on parenting of the Aventuras para Niños study. *American Journal of Preventive Medicine, 38*(2), 154–162.

Ayala, G. X., Vaz, L., Earp, J. A., Elder, J. P., & Cherrington, A. (2010). Outcome effectiveness of the lay health advisor model among Latinos in the United States: An examination by role type. *Health Education Research, 25*(5), 815–840.

Blanck, H. M., Gillespie, C., Kimmons, J. E., Seymour, J. D., & Serdula, M. K. (2008). Trends in fruit and vegetable consumption among U.S. men and women, 1994–2005. *Preventing Chronic Disease, 5*(2), 1–10.

Block, D., & Kouba, J. (2006). A comparison of the availability and affordability of a market basket in two communities in the Chicago area. *Public Health Nutrition, 9*, 837–845.

Bosetti, C., Pelucchi, C., & La Vecchia, C. (2009). Diet and cancer in Mediterranean countries: Carbohydrates and fats. *Public Health Nutrition, 12*(9A), 1595–1600.

Briefel, R. R., & Johnson, C. L. (2004). Secular trends in dietary intake in the United States. *Annual Review of Nutrition, 24*, 401–431.

Brownson, R. C., Seiler, R., & Eyler, A. A. (2010). Measuring the impact of public health policy. *Preventing Chronic Disease, 7*(4), 1–7. Available at http://www.cdc.gov/pcd/issues/2010/jul/09_0249.htm.

Carlson, A., Lino, M., Juan, W.-Y., Hanson, K., & Basiotis, P. P. (2007). *Thrifty food plan, 2006.* (CNPP-19). U.S. Department of Agriculture, Center for Nutrition Policy and Promotion.

Centers for Disease Control and Prevention. (2010a). *A closer look at African American men and high blood pressure control: A review of psychosocial factors and systems-level interventions.* Atlanta, CA: U.S. Department of Health and Human Services.

Centers for Disease Control and Prevention. (2014). National health and nutrition examination survey. Available at http://www.cdc.gov/nchs/nhanes.htm.

Cohen, B. (2002). Community food security assessment toolkit. U.S. Department of Agriculture, Economic Research Service, Publication E-FAN No. (02-013). Available at http://www.ers.usda .gov/publications/efan-electronic-publications-from-the-food-assistance-nutrition-research-program /efan02013.aspx

Cohen, D. J., Clark, E. C., Lawson, P. J., Casucci, B. A., & Flocke, S. A. (2011). Identifying teachable moments for health behavior counseling in primary care. *Patient Education and Counseling*, *85*(2), 8–15.

Copeland, K. A., Neelon, S. E., Howald, A. E., & Wosje, K. S. (2013). Nutritional quality of meals compared to snacks in child care. *Childhood Obesity*, *9*(3), 223-232.

Crespo, N., Elder, J. P., Ayala, G. X., Slymen, D. J., Campbell, N. R., Sallis, J. F., McKenzie, T. L., Baquero, B., & Arredondo, E. M. (2012). Results of a multi-level intervention to prevent and control childhood obesity among Latino children: The Aventuras para Niños study. *Annals of Behavioral Medicine*, *43*(1), 84-100.

Davis, B., & Carpenter, C. (2009). Proximity of fast-food restaurants to schools and adolescent obesity. *American Journal of Public Health*, *99*, 505–510.

Davison, K. K., & Campbell, K. (2005). Opportunities to prevent obesity in children within families: An ecological approach. In D. Crawford & R. W. Jeffery (Eds.), *Obesity prevention and public health* (1st ed.; p. 208). New York, NY: Oxford University Press.

Demark-Wahnefried, W., Aziz, N. M., Rowland, J. H., & Pinto, B. M. (2005). Riding the crest of the teachable moment: Promoting long-term health after the diagnosis of cancer. *Journal of Clinical Oncology*, *23*(24), 5814–5830.

Duerksen, S. C., Campbell, N., Arredondo, E. M., Ayala, G. X., Baquero, B., & Elder, J. P. (2007). Aventuras para niños: Obesity prevention in the homes, schools, and neighborhoods of Mexican American children. In W. D. Brettschneider & R. Naul (Eds.), *Obesity in Europe* (pp. 135–152). Frankfurt A.M.: Peter Lang.

Ebster, C., & Wagner, U., & Neumueller, D. (2009). Children's influences on in-store purchases. *Journal of Retailing and Consumer Services, 16*, 145–154.

Elder, J. P., Ayala, G. X., Campbell, N. R., Arredondo, E. M., Slymen, D. J., Baquero, B., Zive, M., Ganiats, T. G., & Engelberg, M. (2006). Long-term effects of a communication intervention for Spanish-dominant Latinas. *American Journal of Preventive Medicine*, *31*(2), 159–166.

Elder, J. P., Ayala, G. X., Slymen, D. J., Arredondo, E. M., & Campbell, N. R. (2009). Evaluating psychosocial and behavioral mechanisms of change in a tailored communication intervention. *Health Education and Behavior*, *36*(2), 366–380.

Flegal, K.M., Carroll, M.D., Ogden, C.L., & Curtin, L.R. (2010). Prevalence and trends in obesity among US adults, 1999-2008. *JAMA, 303*(3), 235-241.

Frankenfeld, C. L., Lampe, J. W., Shannon, J., Gao, D. L., Ray, R. M., Prunty, J., et al. (2004). Frequency of soy food consumption and serum isoflavone concentrations among Chinese women in Shanghai. *Public Health Nutrition*, *7*(6), 765–772.

French, S. A. (2003). Pricing effects on food choices. *The Journal of Nutrition*, *133*(3), 841S–843S.

Ghirardeli, A., Quinn, V., & Foerster, S. B. (2010). Using geographic information systems and local food store data in California's low-income neighborhoods to inform community initiatives and resources. *American Journal of Public Health*, *100*(11), 2156–2162.

Gordon, A., Hall, J., Zeidman, E., Crepinsek, M. K., Clark, M., & Condon, E. (2007). *School nutrition dietary assessment study–III: Summary of findings.* U.S. Department of Agriculture, Food and Nutrition Service. Alexandria, VA.

Graham, D. J., & Jeffery, R. W. (2011). Location, location, location: Eye-tracking evidence that consumers preferentially view prominently positioned nutrition information. *Journal of the American Dietetic Association,111*(11), 1701–1711.

Graudal, N. A., Hubeck-Graudal, T., & Jurgens, G. (2011). Effects of low-sodium diet versus high-sodium diet on blood pressure, renin, aldosterone, catecholamines, cholesterol, and triglyceride. *Cochrane Database of Systematic Reviews, 11*, CD004022.

Hermans, R. C. J., Larsen, J. K., Herman, C. P., & Engels, R. C. M. E. (2012). How much should I eat? Situational norms affect young women's food intake during meal time. *British Journal of Nutrition, 107*, 588–594. doi:10.1017/S0007114511003278

Horowitz, C. R., Colson, K. A., Hebert, P. L., & Lancaster, K. (2004). Barriers to buying healthy foods for people with diabetes: Evidence of environmental disparities. *American Journal of Public Health, 94*(9), 1549–1554.

IOM (Institute of Medicine). (2011). *Dietary reference intakes for calcium and vitamin D.* Washington, DC: National Academies Press.

Jaenke, R. L., Collins, C. E., Morgan, P. J., Lubans, D. R., Saunders, K. L., & Warren, J. M. (2012). The impact of a school garden and cooking program on boys' and girls' fruit and vegetable preferences, taste rating, and intake. *Health Education & Behavior,39*(2), 131–141.

Kaufman, P. R., MacDonald, J. M., Lutz, S. M., & Smallwood, D. M. (1997). *Do the poor pay more for food? Item selection and price differences affect low-income household food costs.* Washington, DC: U.S. Department of Agriculture. Report no. 759.

Kris-Etherton, P., Eckel, R. H., Howard, B. V., St. Jeor, S., & Bazzarre, T. L. (2001). AHA Science Advisory: Lyon diet heart study. Benefits of a Mediterranean-style, National Cholesterol Education Program/American Heart Association Step I dietary pattern on cardiovascular disease. *Circulation, 103*(13), 1823–1825.

Kubik, M. Y., Lytle, L. A., Hannan, P. J., Perry, C. L., & Story, M. S. (2003). The association of the school food environment with dietary behaviors of young adolescents. *American Journal of Public Health, 93*, 1168–1173.

Laska, M. N., Borradaile, K. E., Tester, J., Foster, G. D., & Gittelsohn, J. (2010). Healthy food availability in small urban food stores: A comparison of four US cities. *Public Health Nutrition, 3*(7), 1031–1035.

Lee, R. E., Heinrich, K. M., Medina, A. V., Regan, G. R., Reese-Smith, J. Y., Jokura, Y., & Maddock, J. E. (2010). A picture of the healthful food environment in two diverse urban cities. *Environmental Health Insights, 4*, 49–60.

Li, F., Harmer, P., Cardinal, B. J., Bosworth, M., & Johnson-Shelton, D. (2009). Obesity and the built environment: Does the density of neighborhood fast-food outlets matter? *American Journal of Health Promotion, 23*(3), 203–209.

McKenzie, T. L., Baquero, B., Crespo, N. C., Arredondo, E. M., Campbell, N. R., & Elder, J. P. (2008). Environmental correlates of physical activity in Mexican American children at home. *Journal of Physical Activity and Health, 5*(4), 579–591.

Michels, K. B. (2003). Nutritional epidemiology—past, present, future. *International Journal of Epidemiology, 32*(4),486–488.

Michie, S., Abraham, C., Whittington, C., McAteer, J., & Gupta, S. (2009). Effective techniques in healthy eating and physical activity interventions: A meta-regression. *Health Psychology, 28*(6), 690–701.

Moore, L. V., Diez Roux, A. V., Nettleton, J. A., & Jacobs Jr., D. R. (2008). Associations of the local food environment with diet quality—a comparison of assessments based on surveys and geographic information systems: The multi-ethnic study of atherosclerosis. *American Journal of Epidemiology, 167*(8), 917–924.

Morland, K., Diez Roux, A. V., & Wing, S. (2006). Supermarkets, other food stores, and obesity: The Atherosclerosis Risk in Communities study. *American Journal of Preventive Medicine, 30*(4), 333–339.

National Cancer Institute. (2012). Dictionary of Cancer Terms. Available at http://www.cancer.gov /dictionary?cdrid=45618.

National Institutes of Health and National Heart, Lung and Blood Institute. (1998). *Clinical guidelines on the identification, evaluation, and treatment of overweight and obesity in adults: The Evidence Report.* NIH Publication No. 98-4083. Available at http://www.nhlbi.nih.gov/guidelines/obesity/ob_gdlns .pdf.

Nestle, M. (2002). *Food politics: How the food industry influences nutrition and health.* Berkeley: University of California Press.

Neuman, W. (2009, October 23). Food label program to suspend operations. *The New York Times.* Retrieved from http://www.nytimes.com/2009/10/24/business/24food.html?_r=1.

New York City Department of Health and Mental Hygiene. (2012). Physical activity and nutrition: Healthy bodega initiative. Available at http://www.nyc.gov/html/ceo/downloads/pdf/BH_PRR.pdf

Nielsen S. J., & Popkin, B. M. (2003). Patterns and trends in food portion sizes, 1977–1998. *Journal of the American Medical Association, 289*(4), 450–453.

Nutrition Environment Measures Survey (NEMS). (2009). University of Pennsylvania. Available at http://www.med.upenn.edu/nems/.

Ogden, C. L., Carroll, M. D., Kit, B. K., & Flegal, K. M. (2014). Prevalence of childhood and adult obesity in the United States, 2011–2012. *Journal of the American Medical Association, 311*(8), 806–814.

Pinson, N. P. (2005). *School soda contracts: A sample review of contracts in Oregon public school districts, 2004.* Community Health Partnership. Portland, OR. Available at http://epsl.asu.edu/ceru/Articles /CERU-0504-147-OWI.pdf.

Powell, L. M., Auld, M. C., Chaloupka, F. J., O'Malley, P. M., & Johnston, L. D. (2007). Associations between access to food stores and adolescent body mass index. *American Journal of Preventive Medicine, 33*(4), S301–S307.

Powell, L. M., Slater, S., Mirtcheva, D., Bao, Y., & Chaloupka, F. J. (2007). Food store availability and neighborhood characteristics in the United States. *Preventive Medicine, 44*(3), 189–195.

Ritchie, L. D., Whaley, S. E., Spector, P., Gomez, J., & Crawford P. B. (2010). Favorable impact of nutrition education on California WIC families. *Journal of Nutrition Education and Behavior, 42*(3S), S2–S10.

Robert Wood Johnson Foundation, Healthy Eating and Research Program. (2007). *Promoting good nutrition and physical activity in child-care settings.* Research Brief May 2007. Available at http://healthyeatingresearch .org/wp-content/uploads/2013/12/HER-Child-Care-Setting-Research-Brief-2007.pdf

Roberto, C. A., Bragg, M. A., Livingston, K. A., Harris, J. L., Thompson, J. M., Seamans, M. J., & Brownell, K. D. (2012). Choosing front-of-package food labeling nutritional criteria: How smart were "Smart Choices"? *Public Health Nutrition, 15*(2), 262–267.

Rose, D., Hutchinson, P. L., Bodor, J. N., Swalm, C. M., Farley, T. A., Cohen, D. A., & Rice, J. C. (2009). Neighborhood food environments and body mass index: The importance of in-store contents. *American Journal of Preventive Medicine, 37*(3), 214–219.

Salvy, S. J., Elmo, A., Nitecki, L. A., Kluczynski, M. A., & Roemmich, J. N. (2011). Influence of parents and friends on children's and adolescents' food intake and food selection. *American Journal of Clinical Nutrition, 93*(1), 87–92.

School Nutrition Dietary Assessment Study (SNDA) III: Data Collection Package. (2007). U.S. Department of Agriculture, Food and Nutrition Service. Available at http://www.fns.usda.gov /sites/default/files/SNDAIII-Vol2.pdf

Sofianou, A., Fung, T. T., & Tucker, K. L. (2011). Differences in diet pattern adherence by nativity and duration of US residence in the Mexican-American population. *Journal of the American Dietetic Association, 111*(10), 1563–1569.

Solfrizzi, V., Panza, F., Frisardi, V., Seripa, D., Logroscino, G., Imbimbo, B. P., & Pilotto, A. (2011). Diet and Alzheimer's disease risk factors or prevention: The current evidence. *Expert Review of Neurotherapeutics, 11*(5), 677–708.

Story, M., Neumark-Sztainer, D., & French, S. (2002). Individual and environmental influences on adolescent eating behaviors. *Journal of the American Dietetic Association, 102*(3), S40–S51.

Taren, D., de Tobar, M., Ritenbaugh, C., Graver, E., Whitacre, R., & Aickin, M. (2000). Evaluation of the Southwest Food Frequency Questionnaire. *Ecology of Food and Nutrition, 38*(6), 515–547.

Thompson, F. F., & Subar, A. F. (2008). Dietary assessment methodology. In A. M. Coulston & C. J. Boushey (Eds.), *Nutrition in the prevention and treatment of disease* (pp. 3–39). Bethesda, MD: National Cancer Institute.

Twiss, J., Dickinson, J., Duma, S., Kleinman, T., Paulsen, H., & Rilveria, L. (2003). Community gardens: Lessons learned from California Healthy Cities and Communities. *American Journal of Public Health,93*(9),1435–1438.

U.S. Department of Agriculture, Economic Research Service. (2011). Briefing rooms: Food security in the United States. Available at http://www.ers.usda.gov/topics/food-nutrition-assistance/food-security -in-the-us.aspx.

U.S. Department of Agriculture, Food and Nutrition Service. (2012). *Nutrition standards in the national school lunch and school breakfast programs, final rule.* Available at http://www.gpo.gov/fdsys/pkg /FR-2012-01-26/pdf/2012-1010.pdf.

U.S. Department of Agriculture, U.S. Department of Health and Human Services. (2010). *Dietary guidelines for Americans, 2010* (7th ed.). Washington, DC: U.S. Government Printing Office.

U.S. Food and Drug Administration, U.S. Department of Health & Human Services. (2011). Food, labeling & nutrition: New menu and vending machine labeling requirements. Available at http://www .fda.gov/Food/IngredientsPackagingLabeling/LabelingNutrition/ucm217762.htm.

Vadiveloo, M. K., Dixon, L. B., & Elbel, B. (2011). Consumer purchasing patterns in response to calorie labeling legislation in New York City. *International Journal of Behavioral Nutrition and Physical Activity, 27*, 8–51.

Valkenburg, P. M., & Cantor, J. (2001). The development of a child into a consumer. *Applied Developmental Psychology, 22*, 61–72.

Ver Ploeg, M., Breneman, V., Farrigan, T., Hamrick, K., Hopkins, D., Kaufman, P., et al. (2009). *Access to affordable and nutritious food—measuring and understanding food deserts and their consequences: report to congress.* Washington, DC: U.S. Department of Agriculture, Economic Research Service, Administrative Publication No. (AP-036).

Viswanathan, M., et al., (2009). *Outcomes of community health worker interventions, in evidence report/technology assessment no. 181.* AHRQ Publication No. 09-E014. Rockville, MD: Agency for Healthcare Research and Quality.

Whitehead, R. D., Ozakinci, G., Stephen, I. D., & Perrett, D. I. (2012). Appealing to vanity: Could potential appearance improvement motivate fruit and vegetable consumption? *American Journal of Public Health, 102*(2), 207–211.

Willett, W., Manson, J., & Liu, S. (2002). Glycemic index, glycemic load, and risk of type 2 diabetes. *American Journal of Clinical Nutrition, 76*(1), 274S–280S.

Wolf, R. L., Lepore, S. J., Vandergrift, J. L., Wetmore-Arkader, L., McGinty, E., Pietrzak, G., & Yaroch, A. L. (2008). Knowledge, barriers, and stage of change as correlates of fruit and vegetable consumption among urban and mostly immigrant black men. *Journal of the American Dietetic Association, 108*(8), 1315–1322.

World Health Organization. (2012). Programs and projects: Trade, foreign policy, diplomacy and health; food security. Available at http://www.who.int/trade/glossary/story028/en/.

Chapter 5

Ernesto Ramirez, MS and Elva M. Arredondo, PhD

PHYSICAL ACTIVITY

Key Terms

appraisal support
basal metabolic rate
domain-specific activity
duration
exercise
formal networks
frequency
informal networks
informational support

instrumental support
intensity
interpersonally focused
  interventions
metabolic equivalent
  (MET)
physical activity
physical activity energy
  expenditure

physical environments
physical fitness
policy
recall bias
social environments
social networks
social support
total energy
  expenditure

Learning Objectives

Upon completion of this chapter, you should be able to:

1. List the four different types of physical activity.
2. Describe three different methods of assessing physical activity.
3. Outline the importance of physical activity for overall health.
4. Describe individual and interpersonal influences on physical activity and methods of intervening.
5. Identify community- and policy-level influences on physical activity and methods of intervening.

6. Describe examples of community wide programs that promote physical activity.
7. Explain the limitations of evaluating community-wide programs.

Chapter Outline

Types of Physical Activity
Assessing Physical Activity
  Subjective Measurement
  Objective Measurement
  Direct Observation
Physical Activity and Health
  Mortality
  Cardiovascular Health
  Metabolic Health and Obesity
  Muscular and Skeletal Health
  Mental Health
  Sedentary Behavior
  Recommendations and Guidelines
Physical Activity Interventions
  Individual-level Interventions
  Interpersonal-Level Interventions
  Environmental-Level Interventions

INTRODUCTION

Humans are designed to move and to be active. Take a minute to look at yourself. Each part of you, from your thumbs to your knees, is an ingenious design to help propel your daily movements. Walking to class, bending down to pick up a dropped book, running after your friends; each of these involves a symphony of biological and mechanical actions. While a discussion of the processes involving human movement and activity would be interesting, this chapter will focus on physical activity within the realm of health.

physical activity is the movement of the human body that increases energy expenditure above resting levels.

Physical activity is a broad term that is meant to encompass all movement that is derived from skeletal muscle contraction that increases energy expenditure above a resting level. Because many different types of movements fit into this broad definition, most public health professionals and organizations limit the use of the term "physical activity" to involve those activities that have health-enhancing benefits (U.S. Department of Health and Human Services, 2008).

Individuals are sometimes confused by the distinctions among physical activity, physical fitness, and exercise. Remember, physical activity can refer to any movement or series of movement that benefits an individual's health. **Physical fitness** is the capacity of an individual's biological systems to carry out physically active tasks. Physical fitness can refer to a number of different activity-related components. For example, cardiorespiratory endurance—the measure of the maximal aerobic capacity—is often an important component of fitness. Other measures include muscular strength and endurance, flexibility, speed, and reaction time. Body composition (measured by percentage body fat and/or percentage muscle mass) is also sometimes used as an indirect measure of physical fitness.

Exercise is a subset of physical activity that is defined by planned, structured, and purposefully done activity in order to improve or maintain one or more of the components of physical fitness. Typically, individuals engage in exercise during their leisure time.

Human energy expenditure or **total energy expenditure** (TEE) is the made up of three major components. **Basal metabolic rate (BMR)** is the amount of energy that is required to support the basic biological process of life such as cell metabolism. An individual's BMR can been determined using indirect calorimetery, a process during which inspired oxygen and expired carbon dioxide are measured, but typically prediction equations based on age, body weight, and gender are used. A small amount of energy is also needed in order to consume and process food. This energy is called the *thermic effect of food* (TEF). In most cases, TEF accounts for approximately 10% of TEE. **Physical activity energy expenditure (PAEE)** refers to the energy expenditure that results from all physical activities. Energy expenditure refers to the amount of caloric expenditure or kilocalories expended due to physical activity. Commonly, the "kilo" prefix is dropped and "calorie" is used to describe the magnitude of energy expenditure.

physical fitness is the body's ability to carry out physically active tasks.

exercise is structured or planned participation in physical activities in order to improve or maintain physical fitness.

total energy expenditure (TEE) is the sum of the three main components of energy expenditure during waking and nonwaking hours. This includes the basal metabolic rate, thermic effect of food, and energy expenditure associated with physical activity.

basal metabolic rate (BMR) is the amount of energy required to maintain the basic biological processes for life.

physical activity energy expenditure (PAEE) refers to the energy expenditure that results from all physical activities.

TYPES OF PHYSICAL ACTIVITY

When addressing how people engage in physical activity, it is common to describe the extent of activity using three factors: *duration*, *frequency*, and *intensity*. The **duration** of activity indicates the length of time (minutes or hours) over which an individual engages in activity. **Frequency** of activity refers to how often the individual is active, usually in days per week. Lastly, **intensity** refers to the level of effort or exertion required to perform the activity. As you have probably guessed, it is fairly easy to estimate and measure the duration and frequency of physical activities. Understanding intensity is slightly more difficult, but it is extremely important, as many health benefits of being active have been shown to be directly related to the intensity of the activity.

One of the most common methods used to understand physical activity intensity is the **metabolic equivalent (MET)**. A MET is the energy cost of physical activity. One MET is equal to consuming 3.5 ml of O_2/kg/min or burning 1 kcal/kg/min. MET values are used instead of other methods such

duration is the length of time, usually in minutes, an individual engages in physical activity.

Frequency is the rate of participation in physical activity, or how often one engages in physical activity.

intensity is the effort required to perform physical activity.

metabolic equivalent (MET) is a unit used to describe physical activity intensity by measuring or estimating the amount of oxygen consumed relative to body weight.

as heart rate or absolute energy expenditure (kcals) because the MET value of an activity is comparable across individuals of different body sizes. Over time, researchers have measured and grouped activities into four different intensity categories.

- *Sedentary behaviors* (1–1.5 METs). This is the class of behaviors that involves little to no movement. Typically this includes behaviors such as sitting, watching television, sitting and working at the computer, and lying down.

- *Light-intensity activities* (1.6–2.9 METs). This is the class of activities that involves little movement. Light activities are commonly referred to as "lifestyle activities." These include activities such as washing and drying dishes, cooking, and slow walking (2.0 mph).

- *Moderate-intensity activities* (3.0–5.9 METs). These are activities that increase heart rate and respiration rate and usually make you start sweating. Walking up and down stairs at a normal pace, leisurely walking (3.0 mph), riding a bicycle (< 10 mph), and general gardening and yard work are all examples of moderate activities.

- *Vigorous-intensity activities* (> 6.0 METs). These are activities that people typically associate with structured exercise or participating in sports. Jogging/running, jumping rope, playing soccer, and stationary rowing are just a few types of activities that are classified as vigorous intensity.

ASSESSING PHYSICAL ACTIVITY

Measuring physical activity and its associated energy expenditure has long been a concern for public health researchers. Numerous tools and methods have been developed and used in laboratory and field studies to determine the duration, frequency, and intensity of physical activity individuals engage in. Almost all methods fit into one of three categories: subjective measurement, objective measurement, or direct observation.

Subjective Measurement

The most common way to assess physical activity participation is through self-report. Many different types of surveys and questionnaires have been developed to understand the physical activity behaviors and patterns of behaviors that individuals engage in. While self-report measures are relatively easy to distribute and analyze, they do suffer from bias. It is difficult for individuals to remember the type of activity, let alone the frequency, duration, and intensity of activity over a specified time frame. This results in **recall bias**—the systematic errors that result because memory does not reflect reality. Recall bias in turn reduces the reliability (consistency) and validity (accuracy) of self-report measures.

recall bias is a description of the error that occurs when individuals use memory to describe past experiences or behaviors.

Model for Understanding

The International Physical Activity Questionnaire (IPAQ) is used throughout the world to conduct population-level physical activity surveillance (Hagströmer, Oja, & Sjöström, 2007). It can be used to understand **domain-specific** (leisure, work, transportation, and domestic) physical activity participation, group individuals into different levels of activity (low, moderate, high), or determine the volume of activity (MET-minutes). The following are a few sample questions:

During the last 7 days, on how many days did you do vigorous physical activities like heavy lifting, digging, heavy construction, or climbing up stairs as part of your work?

Think about only those physical activities that you did for at least 10 minutes at a time.

_____ *days per week*
_____ *No vigorous job-related physical activity*

How much time did you usually spend on one of those days doing vigorous physical activities as part of your work?

_____ *hours per day*
_____ *minutes per day*

Objective Measurement

> **domain-specific** is the grouping of physical activities into distinct environments where they occur throughout the day, such as work and home.

To deal with the reliability and validity issues of physical activity, sensing devices can be used to measure and track physical activity behavior. Although there are many different types of physical activity measurement devices, we will focus on the two most common: pedometers and accelerometers.

Pedometers

The most common equipment used to determine the extent of daily physical activity is a pedometer (see Figure 5-1). Pedometers are usually worn on the hip and

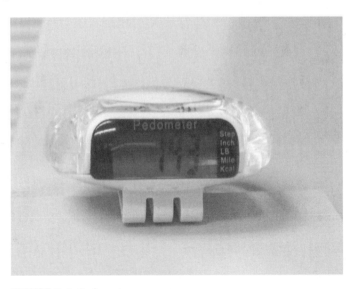

FIGURE 5–1 Pedometer.

usually display the total steps taken during the day and in some cases the amount of time a person spends moving. Most pedometers require little to no technological knowledge or expertise to operate and can be dispersed to a wide range of individuals to track activity. The low cost and ease of use make pedometers ideal tools for many individuals wishing to start a physical activity program and track their progress. Pedometers have limitations that can addressed by more sophisticated sensing technologies. These limitations include issues related to accuracy of derived step counts, the inability to discern intensity of movement, and the lack of daily energy expenditure information (Tudor-Locke, Williams, Reis, & Pluto, 2002).

Accelerometers

Accelerometers (see Figure 5-2) are usually small microchips that contain systems for measuring the gravitational force (g-force) acting on the device. They are usually worn on the hip but can also be worn on the wrist. Typically, accelerometers measure g-force along a given directional axis. Accelerometers are used in combination with microprocessors in movement-sensing devices. These microprocessors help make sense of the g-force readings supplied by the accelerometer. Most devices have proprietary algorithms that take the accelerometer data and translate it into useful movement information, such as (a) the number of steps taken, (b) the time spent moving, (c) the intensity of the movement, (d) the distance traveled, and (e) the user's calorie expenditure. It is important to note here that accelerometers are best used when trying to measure primarily leg-based movements that involve a ground reaction force. These movements, such as walking and running, typically make up the majority of daily human movement (Troiano et al., 2008). Movements that are not captured well are water-based activities such as swimming and activities with little to no ground-reaction force involved, such as cycling and upper body movements, given that the accelerometer measures activity from the waist down (Chen & Bassett Jr., 2005).

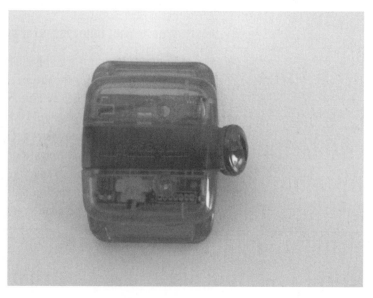

FIGURE 5–2 Accelerometer.

Direct Observation

In some cases, it may be more difficult to gather information about physical activity behavior from self-report or sensing devices such as pedometers and accelerometers. In these instances, such as classifying the physical activity of young children or physical activity behaviors in specific locations like city parks, it may be necessary to use direct observation methods. Direct observation is a technique in which trained observers create a record of the physical activity behaviors of individuals using specific notations and classification systems. The most commonly used direct observation methods tools are the System for Observing Fitness Instruction Time (McKenzie, Sallis, & Nader, 1991) and the System for Observing Play and Leisure Activity in Youth (McKenzie, Marshall, Sallis, & Conway, 2000). The disadvantages of direct observation include that it requires a lot of resources (e.g., staff time) to capture the activity representative in a specific area. Also, there is potential for subject reactivity, people changing their behavior if they realize they are being observed.

PHYSICAL ACTIVITY AND HEALTH

Consistent physical activity plays an important role in the prevention and control of chronic diseases. While most individuals focus on physical activity for its role in helping individuals control their weight, multiple health benefits are derived from engaging in a physically active lifestyle.

Mortality

Premature mortality is a term used to describe death that occurs before an individual meets the current life expectancy. For example, the most current statistics estimate the average life expectancy in the United States to be 77.9 years (Arias, 2011). Numerous studies across many different populations have indicated that participating in regular physical activity decreases an individual's chance of dying prematurely. Findings from a review of 44 studies indicate that engaging in physical activity equal to or exceeding 1,000 kcal per week of energy expenditure is associated with a 20 to 30% reduction in all-cause mortality (Lee & Skerrett, 2001). The dose–response relationship between physical activity participation and physical fitness and mortality appears to follow a linear trend, with larger reduction in risk associated with higher volumes of physical activity or higher levels of physical fitness (Myers, Prakash, & Froelicher, 2002; Paffenbarger, Hyde, Wing, & Hsieh, 1986).

Cardiovascular Health

"Cardiovascular disease" is a commonly used term to refer to the group of diseases that afflict the heart and blood-carrying vessels (arteries and veins). Of these diseases, the most common is coronary heart disease, which includes myocardial infarctions (heart attacks). Heart disease is the number one cause of death in the United States, claiming more than 596,339 lives in 2011 (Hoyert & Xu, 2012). Cardiovascular diseases also includes stroke, a loss of the blood supply to the brain due to blood clots or bleeding. Last, peripheral arterial disease is included in the cardiovascular disease grouping. Atherosclerosis, the narrowing of arteries resulting in constriction and limited blood flow, is the condition that leads to peripheral arterial disease, a disease in which plaque builds up in the arteries that carry blood to your head, organs, and limbs.

For more than 50 years, research has indicated that physical activity is important for both primary and secondary prevention of cardiovascular disease. Most of the research regarding the relationship between physical activity and cardiovascular health can be traced to Dr. Jerry Morris. In his study of London bus drivers and conductors, Dr. Morris and this colleagues conducted a large-scale survey and found that those who were more physically active were less likely to die from heart attacks (Morris, Heady, Raffle, Roberts, & Parks, 1953). This brought about a cascade of research studies that have indicated that physical activity has a dose–response relationship with cardiovascular disease. Across men and women, it appears that participating in light to moderate amounts of regular physical activity, even daily walking, can reduce the risk of developing cardiovascular disease and stroke (Oguma & Shinoda-Tagawa, 2004; Wannamethee & Shaper, 2001).

Metabolic Health and Obesity

Physical activity also affects the function of metabolic systems that are essential for maintaining homeostasis. Physical activity can have an impact on the organs of the digestive and endocrine systems and the hormones and enzymes they produce that help regulate energy production and storage. The primary metabolic disorders that are affected by physical activity are insulin resistance and type 2 diabetes. Insulin resistance occurs when the body no longer responds properly to circulating insulin, therefore causing the pancreas to produce higher-than-normal amounts. Prolonged insulin resistance can lead to abnormally high levels of blood glucose, which can result in a type 2 diabetes diagnosis. Physical activity is an effective treatment and preventive measure for individuals who are diagnosed with insulin resistance or type 2 diabetes. Being physically active helps to consume energy and, in turn, can reduce circulating blood glucose. Additionally, participating in regular physical activity can reduce excess weight—a common condition that increases the risk of developing type 2 diabetes.

Excess weight is one of the leading conditions associated with the onset of many of the aforementioned cardiovascular and metabolic conditions. Approximately 32% of the American adult population is classified as overweight or obese (Ogden et al., 2006). Obesity is defined in terms of body mass index (BMI; height in kg divided by height in meters squared) where adults with a BMI greater than 30.0 are considered obese. For children and adolescents, BMI percentile scales that take into account typical growth patterns are used to determine obesity status. A child with a BMI greater than the 95th percentile for his or her age is considered obese. Participating in regular physical activity across the lifespan from childhood into adulthood greatly reduces the risk of gaining excess weight (Goran, Reynolds, & Lindquist, 1999; Hill & Wyatt, 2005). From an energy balance standpoint, obesity can be traced to a misalignment between the energy (calories) consumed and the energy expended. Physical activity helps to regulate energy balance by providing an opportunity to increase caloric expenditure. When increased activity is combined with decreased consumption through dietary changes, individuals can effectively reduce excess weight.

Muscular and Skeletal Health

Participating in regular physical activity is important for building and preserving the health of the muscles, bones, and joints. This is especially true for young children and adolescents, as physical activity helps to build muscular strength as well as improve motor control and encourages bone growth and strength. Most of the musculoskeletal benefits of physical activity focus on older adults, as muscle and bone health tend to deteriorate with age. As individuals get older, physical activity can become an important preventive health measure for osteoporosis, the loss of bone mineral content and bone strength. Osteoporosis is a common condition in older adults, particularly older adult females, and can lead to increased risk for hip and spine fractures. Adults who lead inactive lifestyles have a much higher risk of developing osteoporosis than those who maintain a physically active lifestyle. Bone health is closely related to the type of physical activity one engages in. The stress placed on the skeletal system during weight-bearing activities, such as running or jumping, can help to strengthen bones and can slow bone loss as adults age.

Regular physical activity can also protect against the proximal cause of osteoporotic fracture—falls. In many cases, older adults suffer from hip and other fractures due to a loss of balance and the subsequent fall. Participating in individual physical activities (e.g., walking) or group activities (e.g., T'ai Chi) has been shown to improve balance and reduce fall risk in older adults (Sherrington, Lord, & Finch, 2004).

Physical activity is also important for maintaining joint health and has even been shown to be a useful treatment for certain types of arthritis. Engaging in low-impact activities like swimming or cycling helps to improve pain management, joint function, and overall quality of life for those with arthritis or rheumatic conditions.

Mental Health

Mental health issues impact the daily lives of millions of Americans. Anxiety disorders affect 18.1% of the population, and mood disorders including depression affect 9.5% (Kessler et al., 2005). In most cases, individuals diagnosed with a mental health problem are treated with either medication or psychotherapy, but over the last 20 years, research evidence indicates that exercise and physical activity are effective methods for reducing the negative effects of anxiety and depression. Meta-analytic reviews of randomized controlled trials examining the usefulness of exercise as treatment for these disorders have found significant positive effects (Rethorst, Wipfli, & Landers, 2009; Wipfli, Rethorst, & Landers, 2008). The usefulness of physical activity as a treatment for mental health issues is especially important when alternative treatments such as exercise, which have few or no negative side effects, are compared to common pharmacological treatments. Treatment via pharmacological agents has come under scrutiny recently, as researchers have found numerous negative side effects associated with their use such as sexual dysfunction, elevated blood pressure, and, in extreme cases, suicidal thoughts (Gardner, Baldessarini, & Waraich, 2005). Furthermore, alternative treatments that are readily available to the general population are greatly needed. Only 21.7% of individuals with depression are adequately treated (Kessler et al., 2003). It stands to reason that a majority of individuals who are experiencing mental health problems are either not seeking adequate treatment or, if being treated with antipsychotic medication, are experiencing unwanted negative side effects.

Sedentary Behavior

Recently, there has been an increased interest in understanding the health effects of sedentary behaviors. Americans spend a majority of their days engaging in sedentary behaviors. Accelerometer data from the 2003 to 2004 National Health and Nutrition Examination Survey indicated that a majority of working-age U.S. adults spent between 7.25 and 8.41 hours per day being sedentary (Matthews et al., 2008). A wealth of research has examined the time spent in sedentary behaviors and its association with a variety of negative health outcomes. The most obvious of these is the relationship between sedentary time and obesity. Time spent in sedentary behaviors invariably negatively affects the energy balance equation and therefore can lead to weight gain (Must & Parisi, 2009; Sugiyama, Healy, Dunstan, Salmon, & Owen, 2008). Additionally, sedentariness has been associated with increased risk for development of cardiovascular disease, metabolic syndrome, type 2 diabetes, ovarian cancer risk, and colon cancer risk (Garabrant, Peters, Mack, & Bernstein, 1984; Hu, Li, Colditz, Willett, & Manson, 2003; Patel, Rodriguez, Pavluck, Thun, & Calle, 2006).

The most common sedentary behavior that contributes to a reduction in total energy expenditure on most days is sitting. In a large prospective study of Canadian adults, time spent sitting was significantly associated with risk of all-cause mortality, cardiovascular disease mortality, and other-cause mortality (Katzmarzyk, Church, Craig, & Bouchard, 2009). This finding is especially important because the significant association of sitting time with mortality was found to be independent of demographic factors (age, sex), negative health behaviors (smoking, alcohol consumption), and positive health behaviors (leisure time physical activity). Additionally, potential relationships between physical inactivity and important biological mechanisms such as lipoprotein lipase regulation have been identified in human and animal models (Hamilton, Hamilton, & Zderic, 2007; Zderic & Hamilton, 2006).

Recommendations and Guidelines

The current guidelines adopted by the U.S. Department of Health and Human Services (2008) recommend adults engage in 150 minutes per week of moderate physical activity, 75 minutes per week of vigorous activity, or any "equivalent combination" of these two intensities. Despite the widespread promotion of these guidelines, there is little evidence that suggests Americans are actually adhering to them. Objective measurements from a large population-based sample indicate that approximately 5% of adults meet these guidelines (Troiano et al., 2008).

PHYSICAL ACTIVITY INTERVENTIONS

It should be apparent that there is a clear need to develop, test, and implement interventions that promote increased physical activity participation. The following section will outline targets of change and intervention methods across four levels of influence: individual, interpersonal, organizational, and environmental (see Chapter 3 for a detailed description).

Individual-level Interventions

self-efficacy within the context of health behavior, is one's perceived confidence in performing a specific health behavior.

Perhaps the most common method of intervening on physical activity behavior is to target individuals. When targeting individuals, interventions typically rely upon health promotion models and determinants of behavior change to guide the development of tools, messages, and mechanisms that are used to encourage behavior change. Many individual-level behavioral targets have been addressed in physical activity interventions. Two of the most common are **self-efficacy**—an individual's perception of his or her ability to perform the behavior—and perceived benefits and barriers related to engaging in the behavior (sometimes referred to as decisional balance). A recent review of methods utilized in physical activity interventions identified 23 unique behavior-change techniques (Abraham & Michie, 2008). Of those 23, 5 "core" behavior-change techniques were identified as being associated with successful interventions (Michie, Abraham, Whittington, McAteer, & Gupta, 2009).

Self-Monitoring

Self-monitoring describes the prompting of individuals to record information about their behavior. In physical activity interventions, this typically corresponds to keeping a log or diary of specific behaviors. One of the most common methods for physical activity self-monitoring relies on individuals wearing a pedometer and recording daily step counts.

Intention Formation

To facilitate behavior change, it is sometimes necessary to prompt individuals to set a broad goal or guideline that they should aim to meet. The Theory of Planned

Behavior (and its predecessor the Theory of Reasoned Action; Ajzen, 1991) is commonly used to understand intention formation for participating in physical activity.

Goal Setting and Review

Prompting an individual to create a plan of action that outlines what they will accomplish along with a time frame for completion can also be an important feature of successful physical activity interventions. Typically, goal setting can be expressed in terms of SMART goals, which are discussed in the program planning chapter (Chapter 2). Because individuals sometimes under- or overestimate their abilities or changes in lifestyle, it is necessary to plan for continual review of goal progress and allow for adaptation when necessary.

Feedback

Providing individuals with information about how they are performing the behavior is also an effective behavior-change strategy. Behavioral feedback can take many different forms. Feedback about an individual's behavior in relation to his or her own historical behavior can motivate individuals to improve. Feedback that references an individual's performance in relation to normative values or others' performance can also be valuable.

Methods for Intervention

There are many different ways to implement these behavior-change strategies for improving physical activity. This section will describe a few of the methods for implementing individual-level physical activity interventions and provide a few examples of intervention implementation.

Face to Face. Face-to-face interventions are still considered the "gold standard" intervention delivery method (Napolitano & Marcus, 2002). Face-to-face interventions typically employ a health counselor or similarly trained individual to deliver intervention materials directly to the participant in a one-on-one setting. The advantages to delivering an intervention in this setting include personal contact and communication, immediate feedback, and the ability to deliver concentrated information. However, face-to-face interventions are time consuming and costly and are only accessible to a small number of individuals.

Tailored Print and Electronic Materials. Delivering interventions to large numbers of individuals requires using tools and techniques that are easily accessible and can provide relevant and important messages based on the aforementioned behavior-change strategies. Using printed materials and electronic materials such as email and web-based systems allows for interventions to simultaneously reach many people at a relatively low cost. Additionally, one of the advantages to using electronic print or web-based materials is the ability to create tailored intervention messages. The level of customization can range from simple personalization (e.g., inserting a participant's name in an automatically sent email message) to complex tailoring that takes into account information about the participant, their historical behavior, and their goals. Highly tailored systems can also leverage this information to provide performance feedback.

Mobile Communication. A new area in physical activity intervention is the use of mobile communication platforms, specifically text messaging (SMS), to deliver tailored messages and prompts to individuals. Current estimates indicate that the majority of

Model for Understanding
The Diabetes Network Internet-Based Physical Activity Study

In this study, a multifaceted, Internet-based intervention designed to increase physical activity participation was compared to a static information-only website. Participants were inactive adults (> 40 yrs) diagnosed with type 2 diabetes. The intervention consisted of four complementary tools accessible via a web-based system. First, participants were assessed for baseline characteristics such as barriers to participating in activity and current level of physical activity. They also reported intentions (how much they intended to increase their activity), identified preferable activities, set goals, and created a specific plan for scheduling activity time. Second, they were given access to an online self-tracking system that allowed them to input information about their daily minutes of physical activity and see visualizations of their progress.

Third, they were given access to an online "coach" who provided them with tailored messages that were based on their baseline assessments. Last, they were encouraged to communicate with other participants by posting messages in an online "support group" area. Participants were encouraged to log on each week during the 8-week intervention. Results indicated that individuals enjoyed using the online intervention system. There was a significant decline in website use over time, with a significantly greater use during the first 2 weeks of the intervention than the last 2 weeks. This led to a finding that indicated that intervention participants who had at least three log-ons increased their moderate to vigorous physical activity MVPA to a greater extent than those who had fewer than three log-ons (McKay, King, Eakin, Seeley, & Glasgow, 2001).

Americans have access to a mobile device that can send and receive text messages. The use of SMS programs for health intervention delivery has grown in popularity in recent years. Using SMS systems has many advantages. It is usually relatively inexpensive, and the system can interact with participants by both pushing information (sending messages) and pulling information (asking for responses).

Model for Understanding
Text Messaging for Increasing Physical Activity

In a 9-week trial conducted by Hurling and colleagues (2007), 77 healthy adults received a tailored SMS program to increase physical activity levels. These messages offered participants solutions for perceived barriers and included scheduled reminders for weekly physical activity. Researchers supplemented the SMS program with email messages, an interactive website with a feedback facility, and wrist accelerometers for self-monitoring. This text message program helped

increase moderate-intensity physical activity by approximately 2.25 hours per week. In another trial conducted by Shapiro and colleagues (2008), 58 children and their parents used SMS to self-monitor physical activity levels. For 8 weeks, the children and parents were instructed to send two messages a day denoting their physical activity, and for each message they received automated SMS feedback. The results showed that using SMS improved adherence to self-monitoring physical activity.

Critical Thinking

What are some of the limitations of intervening on the individual level?

Interpersonal-Level Interventions

Human beings are social creatures who are influenced by interactions with other people. Studies have found that people who report having social relationships tend to report better health than people who do not (Ayotte, Margrett, & Hicks-Patrick, 2010; Driver, 2005; Duncan & Mummery, 2005). There is not a theory that comprehensively and adequately accounts for the mechanisms between social relations and health; however, several conceptual models have been proposed to explain the influence of social relations on health behavior. The terms "social networks" and "social support" are sometimes used interchangeably. However, the term "**social networks**" refers to the social structure composed of individuals (or organizations) called "nodes," which are tied (connected) by one or more specific types of interdependency, such as friendship, kinship, common interest, financial exchange, dislike, or intimate relationships or relationships involving specific beliefs, knowledge, or prestige that consider the number or frequency of contacts with family members, relatives, friends, and colleagues (Due, Holstein, Lund, Modvig, & Avlund, 1999). Social support and relationships are subconcepts of social networks. **Social support** is a social network function (as it provides aid and assistance) given by members in a social network. The provision of *social support* is an important function of social relationships (Burg & Seeman, 1994; House, 1981; Israel, 1982). Social support can encourage individuals to initiate and maintain physical activity through psychological mechanisms such as motivation and self-efficacy and by providing tangible resources such as access to information that can help individuals find a place to be active. The most common types of social support given are emotional, instrumental, informational, and appraisal support. Emotional support refers to the amount of sympathy, care, and understanding provided by others. **Instrumental support** is defined as help, aid, or assistance with material resources like providing a ride to a gym, paying bills, and cleaning. **Appraisal support** refers to the type of support that helps with decisions, such as providing appropriate feedback or helping decide which course of action to take. **Informational support** refers to the provision of advice or information related to the need.

Many cross-sectional and epidemiologic studies provide evidence for the role of social support on individuals' health practices and physical activity (Trost, Owen, Bauman, Sallis, & Brown, 2002). Findings from a literature review suggest that individuals who reported low levels of social support from friends or family were 20 to 55% more likely to be insufficiently active compared to those who reported receiving more social support (Trost, et al., 2002). Among children, parent

social networks refer to the social structure composed of individuals (or organizations) called "nodes," which are tied (connected) by one or more specific types of interdependency, such as friendship, kinship, common interest, financial exchange, dislike, intimate relationships, or relationships involving specific beliefs, knowledge, or prestige.

social support is a social network function (as it provides aid and assistance) given by members in a social network.

instrumental support is defined as the help, aid, or assistance with material resources like providing a ride to a gym, paying bills, and cleaning.

appraisal support refers to the type of support that involves helping with decisions, providing appropriate feedback, or helping decide which course of action to take.

informational support refers to the provision of advice or information related to the need.

support for physical activity also influences children's physical activity (Sallis, Prochaska, & Taylor, 2000). Furthermore, research suggests that the type of social support may have differential effects among those who are considering starting a physical activity program or have recently started compared to those who have been physically active for some time. Emotional, appraisal, instrumental, and informational support can positively influence motivation to *initiate* physical activity and confidence to perform it (Oliveira et al., 2011). In comparison, for those who have *maintained* activity, practical aspects like access to appropriate materials (i.e., informational support) or locations (i.e., instrumental support) appear to be an important predictor of maintaining activity.

Interpersonal Methods of Promoting Physical Activity

There is strong evidence suggesting that interpersonally focused interventions can influence compliance and adherence to physical activity among diverse populations. One reason these types of interventions are effective in promoting physical activity is that individuals have a fundamental need to belong and be connected to others (Baumeister & Leary, 1995). There are several ways in which **interpersonally focused interventions** can enhance social support and, in turn, increase people's physical activity. An interpersonally focused intervention can be offered through **informal networks** (e.g., family, friends, etc.) and more **formal networks** (e.g., health coaches, health care providers, community health workers, etc.). By providing information and enhancing existing networks, health promotion interventions can provide skills and influence the attitude and behavior of the recipient. Despite emerging evidence showing an influential role of social relations on health, the evidence has been more compelling with women than men (Molloy, Dixon, Hamer, & Sniehotta, 2010).

Health promotion interventions involving health coaches, community health workers (CHW) (or indigenous natural helpers), counselors, or other paraprofessionals have been effective in promoting physical activity. When working with minority communities, the involvement of CHWs has been found to be effective in promoting health practices because they are trusted leaders whom community members can identify with and turn to for advice, support, and other types of aid (Eng, Parker, & Harlan, 1997; Eng & Young, 1992). Community health workers can provide informational, emotional, and instrumental support. Community health workers can provide these types of support through one-on-one or group interactions. Previous studies involving Community health workers have been effective in promoting physical activity. In *Pasos Adelante* (Steps Forward), Staten and colleagues involved CHWs to help promote physical activity among residents living in a United States–Mexico border region (Staten, Scheu, Bronson, Peña, & Elenes, 2005). The CHW in this project not only provided important information about physical activity but also supported participants' efforts by problem solving barriers to physical activity and encouraging participants who were not feeling motivated to attend the group exercise classes. As a result, the physical activity of program participants increased over time. These studies provide further evidence that social support is likely to facilitate physical activity.

interpersonally focused interventions can increase intangible (e.g., coping) and tangible (e.g., money) resources that lead to positive health behaviors (e.g., physical activity) and health outcomes.

informal networks are social networks of individuals and/or groups without formal structures, linked together by one or more social relationships, such as kinship and friendship.

formal networks are networks of individuals that have formal structures (e.g., sporting or recreational clubs, and political parties).

Environmental-Level Interventions

Extending the interpersonal level of the Social Ecological Framework includes the community and policy levels. Individuals and groups are influenced by the physical and social environment (Sallis & Owen, 1996). The **physical environment** refers to environments that are human modified, including homes, schools, workplaces, air pollution, the transportation system, highways, urban sprawl, and other design features that may provide opportunities for travel and physical activity. The **social environment** considers the economic climate, power relations, social inequalities, cultural practices, religious institutions, and political and societal forces that shape the availability and choices for physical activity. Although the evidence is not consistent, many studies show a link between the type of environment people live in and physical activity patterns. For example, research has found that neighborhoods with poor access to parks have residents who engage in less physical activity (Babey, Hastert, Yu, & Brown, 2008).

The association between individuals' physical activity and the environment they live in varies depending on the characteristics of the environment considered, the level of activity, and the way these factors have been assessed (objective vs. self-report). Some of these studies show that the presence of recreational resources (e.g., exercise facilities at work, etc.) but not aspects of neighborhood design are positively associated with vigorous physical activity (De Bourdeaudhuij, Sallis, & Saelens, 2003). Also, research has found that minutes of walking and moderate activity are associated with accessibility of public transportation and other neighborhood facilities. Other study findings have shown that neighborhood characteristics including access to parks, presence of sidewalks, enjoyable scenery, heavy traffic, and hills were positively related to physical activity (Brownson, Baker, Housemann, Brennan, & Bacak, 2001). The findings of a more recent literature review showed consistent associations between access to physical activity facilities, high residential activity, convenient access to destinations, and measures of physical activity (Bauman & Bull, 2007). The link between the environment and physical activity has been found in studies that have included adults and children (Ferreira et al., 2007).

Most studies that examine the link between the environment and physical activity have been correlational; therefore, it is not clear whether people who are physically active move to neighborhoods with more access to physical activity opportunities or the reverse is true. Experimental and longitudinal studies are needed to evaluate the causal link between the environment and physical activity. These studies are difficult to conduct because of the high cost and lack of practicality (e.g., hard to randomly assign people to neighborhoods, etc.).

Critical Thinking

Why would a physical activity intervention target one level of the Social Ecological Framework rather than another? What should be considered?

Methods of Promoting Physical Activity Through the Environment

An environmentally focused intervention may improve parks, add trails, reduce crime, improve sidewalks, and use promotional messages to promote physical activity. Promoting stair use in work settings or in the larger community by adding promotional materials such as posters to prompt using stairs instead of using the escalator or elevator has been associated with increases of physical activity. Webb, Eves, and Kerr conducted a review summarizing the effectiveness of mall-based stair-climbing interventions while adjusting for possible moderators (Webb, Eves, & Kerr, 2011). Their findings suggest that individuals who were prompted to use the stairs were more likely to use them compared to those who were not prompted. Differences were noted in the sexes in that men were more likely to use the stairs than women were. Despite the immediate effects that environmentally focused interventions have had on stair use, their long-term impact has been questioned. In other words, when the prompts are removed, people often revert to the previous behavior (i.e., taking the escalator or elevator).

The impact of environmentally focused interventions on people's physical activity has been evident in other studies. Linenger and colleagues (Linenger, Chesson, & Nice, 1991) found that fitness levels increased after increasing physical activity opportunities by adding a gymnasium, organizing running clubs, and so forth in a military base. A more recent study has found that the vigorous activity of military personnel in the environmental intervention group increased from 46% to 55% compared to the 4% increase in the group that did not receive the environmental intervention (Peel & Booth, 2001). Although the impact of environmentally focused interventions appears to be moderate, these types of studies provide some evidence that modifying the environment is likely to influence the physical activity of individuals.

Policy and the Environmental Level

Often considered part of the environmental level is the policy level. Environmental and policy factors have the potential for making profound changes at the population level. **Policy** refers to the legislative, regulatory actions taken by local, state, or federal governments that are meant to influence behavior by demanding specific behaviors or inhibiting others; policies may be implicit (e.g., informal policy at work) or explicit (Schmid, Pratt, & Witmer, 2006), and policy interventions require public support. Policies can indirectly influence physical activity by influencing the safety of neighborhoods, adding more public transportation, creating and supporting physical activity programs, and increasing access to physical activity opportunities, but they also can impact physical activity directly by encouraging people to use structures in the environment that facilitate physical activity. Policies can also influence the design of a city, which can consequently facilitate physical activity by adding or improving parks and walking and bicycle trails.

Policy and Physical Activity. There have been limited studies showing changes in physical activity following the implementation of policies promoting physical activity. One published review of studies on physical activity interventions for children and adolescents found that interventions focusing on increasing the amount of physical activity during regular physical education were more effective than

policy refers to the legislative, regulatory actions taken by local, state, or federal governments that are meant to influence behavior by demanding specific behaviors or inhibiting others; policies may be implicit (e.g., informal policy at work) or explicit and policy interventions require public support.

interventions targeting overall levels of physical activity (Ringuet & Trost, 2001). There is strong evidence to support policies focused on promoting physical education in schools, with the strongest evidence deriving from policy-related interventions that are multicomponent in nature like improving the school environment and incorporating faculty/staff health promotion and family involvement (Pate, Trilk, Wonwoo, & Jing, 2011). Programs that have increased the quality and quantity of PE classes, providing physical activity–related health education, and improving the school environment have increased the physical activity of children (Webber et al. 2008). Currently, 50 states have state standards for PE, 26 states require student assessment of PE, 14 states require fitness assessments, and 28 states require PE grades to be included in students' GPA (Shape of the Nation Report, 2012). Based on a CDC report (School Health Policies and Programs Study; Lee, Burgeson, Fulton, & Spain, 2007), physical education was taught only by a physical education teacher or specialist in 80.1% of elementary schools. In 73.3% of middle schools and 66.3% of high schools, physical education was taught only by a physical education teacher.

Policy and Environmentally Focused Interventions. Many government-supported programs that promote physical activity have successfully encouraged community members to be more physically active. The types of policies that governments can pass have the potential to increase physical activity among community members by increasing the safety of parks, working with urban planners to ensure the addition of parks in city planning, and adding park amenities (e.g., walking paths), among other efforts that can increase the opportunities to be physically active. Two programs promoting physical activity that have received government support have taken place in Brazil and Colombia. The governments in these two countries have allocated financial resources to support and implement programs that promote physical activity. Details about program components and findings from their evaluation efforts are provided in the case studies at the end of the chapter.

Summary

There are strengths and limitations to assessing physical activity via self-report (e.g., survey) and through more objective methods like using accelerometers. Researchers may need to consider using both these methods to better understand the type (e.g., leisure time) and level (e.g., moderate) of physical activity that participants engage in. When assessing physical activity through self-report or accelerometers is not feasible, researchers may want to consider using observational methods. Intervention researchers can evaluate the impact of their program on changes in type and level of physical activity.

Researchers have argued that interventions should be most effective when targeting multiple levels of the Social Ecological Framework. The majority of the research has included studies examining the influences of individual and interpersonal factors on physical activity. Recently, there has been more enthusiasm to examine the impact of the environment on behavior because of its potential to change the behavior of large sets of people. However, many argue that in order to maximize the effects of an environmentally focused intervention, structured programs promoting physical activity should also be implemented (Sallis, Bauman, & Pratt, 1998).

Furthermore, little is known about how the levels of the Social Ecological Framework influence each other. The potential influences of social networks and social support on organizational and community factors (e.g., competence) is not well understood. It may be that strengthening social networks and enhancing the exchange of social support may influence a community's ability to garner its resources and solve problems. Therefore, it is unclear the impact that each level has in influencing physical activity because the interactions are difficult to disentangle.

5-1 CASE STUDY   Physical Activity Promotion in Brazil

As the largest country in Latin America, Brazil has developed comprehensive programs to promote physical activity in three cities: Curitiba, Recife, and Sao Paulo. In Curitiba, a program called CuritibAtiva promotes physical activity conditioning, gymnastics, water activities, community entertainment, dancing, running, and school games in parks, squares, schools, parking lots, and sports centers. Findings from their studies evaluating the impact of the CuritibAtiva on the physical activity of community members suggest that people who reported being familiar with the program were more likely to be physically active (Reis et al., 2010; Ribeiro et al., 2010).

In Recife, Academia da Cidade (ACP) promotes leisure-time physical activity throughout the city. In response to community demands, the government funded ACP to promote supervised leisure-time physical activity for community members in 21 public spaces of Recife (e.g., parks). At ACP sites (see Figure 5-3), physical education teachers contracted by the city offer free supervised leisure-time physical activity sessions and nutrition, education, and health monitoring (i.e., blood pressure measurements, anthropometric and nutrition assessments). As a result, there has been a higher prevalence of moderate to high levels of leisure-time physical activity among former and current ACP participants compared to people who were not exposed to the program. Simoes and colleagues concluded that community-level professionally supervised and publicly available programs such as ACP are likely to be effective strategies for increasing levels of leisure time PA (Simoes et al., 2009).

In Sao Paulo, Agita Sao Paulo programs are designed to increase the population's knowledge of the benefits of moderate physical activity participation with a particular focus on students and elderly (Matsudo et al., 2003). The partnerships involved in these efforts are governmental and nongovernmental sectors; at the beginning of the program, a board was created involving different sectors like education (federal, state, and private universities), sports, health, industry, commerce, and services to inform the development and implementation of the physical activity program. Furthermore, the program involves students to help develop special events where they discussed the benefits of physical activity during festivals and communitywide events. Agita Sao

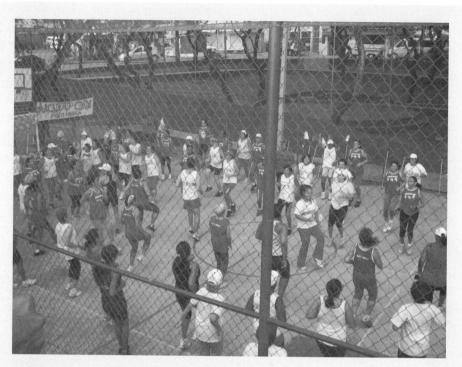

FIGURE 5–3 Academia da Cidade.

Paulo also uses the media to promote physical activity as well as special promotional activities like samba during Carnival. Findings from their evaluation efforts suggest improvements in activity among individuals who had been exposed to the program (Matsudo, Matsudo, Andrade, Araújo, & Pratt, 2006).

Thought Questions

1. If a baseline questionnaire is not administered prior to beginning a community intervention (to compare pre- and postsurvey results), how would one assess the impact of a program?

2. How can policy influence the implementation of a program?

5-2   **CASE STUDY**   Physical Activity Promotion in Colombia

Similar to Brazil, Colombia has also made significant advancements in promoting physical activity in Bogota. Muevete Bogota is an example of another successful program that uses multisectoral strategies to promote physical activity in urban regions. The development of the program was informed by the guidelines proposed by the CDC and the American College of Sports Medicine (Pate et al., 1995) as well as input from physical activity programs developed in other countries like the Agita Sao Paulo program in Brazil (Matsudo et al., 2003). To market the physical activity program in the community, Muevete Bogota used media campaigns through work sites, schools, health care centers, and community settings. The program used three main strategies in its efforts: (1) building program awareness and recruiting partners, (2) educating and training program implementers, and (3) delivering the intervention to the sites. The program implemented "Healthy and Active" stations that involved measurement of physical fitness at various sites, increasing capacity among leaders who promote physical activity, activities, and competitions of employees through participating companies and various initiatives like Active Workers Week. The support of the government has been one reason the program has been sustained over the years. The evaluation efforts focused primarily on refining and improving program activities by evaluating whether performance indicators were being met and whether additional efforts were needed to promote physical activity in the community.

Thought Questions

1. How can researchers evaluate the impact of a marketing program on the activity level of the community?

Review Questions

1. Which of the following best describes physical activity?

    a. The body's ability to carry out active tasks
    b. The amount of energy required to maintain basic biological processes needed for life
    c. Structured activity that is used to improve fitness
    d. Movement of the human body that increases energy expenditure above resting levels
    e. Movement that makes you sweat or breathe hard

2. Which of the following is not one the four levels used to describe physical activity intensity?

    a. Sedentary
    b. Basal
    c. Light
    d. Moderate
    e. Vigorous

3. What type of measurement best describes the act of asking participants what type of physical activity they have done over the past week?

    a. Subjective measurement
    b. Objective measurement
    c. Direct observations
    d. Recall bias

4. Which of the following health conditions is NOT related to physical activity behavior?

   a. Heart disease
   b. Obesity
   c. Depression
   d. Arthritis
   e. None of the above

5. Which of the following is NOT one of the five "core" physical activity behavior change strategies?

   a. Goal setting
   b. Goal review
   c. Social support
   d. Intention formation
   e. Self-monitoring

6. How can community health workers promote physical activity?

   a. By providing emotional support
   b. By providing informational support
   c. By providing instrumental support
   d. By providing appraisal support
   e. All of the above

7. What are some of the limitations of the studies that examine the relationship between the built environment and physical activity?

   a. Difficult to examine causal relationships
   b. Difficult to define the physical environment
   c. Challenging to motivate people to be physically active
   d. None of the above

8. The following environment is human modified, which includes homes, schools, workplaces, and other design features that may provide opportunities for travel and physical activity.

   a. Built environment
   b. Social environment
   c. Political environment
   d. None of the above

9. The following environment considers the economic climate, power relations, social inequalities, cultural practices, religious institutions, and political and societal forces that shape the availability and choices for physical activity.

   a. Built environment
   b. Social environment
   c. Political environment
   d. None of the above

10. _____ refers to the legislative, regulatory actions taken by local, state, or federal governments that are meant to influence behavior by demanding specific behaviors or inhibiting others.

    a. Environmental support
    b. Policy
    c. Community support
    d. None of the above

Web Resources

Visit the following websites to learn more about some of the topics presented in this chapter.

The Centers for Disease Control and Prevention's benefits of walkable communities as they relate to health, the environment, and social interaction. http://www.cdc.gov/healthyplaces/healthy_comm_design.htm

The Centers for Disease Control and Prevention's National Health and Nutrition Examination Survey (NHANES) http://www.cdc.gov/nchs/nhanes.htm

The Centers for Disease Control and Prevention's Transportation and Health http://www.cdc.gov/healthyplaces/healthtopics/transportation/default.htm

References

Abraham, C., & Michie, S. (2008). A taxonomy of behavior change techniques used in interventions. *Health psychology: Official journal of the Division of Health Psychology, American Psychological Association, 27*(3), 379–387.

Ajzen, I. (1991). The theory of planned behavior. *Organizational Behavior and Human Decision Processes, 50*(2), 179–211.

Arias, E. (2011). United States life tables, 2007. *National vital statistics reports: From the Centers for Disease Control and Prevention, National Center for Health Statistics, National Vital Statistics System, 59*(9), 1–60.

Ayotte, B. J., Margrett, J. A., & Hicks-Patrick, J. (2010). Physical activity in middle-aged and young-old adults: The roles of self-efficacy, barriers, outcome expectancies, self-regulatory behaviors and social support. *Journal of Health Psychology, 15*(2), 173–185.

Babey, S. H., Hastert, T. A., Yu, H., & Brown, E. R. (2008). Physical activity among adolescents. When do parks matter? *American Journal of Preventive Medicine, 34*(4), 345–348.

Bauman, A., & Bull, F. C. (2007). *Environmental correlates of physical activity and walking in adults and children: A review of reviews.* London, UK:

Baumeister, R. F., & Leary, M. R. (1995). The need to belong: Desire for interpersonal attachments as a fundamental human motivation. *Psychological Bulletin, 117*(3), 497–529.

Brownson, R. C., Baker, E. A., Housemann, R. A., Brennan, L. K., & Bacak, S. J. (2001). Environmental and policy determinants of physical activity in the United States. *American Journal of Public Health, 91*(12), 1995–2003.

Burg, M. M., & Seeman, T. E. (1994). Families and health: The negative side of social ties. *Annals of Behavioral Medicine, 16*(2), 109–115.

Chen, K. Y., & Bassett Jr., D. R. (2005). The technology of accelerometry-based activity monitors: Current and future. *Medicine & Science in Sports & Exercise, 37*(11 Suppl), S490–S500.

De Bourdeaudhuij, I., Sallis, J. F., & Saelens, B. E. (2003). Environmental correlates of physical activity in a sample of Belgian adults. *American Journal of Health Promotion, 18*(1), 83–92.

Driver, S. (2005). Social support and the physical activity behaviours of people with a brain injury. *Brain Injury, 19*(13), 1067–1075.

Due, P., Holstein, B., Lund, R., Modvig, J., & Avlund, K. (1999). Social relations: Network, support and relational strain. *Social Science & Medicine, 48*(5), 661–673.

Duncan, M., & Mummery, K. (2005). Psychosocial and environmental factors associated with physical activity among city dwellers in regional Queensland. *Preventive Medicine, 40*(4), 363–372.

Eng, E., Parker, E., & Harlan, C. (1997). Lay health advisor intervention strategies: a continuum from natural helping to paraprofessional helping. *Health Education & Behavior, 24*(4), 413–417.

Eng, E., & Young, R. (1992). Lay health advisors as community change agents. *Family & Community Health: The Journal of Health Promotion & Maintenance, 15*(1), 24–40.

Ferreira, I., van der Horst, K., Wendel-Vos, W., Kremers, S., van Lenthe, F. J., & Brug, J. (2007). Environmental correlates of physical activity in youth—a review and update. *Obesity Reviews, 8*(2), 129–154.

Garabrant, D. H., Peters, J. M., Mack, T. M., & Bernstein, L. (1984). Job Activity and Colon Cancer Risk. *American Journal of Epidemiology, 119*(6), 1005.

Gardner, D. M., Baldessarini, R. J., & Waraich, P. (2005). Modern antipsychotic drugs: A critical overview. *Canadian Medical Association Journal, 172*(13), 1703–1711.

Goran, M. I., Reynolds, K. D., & Lindquist, C. H. (1999). Role of physical activity in the prevention of obesity in children. *Obesity, 23*(Suppl 3), S18–S33.

Hagströmer, M., Oja, P., & Sjöström, M. (2007). The International Physical Activity Questionnaire (IPAQ): A study of concurrent and construct validity. *Public Health Nutrition, 9*(06), 755–762.

Hamilton, M. T, Hamilton, D. G., & Zderic, T. W. (2007). Role of low energy expenditure and sitting in obesity, metabolic syndrome, type 2 diabetes, and cardiovascular disease. *Diabetes*, 56, 2655–2667.

Hill, J. O., & Wyatt, H. R. (2005). Role of physical activity in preventing and treating obesity. *Journal of Applied Physiology*, *99*(2), 765–770.

House, J. S. (1981). *Work stress and social support*. Reading, MA:Adison-Wesley.

Hu, F. B., Li, T. Y., Colditz, G. A., Willett, W. C., & Manson, J. E. (2003). Television watching and other sedentary behaviors in relation to risk of obesity and type 2 diabetes mellitus in women. *JAMA*, *289*(14), 1785–1791.

Israel, B. A. (1982). Social networks and health status: Linking theory, research, and practice. *Patient Counselling & Health Education*, *4*(2), 65–79.

Katzmarzyk, P. T., Church, T. S., Craig, C. L., & Bouchard, C. (2009). Sitting time and mortality from all causes, cardiovascular disease, and cancer. *Medicine and Science in Sports and Exercise*, *41*(5), 998–1005.

Kessler, Ronald C, Demler, O., Frank, R. G., Olfson, M., Pincus, H. A., Walters, E. E., Wang, P., et al. (2005). Prevalence and treatment of mental disorders, 1990 to 2003. *The New England Journal of Medicine*, *352*(24), 2515–2523.

Kessler, R. C., Berglund, P., Demler, O., Jin, R., Koretz, D., Merikangas, K. R., Rush, A. J., et al. (2003). The epidemiology of major depressive disorder. *JAMA*, *289*(23), 3095.

Lee, I. M., & Skerrett, P. J. (2001). Physical activity and all-cause mortality: What is the dose-response relation? *Medicine and Science in Sports and Exercise*, *33*(6 Suppl), S459–S471.

Lee, S. M., Burgeson, C. R., Fulton, J. E., & Spain, C. G. (2007). Physical education and physical activity: results from the School Health Policies and Programs Study 2006. *Journal of School Health*, *77*(8), 435–463.

Linenger, J. M., Chesson, C. V., 2nd, & Nice, D. S. (1991). Physical fitness gains following simple environmental change. *American Journal of Preventive Medicine*, *7*(5), 298–310.

Matsudo, S. M., Matsudo, V. K. R., Andrade, D. R., Araújo, T. L., & Pratt, M. (2006). Evaluation of a physical activity promotion program: The example of Agita São Paulo. *Evaluation & Program Planning*, *29*(3), 301–311.

Matsudo, S. M., Matsudo, V. R., Araujo, T. L., Andrade, D. R., Andrade, E. L., de Oliveira, L. C., et al. (2003). The Agita São Paulo Program as a model for using physical activity to promote health. *Revista Panamericana De Salud Pública*, *14*(4), 265–272.

Matthews, C., Chen, K., Freedson, P., Buchowski, M., Beech, B., Pate, R., & Troiano, R. (2008). Amount of time spent in sedentary behaviors in the United States, 2003–2004. *American Journal of Epidemiology*, *167*(7), 875–881.

McKay, H. G., King, D., Eakin, E. G., Seeley, J. R., & Glasgow, R. E. (2001). The diabetes network internet-based physical activity intervention: A randomized pilot study. *Diabetes Care*, *24*(8), 1328–1334.

McKenzie, T., Sallis, J., & Nader, P. (1991). SOFIT: System for observing fitness instruction time. *Journal of Teaching in Physical Education*, *11*(2), 195–205.

McKenzie, T. L., Marshall, S. J., Sallis, J. F., & Conway, T. L. (2000). Leisure-time physical activity in school environments: An observational study using SOPLAY. *Preventive Medicine*, *30*(1), 70–77.

Michie, S., Abraham, C., Whittington, C., McAteer, J., & Gupta, S. (2009). Effective techniques in healthy eating and physical activity interventions: A meta-regression. *Health Psychology*, *28*(6), 690–701.

Molloy, G. J., Dixon, D., Hamer, M., & Sniehotta, F. F. (2010). Social support and regular physical activity: Does planning mediate this link? *British Journal of Health Psychology*, *15*(Pt 4), 859–870.

Morris, J., Heady, J., Raffle, P., Roberts, C., & Parks, J. (1953). Coronary heart disease and physical activity of work. *The Lancet*, *262*(6795), 1053–1057.

Must, A., & Parisi, S. M. (2009). Sedentary behavior and sleep: Paradoxical effects in association with childhood obesity. *International Journal of Obesity (2005)*, *33 Suppl 1*(S1), S82–S86.

Myers, J., Prakash, M., & Froelicher, V. (2002). Exercise capacity and mortality among men referred for exercise testing. *New England Journal of Medicine*, *346*(11), 793–801.

Napolitano, M. A., & Marcus, B. H. (2002). Targeting and tailoring physical activity information using print and information technologies. *Exercise and Sport Sciences Reviews*, *30*(3), 122–128.

Ogden, C. L., Carroll, M. D., Curtin, L. R., McDowell, M. A., Tabak, C. J., & Flegal, K. M. (2006). Prevalence of overweight and obesity in the United States, 1999–2004. *JAMA*, *295*(13), 1549–1555.

Oguma, Y., & Shinoda-Tagawa, T. (2004). Physical activity decreases cardiovascular disease risk in women: Review and meta-analysis. *American Journal of Preventive Medicine*, *26*(5), 407–418.

Oliveira, A. J., Lopes, C. S., de Leon, A. C. P., Rostila, M., Griep, R. H., Werneck, G. L., et al. (2011). Social support and leisure-time physical activity: Longitudinal evidence from the Brazilian Pró-Saúde cohort study. *The International Journal of Behavioral Nutrition and Physical Activity*, 8, 77.

Paffenbarger, R., Hyde, R., Wing, A., & Hsieh, C. (1986). Physical activity, all-cause mortality, and logevity of college alumni. *New England Journal of Medicine*, *314*(10), 605–613.

Pate, R. R., Pratt, M., Blair, S. N., Haskell, W. L., Macera, C. A., Bouchard, C., et al. (1995). Physical activity and public health. A recommendation from the Centers for Disease Control and Prevention and the American College of Sports Medicine. *JAMA: The Journal of the American Medical Association*, *273*(5), 402–407.

Pate, R. R., Trilk, J. L., Wonwoo, B., & Jing, W. (2011). Policies to increase physical activity in children and youth. *Journal of Exercise Science & Fitness*, *9*(1), 1–14.

Patel, A. V., Rodriguez, C., Pavluck, A. L., Thun, M. J., & Calle, E. E. (2006). Recreational physical activity and sedentary behavior in relation to ovarian cancer risk in a large cohort of US women. *American Journal of Epidemiology*, *163*(8), 709–716.

Peel, G. R., & Booth, M. L. (2001). Impact evaluation of the Royal Australian Air Force health promotion program. *Aviation, Space, and Environmental Medicine*, *72*(1), 44–51.

Reis, R. S., Hallal, P. C., Parra, D. C., Ribeiro, I. C., Brownson, R. C., Pratt, M., et al. (2010). Promoting physical activity through community-wide policies and planning: Findings from Curitiba, Brazil. *Journal of Physical Activity & Health*, 7Suppl 2, S137–S145.

Rethorst, C. D., Wipfli, B. M., & Landers, D. M. (2009). The antidepressive effects of exercise: A meta-analysis of randomized trials. *Sports Medicine*, *39*(6), 491–511.

Ribeiro, I. C., Torres, A., Parra, D. C., Reis, R., Hoehner, C., Schmid, T. L., et al. (2010). Using logic models as iterative tools for planning and evaluating physical activity promotion programs in Curitiba, Brazil. *Journal of Physical Activity & Health*, 7 Suppl 2, S155–S162.

Ringuet, C. J., & Trost, S. G. (2001). Effects of physical activity intervention in youth: A review. *International SportsMedicine Journal, 2*(5), 1.

Sallis, J. F., Bauman, A., & Pratt, M. (1998). Environmental and policy interventions to promote physical activity. *American Journal of Preventive Medicine, 15*(4), 379–397.

Sallis, J. F., & Owen, N. (1996). Health behavior and health education: Theory, research, and practice, 2nd ed. In K. Glanz, F. Lewis & B. Rimer (Eds.): Jossey-Bass.

Sallis, J. F., Prochaska, J. J., & Taylor, W. C. (2000). A review of correlates of physical activity of children and adolescents. *Medicine and Science in Sports and Exercise, 32*(5), 963–975.

Schmid, T. L., Pratt, M., & Witmer, L. (2006). A framework for physical activity policy research. *Journal of Physical Activity & Health,* 3 (Suppl1), S20–S29.

Shapiro, J. R., Bauer, S., Hamer, R. M., Kordy, H., Ward, D., & Bulik, C. M. (2008). Use of text messaging for monitoring sugar-sweetened beverages, physical activity, and screen time in children: a pilot study. *Journal of Nutrition Education and Behavior, 40*(6), 385–391.

Sherrington, C., Lord, S. R., & Finch, C. F. (2004). Physical activity interventions to prevent falls among older people: Update of the evidence. *Journal of Science and Medicine in Sport, 7*(1 Suppl), 43–51.

Simoes, E. J., Hallal, P., Pratt, M., Ramos, L., Munk, M., Damascena, W., et al. (2009). Effects of a community-based, professionally supervised intervention on physical activity levels among residents of Recife, Brazil. *American Journal of Public Health, 99*(1), 68–75.

Staten, L. K., Scheu, L. L., Bronson, D., Peña, V., & Elenes, J. (2005). Pasos Adelante: The effectiveness of a community-based chronic disease prevention program. *Preventing Chronic Disease, 2*(1), A 18.

Sugiyama, T., Healy, G. N., Dunstan, D. W., Salmon, J., & Owen, N. (2008). Joint associations of multiple leisure-time sedentary behaviours and physical activity with obesity in Australian adults. *International Journal of Behavioral Nutrition and Physical Activity,* 6, 1–6.

Troiano, R. P., Berrigan, D., Dodd, K. W., Mâsse, L. C., Tilert, T., & Mcdowell, M. (2008). Physical activity in the United States measured by accelerometer. *Medicine & Science in Sports & Exercise, 40*(1), 181–188.

Trost, S. G., Owen, N., Bauman, A. E., Sallis, J. F., & Brown, W. (2002). Correlates of adults' participation in physical activity: Review and update. *Medicine and Science in Sports and Exercise, 34*(12), 1996–2001.

Tudor-Locke, C., Williams, J. E., Reis, J. P., & Pluto, D. (2002). Utility of pedometers for assessing convergent validity. *Sports Medicine, 32*(12), 795–808.

U.S. Department of Health and Human Services. (2008). *2008 Physical Activity Guidelines for Americans.* Washington, DC:Author.

Wannamethee S. G., & Shaper, A. G. (2001). Physical activity in the prevention of cardiovascular disease: An epidemiological perspective. *Sports Medicine, 31*(2), 101–114.

Webb, O. J., Eves, F. F., & Kerr, J. (2011). A statistical summary of mall-based stair-climbing interventions. *Journal of Physical Activity & Health, 8*(4), 558–565.

Webber, L. S, Catellier, D. J., Lytle, L. A., Murray, D. M., Pratt, C. A., Young, D. R., Elder, J. P., Lohman, T. G., Stevens, J., Jobe, J. B., & Pate, R. R. (2008). Promoting physical activity in middle school girls: Trial of Activity for Adolescent Girls (TAAG). *American Journal Preventive Medicine, 34*(3), 173–84. doi: 10.1016/j.amepre.2007.11.018

Wipfli, B. M., Rethorst, C. D., & Landers, D. M. (2008). The anxiolytic effects of exercise: A meta-analysis of randomized trials and dose-response analysis. *Journal of Sport & Exercise Psychology*, *30*(4), 392–410.

Zderic, T. W., & Hamilton, M. T. (2006). Physical inactivity amplifies the sensitivity of skeletal muscle to the lipid-induced downregulation of lipoprotein lipase activity. *Journal of Applied Physiology*, *100*(1), 249–257.

Chapter 6

Reem Daffa, MPH and Hala Madanat, PhD

TOBACCO

Key Terms

carcinogens

cognitive-behavioral therapy

community-level tobacco interventions

economic interventions

environmental tobacco restrictions

excise taxes

health behavior

health education

interpersonal networks

interventions

large-scale programs

multilevel interventions

nicotine

nitrosamines

occasional smoker

organizational interventions

passive smoking

public education campaigns

public policy interventions

recreational tobacco consumption

regular smoker

sales restrictions

smokeless tobacco

smokeless zones

smoking bans

smoking cessation

tobacco advertising

Learning Objectives

Upon completion of this chapter, you should be able to:

1. Understand statistics regarding tobacco use, including prevalence rates in the United States and health risks associated with tobacco use.
2. Identify factors associated with tobacco initiation, use, and cessation.
3. Describe the Social Ecological Framework for understanding tobacco control interventions.
4. Compare various methods for conducting tobacco control intervention and their strengths and weaknesses.
5. Explain how various intervention methods can work together to create a comprehensive approach to tobacco control interventions.

Chapter Outline

INTRODUCTION

This chapter begins with an overview of the history of tobacco use, rates of use among various individuals, and the associated health risks of tobacco use. Following this, intervention strategies are explored that seek to prevent and stop use, including individual, organizational, community, and policy interventions.

HISTORY OF TOBACCO USE

The use of tobacco can be traced back to 5,000 to 3,000 B.C. Its use has varied widely across cultures and time. Some civilizations used the leaf as an intoxicant in medicinal remedies, while others burned tobacco as incense during religious ceremonies (Gately & Iain, 2004).

Although already in use in the Americas prior to the arrival of the European settlers (Grim, 2009), it was only after Columbus's arrival from the Americas that tobacco use was introduced to Europe. It gained popularity and became a heavily-prized trade item (Borio, 2007). Over the centuries, **recreational tobacco consumption**, or using tobacco solely for its effects as an intoxicant, grew and spawned many different methods of delivery. In the 18th century, snuff was the most prevalent form of tobacco. In manufacturing snuff, tobacco leaves were processed to produce a smokeless, fine, dry substance that was inhaled through the nose (Porter & Teich, 1997). Later in the 19th century, pipe smoking and cigars were the preferred method of tobacco use (Taylor II, 2014), before tobacco was industrialized through the mass production of cigarettes in the 20th century (Goodman, 1993). It was this industrialization that was primarily responsible for the rapid, worldwide adoption of cigarettes as the recreational tobacco of choice.

> **recreational tobacco consumption** involves ingesting tobacco for its intoxicating effects rather than for medicinal or religious purposes.

In recent years, the spread of hookah or waterpipe lounges in the United States has introduced a new method of tobacco use (Maziak et al., 2004). Hookah smoking has gained popularity among adolescents and college students (Smith et al., 2011). Waterpipes burn a flavored tobacco whose smoke is passed through water before it is inhaled. Yet, for all their presumed stylishness, waterpipes are far from innocuous. A single waterpipe session, which usually lasts about 40 minutes, may expose the user to three to nine times the amount of carbon monoxide and nearly twice the amount of nicotine as a single cigarette (Fromme et al., 2009). The smoke retains most of the same toxins contained in regular cigarette smoke, including volatile organic compounds, polycyclic aromatic hydrocarbons, and metals. Like cigarette smoke, the compounds found in waterpipe smoke expose other people to secondhand smoke with its associated health risks. Additionally, the practice of communally sharing a single pipe increases the risk of communicable or infectious diseases, as well as germ and bacterial transmission. Furthermore, the waterpipe stimulates the same addictive and dependent behavior as cigarettes and can hinder cessation of tobacco use by providing smokers with a substitute means of ingesting nicotine. Use of a waterpipe may also serve as a catalyst for smoking initiation (Maziak, 2010).

Current Tobacco Use Trends

The Centers for Disease Control and Prevention (CDC) closely monitors tobacco use across several demographic categories: both the forms in which tobacco is used and by whom. The prevalence and type of tobacco use varies depending on a host of cultural and societal norms, as well as socioeconomic status and gender.

Generally, a larger percentage of young people use tobacco alternatives like cigars and smokeless tobacco than adults do. However, cigarette smoking is still the most dominant form of tobacco use among both adults and young people. In fact, cigarette smoking is also the most common form of tobacco use across all racial, ethnic, and age demographic categories. According to CDC, more than 45.3 million American adults smoked cigarettes in 2010, approximately 19% of all adults; 21.5% of adult men and 17.3% of adult women smoke cigarettes (CDC, 2011a). Furthermore, 19.5% of high school students and 5.2% of middle school students smoke at least one cigarette per month (CDC, 2009a). This chapter will later discuss racial and ethnic differences in smoking cigarettes and other tobacco products.

The next most common form of tobacco use is cigar smoking. In 2009, 5.4% of adults smoked cigars with 9.1% of American adult men being cigar smokers, and only 1.9% of adult females (CDC, 2009b) smoking cigars. However, cigar use was actually higher among youth under 18. In 2009, 14% of high school students and about 4% of middle school students were cigar smokers (CDC, 2009a).

Smokeless tobacco is the next most common form of tobacco use. In 2008, the CDC estimated that 3.5% of adults used smokeless tobacco. Again, smokeless tobacco use was more prevalent by youth under 18 years of age than with adults; approximately 6% of high school students and nearly 3% of middle school students used smokeless tobacco. The two most common types of smokeless tobacco were snuff and chewing tobacco, that is, treated tobacco that may be held between the cheek and gums, ingested orally, or inhaled through the nostrils (CDC, 2009c).

The CDC also measures the rates of use of more exotic tobacco products, including hookahs, bidis, and kreteks. Hookahs are waterpipes commonly used in the Middle East and India that utilize a flavored loose-leaf tobacco. Bidis are slender cigarettes from Southeast Asia wherein flavored or unflavored tobacco is hand rolled in the leaves of either the tendu or temburni plant, which are native to Southeast Asia. Kretek cigarettes are also from Southeast Asia, namely Indonesia, and include cloves or other additives mixed in with the tobacco (CDC, 2009d, 2009e).

History of Tobacco Advertising

The history of tobacco advertising in the media is long and complex. The first tobacco advertisements in the United States appeared in 1789, long before the health effects of tobacco use were known (James & Olstad, 2009). Given the difficulty of importing tobacco products at this time, mass marketing of these products did not go into effect until after the Civil War, when the Bull Durham Tobacco Company was founded (James & Olstad, 2009). The changing economic climate of post–Civil War America, along with the invention of tools to mass produce cigarettes, also increased advertising, as companies were able to create more product faster and for less money.

Tobacco advertising gained further prominence during the World Wars. In 1918, the War Department bought out Bull Durham Tobacco and issued soldiers cigarette rations (Borio, 2007). Cigarettes were again distributed to soldiers during World War II, with an increase in the prominence of tobacco advertising following soldiers' return home (James & Olstad, 2009). Tobacco companies sponsored television shows, radio programs, and other media in an attempt to create brand loyalty, and smoking was seen in movies and other media, including media geared toward children.

In 1961, the Surgeon General's report on smoking outlined the health risks of tobacco, and restrictions were put into place (Rongey, 2001). Health warnings appeared on cigarette packages beginning with the Federal Cigarette Labeling and Advertising Act of 1965, and in 1967 the Federal Communications Commission (FCC) required television and radio programs that contained cigarette commercials to disclose the health risks of smoking (Rongey, 2001). The FCC also required media channels to provide one public service announcement (PSA) about the dangers of smoking for every three paid cigarette commercials. During this time, per-capita cigarette sales decreased by 6.9% (Rongey, 2001). Given these drops in sales, in 1970, the tobacco industry agreed to remove radio and television advertisements for their products, citing that the required PSAs were damaging sales.

On November 23, 1998, tobacco companies and various states entered into the Master Settlement Agreement (MSA). The MSA responded to litigation by states seeking reimbursement related to costs spent for health care due to smoking-related illnesses. Under the MSA, the states and tobacco companies agreed to undertake efforts to reduce youth smoking, begin new public health initiatives, and regulate tobacco business (Rongey, 2001). The MSA also strictly limited the ways tobacco companies could advertise, including banning advertising aimed at youth, removing tobacco ads from stadiums and mass transit, removing tobacco licenses from media catering to youth, and removing tobacco product promotions in venues accessible to youth (Rongey, 2001). The MSA greatly limited where and how tobacco companies could advertise in hopes of reducing smoking, especially among youth.

In 2009, President Barack Obama signed the Tobacco Regulation Bill, also known as the Family Smoking Prevention and Tobacco Control Act, into law. This bill grants the Food and Drug Administration (FDA) power over the sale, production, and marketing of tobacco products and induces provisions aimed at decreasing youth smoking. Among the bill's requirements are that cigarette companies must disclose product ingredients to the FDA and are prohibited from labeling products in such a way as to minimize health risks (i.e., cigarettes cannot be marketed as "safe" if they are organic, light, or low tar). Among other restrictions, the bill also bans cigarettes in youth-friendly flavors, and cigarette companies are no longer allowed to advertise near schools (Snowden, 2009). The Tobacco Regulation Bill represents the FDA's "most expansive authority over the tobacco industry to date" (James & Olstad, 2009).

FACTORS ASSOCIATED WITH TOBACCO USE

There are several well-known factors associated with tobacco use; one example is gender. Gender differences in smoking prevalence may be attributed to historical cultural norms. Cigars, for instance, have been stereotypically associated with power and masculinity and are therefore a popular choice among men who seek to establish these characteristics as part of their self-image. In adolescence, smoking or **smokeless tobacco** (e.g., snuff or chewing) use may be perceived as a sign of implicit rebellion against parents. Cigarette smoking is also viewed as an effective social tool for starting conversations with strangers and reaffirming social status.

smokeless tobacco is tobacco that is chewed or held in the mouth rather than smoked.

Additionally, racial and ethnic differences exist. While only 9% of Asians and 12.5% of Hispanics smoke cigarettes, approximately 20% of both Black and non-Hispanic Whites and more than 30% of Indian or Alaskan Natives smoke cigarettes. African Americans, Native Alaskans, and American Indians have the highest adult rates of cigar smoking, 7.7% and 7.2% respectively (Native Alaskans and American Indians were counted as a single group). These groups are followed by Whites and Hispanic adults; 5.3% of White adults and 4.9% of Hispanic adults smoke cigars. Asian adults have the lowest rate of cigar use at just 1.5%. Youth cigar smoking rates are higher than those of adults: 15% of male and 6.7% of female high schools students smoke cigars—a total of 10.9% of all high school students. Furthermore, almost 4% of middle school students smoke cigars: 4.5% of male and 3.2% of female students (CDC, 2009b).

Education and income are perhaps the strongest indictors of the tendency to smoke cigarettes. While 9.9% of college graduates and 6.3% of postgraduate degree holders are cigarette smokers, cigarette smoking rates are much higher among those individuals with lower levels of education (CDC, 2011a). For those people who are not college graduates, the rates of smoking are as follows: 45.2% of adults who hold only a GED smoke, 33.8% of adults who have completed 9 to 11 years of education smoke, and 23.8% who are only high school graduates smoke. Furthermore, almost 30% of adults living in poverty smoke, compared with 18.3% of adults living at or above the poverty line (CDC, 2011a).

In the United States, each of the three youngest age brackets has approximately equal rates of cigarette smoking: approximately 20% of individuals aged 18 to 24, 25 to 44, and 45 to 64 are smokers. In contrast, 9.5% of adults 65 and older smoke. In addition, data show that more than 80% of adult smokers became addicted to tobacco products before the age of 18. Using data from 2009, the CDC estimated that 17.2% of all high school students are **regular smokers**, or smoke every day: 19.6% of males and 14.8% of females. Rates of use by **occasional smokers**, or those who do not smoke every day, are higher; 19.5% of high school students smoked at least one cigarette per month. In fact, a CDC study revealed that 19.8% of male and 19.1% of female high school students smoked one or more cigarettes in the month preceding the study. Additionally, 5.2% of all middle school students are regular smokers: 5.6% of males and 4.7% of females (CDC, 2009a).

Among high school students, non-Hispanic Whites have the highest cigarette smoking rate (19.4%), followed by Hispanics (19.2%), Asian Americans (9.7%), and Blacks (7.4%). In middle school, Hispanic youth have the highest cigarette smoking rate (6.7%), followed by Blacks (5.2%), Whites (4.3%), and Asian Americans (2.5%; CDC, 2009a). Rates of use for hookahs, bidis, and kreteks are generally lower, and the CDC does not maintain consistent data collection or rate estimates on their usage. However, the CDC does note that rates of bidi and kretek use by middle school students are below 3% (CDC, 2009d).

> A **regular smoker** is someone who smokes daily.
>
> An **occasional smoker** is someone who smokes less frequently than daily.

HEALTH EFFECTS OF TOBACCO USE

Studies have shown that smoking tobacco and using tobacco-based products have a variety of adverse health ramifications. In the United States alone, smoking is responsible for 443,000 deaths, or one in every five, each year (CDC, 2010). Furthermore, the U.S. Surgeon General (2010) reported that for every tobacco-related death, an additional 20 Americans suffer from at least one severe or chronic tobacco-related illness.

Cigarette smoke contains 7,000 chemicals and compounds, at least 200 of which are toxic, either alone or in combination with one another (Vardavas & Panagiotakos, 2009). Sixty-nine are known **carcinogens**, or cancer-causing agents, including carbon monoxide, which puts the smoker at a higher risk for diseases such as lung, larynx, and pancreatic cancer (USDHHS, 2010). In a 2010 report, the U.S. Surgeon General indicated that even brief, secondhand, or intermittent exposure to cigarette smoke can have immediate and long-term adverse health consequences. The smoke first impacts the lungs, where it can cause inflammation or impaired lung function, which can lead to chronic pulmonary diseases, chronic bronchitis, heart attack, or stroke. From the lungs, chemicals from the smoke pass into the bloodstream and are distributed to every organ and tissue system in the body, where

> **carcinogens** are cancer-causing agents or substances. Tobacco products contain a wide array of carcinogens that are damaging to the human body.

they may damage DNA, weaken the immune system, increase risk for cancers such as those of the pancreas (Tranah, Holly, Wang, & Bracci, 2011) and lungs, and aggravate existing conditions, such as diabetes or cancer (USDHHS, 2010).

nitrosamines are among the most harmful carcinogens found in tobacco products.

Additionally, the tobacco fermentation process produces specific forms of **nitrosamines**, which are among the most harmful carcinogens (Richter et al., 2008). Thus, even smokeless tobacco, though free of tar and potentially lethal gases, can still increase the risk of oral cancer (as with chewable tobacco) or nasopharyngeal cancer (with the use of snuff). The CDC (2011b) reported that smokeless tobacco still contains 28 carcinogens and places users at increased risk of developing cancers of the oral cavity, as well as tooth, gum, and soft tissue disease. Both smoking and smokeless tobacco product use are also known to adversely affect both male and female reproductive systems. Research has shown that smoking during advanced prenatal stages can hinder cognitive development in fetuses and even infants (Stanton, Martin, & Henningfield, 2005). **Nicotine**, the stimulant in tobacco that causes addiction, and the other toxins found in tobacco products, are especially harmful to the ovaries, where they may interfere with estrogen production and regulation, and fallopian tubes, which may increase smokers' risk of ectopic pregnancies, miscarriages, premature births, and low birth weight babies (CDC, 2011a; Dechanet et al., 2011; USDHHS, 2010). Tobacco toxins, both smoke-based and smokeless varieties, may also damage sperm-borne DNA, which can contribute to problematic fetal development or birth defects as well as infertility (CDC, 2011b; USDHHS, 2010). Compared to cigarette smoke, the prevalence of smokeless tobacco products is relatively low in the general population. According to data reported in 2009, the CDC (2011b) estimated that 3.5% of all adults, 6.1% of all high school students, and 2.6% of all middle school students used some form of smokeless tobacco product.

Nicotine is the stimulant in tobacco that is responsible for its addictive nature.

passive smoking also known as secondhand smoking or environmental tobacco smoking, occurs when a person other than the individual smoking a tobacco product inhales tobacco smoke.

Passive smoking, also known as secondhand smoking (SHS) or environmental tobacco smoking (ETS), is also a major cause of smoking-related health problems, including disease, disability, and even death (U.S. Surgeon General, 2006). In passive smoking, people other than the smoker inhale tobacco smoke and can receive its harmful health effects. Specifically, secondhand smoke can increase nonsmokers' risk of developing lung cancer by 20% to 30% and heart disease by 25% to 30% (USDHHS, 2006). Other studies have found that exposure to passive smoking may produce nearly the same 70% to 80% increased risk of coronary heart disease presented by light smoking (Vardavas & Panagiotakos, 2009). Significant exposure to passive smoking has also been shown to increase the risk of non-Hodgkin and follicular lymphoma in lifetime nonsmokers (Lu et al., 2011). CDC data show that as a result of exposure to secondhand smoke, 46,000 nonsmokers die from heart disease and 3,400 nonsmokers die from lung cancer annually in the United States (Tynan, Babb, MacNeil, & Griffin, 2011). Even thirdhand smoking, caused by residual contamination of smoke-borne toxins on surfaces, carpets, and clothing, among other things, long after the cigarette has been extinguished, may prove to be a possible health hazard (Sleiman et al., 2010).

In addition to health effects, the use of tobacco products also has an associated financial cost, both for the individual (cost of the products themselves and the costs of the attendant health problems) and for society. According to the U.S.

Department of Health and Human Services, cigarette smoking in the United States adds up to nearly $133 billion a year in health care costs alone, not including a comparable $156 billion in lost productivity (USDHHS, 2014). While secondhand smoking does not cost nearly as much, it does total nearly $10 billion per year in health care expenditures (Behan, Eriksen, & Lin, 2005).

Measurement

There are various measurements for smoking exposure and health risks that can be used to gauge prevalence and problems. Subjectively, smokers can self-report smoking and its health effects or take self-administered surveys. Estimates of tobacco consumption in most population surveys are usually based on self-reported information, which is generated from standard questions such as: Are you a current or former smoker? Have you ever smoked? Do you now smoke every day, some days, or not at all? How many packets of cigarettes do you smoke per day? However, studies show that self-reported estimates may underestimate true smoking prevalence (Coultas, Howard, Peake, Skipper, & Samet, 1988; Lewis et al., 2003; Tyrpien, Bodzek, & Manka, 2001). Alternatively, scientists may choose to use biochemical tests to objectively measure tobacco use and exposure. Objective measures include measuring nicotine levels in blood, hair, and urine (Al-Delaimy, Crane, & Woodward, 2002; Benowitz, Hukkanen, & Jacob III, 2009). These measures have proven effective in controlling for the biases of self-reported tobacco use rates but may not be feasible for measurement in large-scale studies (Connor-Gorber, Schofield-Hurwitz, Hardt, Levasseur, & Tremblay, 2009).

OVERVIEW OF TOBACCO CONTROL INTERVENTIONS

As previously mentioned, the Social Ecological Framework considers the environmental, political, and social factors that impact people's experiences and behavior (Sullivan, 2009). For tobacco control interventions, this perspective provides a comprehensive approach to understanding the determinants of tobacco use, the challenges to intervention development, and best approaches to implementation of interventions.

It provides a practical framework for communicating the implications of tobacco addiction, initiation, and maintenance. Societal and social influences are broken into levels and clarified through a scalar system approach as well (Corbett, 1999; Green, Richard, & Potvin, 1996; Levesque, Richard, & Potvin, 2000; Stokols, 1996).

Tobacco-related behaviors occur in particular contexts and are continuously changing due to multilayered challenges associated with culture, economics, health, government and private-sector policies, laws and regulations, and the behavior of the tobacco industry at large (Houston & Kaufman, 2000). Researchers have recently switched gears from employing approaches that are primarily directed toward modifying individuals' behavior to addressing larger social and environmental factors that influence tobacco use initiation. These span from intra-individual factors to factors that would influence ease of access and demand, including individual, interpersonal, organizational, and even population factors. Some examples include educational programming in schools; strict tobacco-free policies that govern hospitals, public schools and universities, and public housing complexes; individual counseling via telephone hotlines; and public signs and notices that highlight the dangers of smoking or publicize smoke or tobacco-free zones (Ferketich et al., 2010; McGoldrick & Boonn, 2010). The remainder of this chapter will address interventions at each level of the Socio-Ecological Framework.

Individual Interventions

health education involves informing people of the harmful effects of smoking. In the tobacco context, health education focuses on detecting and preventing smoking-related diseases, helping smokers make educated decisions about smoking cessation aids, and empowering them to manage their addiction to nicotine.

cognitive-behavioral therapy are interventions that address thoughts and behaviors associated with problems.

At the individual level, the classical approach to preventing tobacco use is **health education**, which seeks to educate people about the dangers of tobacco use. There are no school-based initiatives that would ensure unequivocal avoidance of experimental or habitual tobacco use among children. However, scientifically and theoretically based programs that are geared toward youth are available. These programs aim to help vulnerable youth build the necessary skills, knowledge, and attitudes to resist the temptation to use tobacco (Corbett, 2001).

For high-risk groups including racial and ethnic minorities, gay, lesbian, bisexual, and transgender youth, youth with low socioeconomic status, or youth who have engaged in other risk behaviors such as drug or alcohol abuse, clinical intervention and **cognitive-behavioral therapy** (interventions that address the thoughts, behaviors, and social pressures that influence tobacco use) prove appropriate for meeting their needs. This is especially true in a clinical or an educational context. In fact, effective, carefully implemented school programs may, at the very least, postpone the adoption of tobacco use. However, there is some evidence that poorly designed or implemented school-based programs have been detrimental to efforts to prevent or delay tobacco use initiation, especially in schools where smoking was already prevalent (Aguilar & Pampel, 2006; CDC, 2009a; Curry et al, 2010; Poulin, 2007). In fact, the presence of a school-based smoking ban was not correlated with smoking initiation. Rather, other factors, such as poor academic performance and low socioeconomic status of individual students, were the strongest corollaries (Poulin, 2007).

The more effective of these programs can delay or prevent smoking in 20% to 40% of participating youth (CDC, 2000). Their effectiveness stems from the fact that they employ multiple strategies and are often coupled with policy approaches targeted toward individual transactions and individuals' relationship with tobacco. These approaches bolster the protection of communities via policies that limit the opportunities for tobacco use, such as pricing that would render tobacco products too costly for youth, and countering the tobacco industry's perception-skewing messages through educational media that aim to combat misinformation.

Another approach for addressing tobacco use at the individual level, especially for high-risk individuals and their families, is health education through health care providers. Health care service has changed over time to the point where it has forced providers to emphasize health education in public health clinics, physicians' offices, and hospitals (Grol et al., 2007), particularly since it provides the opportunity to reach a significant number of people (Campbell, 1993; Glanz et al., 1990).

In a tobacco-related context, health education focuses on detecting and preventing smoking-related diseases and helping smokers make educated decisions about **smoking cessation** aids as well as empowering them to manage their addiction to nicotine.

Health education through health care providers is an underused method of addressing tobacco use in youth. A national study of Canadian youth found that 20% of young people had discussed tobacco use with their physician or dentist, and just 25% of respondents reported their physicians attempted to broach the subject with them (Snider & Brewster, 2002). In 1999, the National Youth Tobacco Survey asked youth if they had seen a health care provider in the previous year and whether they were given any advice related to tobacco use (Faulkner & Thomas, 2001). Only approximately one third reported that they had. Even though pediatricians have been pressured to encourage young smokers to quit, few have taken the initiative to provide any such encouragement (Benuck, Gidding, & Binns, 2001; Slade, 1993; Stein et al., 2000). Studies are needed to establish appropriate roles for health professionals to prevent tobacco use.

> **smoking cessation** means ceasing to use or quitting tobacco products. Cessation programs can take many forms, including quitting "cold turkey," cutting down, or replacing tobacco products with a variety of substances such as patches, gums, electronic cigarettes, and so on.

Interpersonal Interventions

Interpersonal interventions discussed at this level include family and peer **interventions** and interventions by health care providers, health coaches, promotores(as) (community health workers), and youth leaders. Only family, peer, and health care provider interventions will be described here. **Interpersonal networks** include peers and family members.

> A health **intervention** is an effort to modify health-related behaviors. Interventions can take many forms, including individual, organizational, social, economic, and political.
>
> **interpersonal networks** are spheres of influence from a personal social network of peers, family members, and health care providers, among others. Interpersonal networks can be drawn on to support the prevention and control of tobacco use.

Family Influence

Home smoking bans also offer family members leverage to confront the smoker about quitting as well as resources to help family smokers maintain cessation pledges and prevent relapses (Gilpin, White, Farkas, & Pierce, 1999). Furthermore, household smoking bans force smokers to alter their behavior, including reducing the overall number of cigarettes smoked per day and increasing the number of attempts to quit, as well as strengthening smokers' intentions to stop and extending the time interval between relapses (Gilpin et al., 1999; Shelley, Nguyen, Yerneni, & Fahs, 2008).

Parental Influence

Modeling and similar factors are likely to play a role in tobacco initiation. Parental smoking is one of the strongest influences associated with child smoking initiation. Specifically, in households where parents smoked regularly, children were twice as likely to smoke. Additionally, the children of regular smokers were more likely to start smoking earlier in life and were more likely to become heavy smokers. Notably, maternal smoking was a stronger influence than paternal smoking (Melchior, Chastang, Mackinnon, Galera, & Fombonne, 2009).

The presence of a smoker living in a household signals a tacit endorsement of smoking to other occupants, particularly children and adolescents, which may be mitigated by adherence to a household smoking ban. Whereas some studies have reported that the presence of a smoking parent or parental disapproval of smoking are correlated with the initiation of adolescent smoking behavior, adolescents living with household smoking bans perceive both lower social acceptability of smoking and lower community-wide prevalence of smoking (Conley Thomson, Siegel, Winickoff, Biener, & Rigotti, 2005). That is, household smoking bans communicate more negative social acceptance of smoking than does verbal discouragement or condemnation. For example, a California study found that smokers who live with a nonsmoking adult or child were six times more likely to institute a home smoking ban than smokers who lived in households without a child or nonsmoking adult. Furthermore, smokers who reported they believe secondhand smoke was dangerous were five times more likely to initiate a home smoking ban (Binns, O'Neil, Benuck, & Ariza, 2009; Gilpin et al., 1999).

However, the parental influence is neither overt nor omnipotent. For example, household smoking bans did not necessarily produce the same deterrent effect on adolescent smokers that was observed in studies concerning adults. Albers, Biener, Siegel, Cheng, and Rigotti (2008) found that household smoking bans did not produce a demonstrable difference in smoking patterns or behavior in established smokers; neither did they slow the progression toward established smoking or prevent smoking initiation. However, they did help foster negative attitudes toward smoking. Notably, youth in homes with nonsmokers were more likely to have slowed progression toward cigarette experimentation if they lived with a home smoking ban than if they lived without one (Albers et al., 2008).

Interventions by Health Care Providers

Discussions with health care professionals have produced mixed research results. Binns, O'Neil, Benuck, and Ariza (2008) found that counseling by pediatric health care professionals was associated with a lower likelihood of adopting a home smoking ban. Queries by pediatric health professionals regarding home smoking bans were most commonly recalled by low-income parents, Black and Hispanic parents, and parents with a high school diploma or less. However, the researchers acknowledged that respondent rates of recalled conversations may have been skewed because individuals were more likely to remember a conversation that resulted in a disagreement. For instance, physician-initiated health consultations with adult smokers were more commonly recalled and they also lasted longer than those reported as pediatric consultations (Binns et al., 2008).

Organizational Interventions

organizational interventions are interventions performed in the workplace, school, church, or other organizational locations.

Workplace smoking regulations and bans are the most common **organizational interventions**. However, the organizational level encompasses many social and organization-oriented groups that may be outside the workplace. It addresses rules and regulations in youth clubs, sports, school curricula, and settings where clinical and health services are provided. In these cases, organizational intervention implementation may take the form of tobacco-free campus policies where implementation and enforcement are required to effect the policy changes. For example, a smoke-free hospital policy is useless unless hospital managers ensure adequate signage is placed around the facility and staff are instructed to confront individuals who violate the policy (McGoldrick & Boonn, 2010).

Some useful approaches at this level take place in more local settings. Some of these include practices and policies enforced in a wide array of community-based organizations, in addition to the respective roles health care professionals, educators, leaders, religious clerics, and politicians play in these organizations. Restrictions enforced in settings that are primarily accessed by youth are likely to influence tobacco-related behaviors, just as smoking bans undertaken at a youth's home are associated with lower rates of tobacco use. In public settings, bans have been shown to discourage smoking initiation (Farkas et al., 2000; Wakefield et al., 2000).

At the workplace, programs and initiatives that aim to restrict smoking have resulted in significant reductions in smoking (Brownson, Hopkins, & Wakefield, 2002). Specifically, researchers have found that workplace smoking bans resulted in decreased daily cigarette consumption during work hours, particularly among heavy smokers (Chapman et al., 1999; Gilpin et al., 1999).

Though workplace bans were correlated with decreases in daily cigarette consumption in most studies, results concerning long-term cessation and overall prevalence are mixed (Levy & Friend, 2003; Rose et al., 2011). Some studies have reported smoke-free workplaces had cessation rates 10% to 15% higher than similar workplaces without smokeless policies; other studies have been unable to conclusively prove there is a statistically significant change from smoke-free policies (Levy & Friend, 2003).

Bans carry implicit messaging that influence individuals' attitudes toward smoking and their own behavior. Bans create expectations for behavior as well as opportunities for social approval and sanctioning. In this way, coworker attitudes can help motivate or shape smokers' behavior. Home and workplace smoking bans are associated with attempts to quit regardless of adult smokers' prior intentions to quit but are not necessarily effective in helping smokers maintain cessation intentions. While results were strongest when both bans coexisted, home bans seem to be the more important of the two because they may inspire cessation attempts where the intention to quit did not previously exist. Furthermore, workplace smoking bans alone may not be sufficiently powerful to motivate cessation (Rose et al., 2011). Unfortunately, many workplace insurance plans, both public and private, do not contain full coverage for tobacco cessation programs, and there are few public resources or programs that individuals can access for little to no cost (McGoldrick & Boonn, 2010).

Community Interventions

There are a number of effective approaches for **community-level tobacco interventions**. These include laws to regulate tobacco, enforcement of restrictions on tobacco access, and efforts on the part of community leaders and institutions to influence community behavior. Some of these include community-based public education, behavior modification, and tobacco control initiatives that use multi-faceted strategies and may employ multiple channels of communication to reach target audiences.

community-level tobacco interventions include laws to regulate tobacco, enforcement of restrictions on tobacco access, and efforts on the part of community leaders and institutions to influence community behavior.

Community-based initiatives where participation is encouraged have been successful in a range of settings, including low-income districts (Fisher et al., 2004). One effort at community-level interventions is to limit tobacco advertising, especially to youth. Duke and colleagues (2009) found that antitobacco ads broadcast on national media networks were extremely effective at introducing and reinforcing tobacco control messages, especially to young people in rural and low-population-density areas. In a study of one particular media campaign, national media broadcasts successfully introduced these concepts to 35% of youth who were previously unaware. For students who were already acquainted with the antitobacco concepts, the national media campaign served to increase the perception that the campaign messages were true, from 40% to 71%. Furthermore, young people in rural and low-population-density communities were receptive to the media message vehicle.

Multiple studies have shown that tobacco interventions directed toward social influence have short-term effectiveness (Botvin, Epstein, & Botvin, 1998; CDC, 2000; Flay, McFall, Burton, Cook, & Warnecke, 1993). They address well-established norms associated with tobacco use among youth, including peer attitude, social affirmation that would encourage use, and several other reasons an adolescent would begin smoking. These norms can have varying degrees of influence over the different stages of initiation, from experimentation to eventual, habitual use of tobacco. For example, the presence of home and workplace **smoking bans** strengthens tobacco-free norms (Jones, Kann, Pechacek, 2011; Poulin, 2007). In contrast, researchers have long known that **tobacco advertising** and media messaging have created specific cultural perceptions and attitudes about youth smoking (Luke, Ribisl, Smith, & Sorg, 2011). There are also potential negative consequences, including inwardly directed feelings of social undesirability and building a resistance to any possible positive associations with tobacco, such as smoking role models.

smoking bans involve outlawing smoking in a particular environment, such as indoors, at restaurants, at work, and the like.

tobacco advertising is media messaging that creates specific cultural perceptions and attitudes about smoking. It is of particular concern in relation to youth tobacco use.

Most community-based smoking interventions share similar strategies, including distributed responsibility, multiple-level policy changes, and targeted, multiple-site engagement (Sinha, Singh, Jha, & Singh, 2003). Future programs can also draw inspiration from past successes. For example, theoretically based, multilayered school programs have been shown to be the most effective at preventing tobacco use. The overall impacts of these school-based programs are almost immediate and are more likely to have a lasting effect through successive interventions and educational inputs (Botvin et al., 1998; Lantz et al., 2000; USDHHS, 1994). They also foster a proper foundation of understanding, self-influence, and resistance skills. Additionally, they become exponentially more effective when integrated into the school's curricula and administered on several occasions over the course of the academic year. If they are directed toward individuals, they can be further enhanced if they are combined with additional approaches, such as public announcements from health care providers, increases in tobacco prices, and the enforcement of restrictions on using tobacco publicly (Orleans & Cummings, 1999).

Model for Understanding

The Respiratory Health Association of Metropolitan Chicago partnered with the Chicago Department of Public Health to implement the Chicago Tobacco Prevention Project, a multitactic program targeted toward high-risk groups. The project incorporated media outreach, policy initiatives, and direct programming to reduce tobacco use and secondhand smoke. The media components educated the public on the dangers of smoking and publicized a smoking helpline. The policy aspect of the program created tobacco-free policies at several public housing complexes and hospital, treatment facility, and school campuses. The project also awarded 30 grants to community groups, cultural centers, health centers, and nonprofit organizations to fund tobacco prevention and cessation programs as well as policy and environmental measures targeted toward the nine local demographic populations thought to be most vulnerable to the health risks associated with first- and secondhand smoke, those who may have particular susceptibility to smoking initiation, or those who may have the most trouble quitting (Eisenberg, n.d.). The county of Santa Clara, California, has a similar program, which focuses on media campaigns specifically targeted to youth and young adult audiences, and educational programs designed to reduce the existence of secondhand smoke around public housing facilities, schools, parks, colleges, and hospitals (County of Santa Clara, n.d.). The Southern Nevada Health District Tobacco Control Program takes a holistic approach, combining local laws and ordinances with public education and smoking prevention and cessation programs. The goal of this multilevel, multiapproach program is to act on as many societal levels as possible to eliminate smoking and secondhand smoke in all homes, cars, and public places in the area (Get Healthy Clark County, 2008).

Regulating Youth Access to Tobacco Products

environmental tobacco restrictions are restrictions placed on where tobacco can be advertised, sold, or used. These can include designated areas for smoking and outright smoking bans.

sales restrictions are restrictions placed on where and to whom cigarettes can be sold. These can include other ways of limiting access to tobacco products, including a consideration of advertising.

At this scope, the community would also benefit greatly from **environmental tobacco restrictions** that would reduce tobacco acquisition among youth. For example, these restrictions can include a ban on tobacco sales. Limiting opportunities for tobacco use can be achieved by placing prohibitions in public settings and therefore delaying any possible initiation and dependence on smoking (Wakefield et al., 2000).

When it comes to minors, placing restrictions on tobacco sales can reduce the accessibility and convenience of obtaining tobacco. These **sales restrictions** may even have an effect on tobacco initiation and overall use, particularly in adolescents (Ferketich et al., 2010). School policies that enforce strong smoking restrictions on school property, as well as similar policies in public buildings, workplaces, restaurants, and at sporting events, also have a measured effect on discouraging tobacco access (Rigotti et al., 1997).

It is also imperative that the sources of tobacco products are addressed. Policies can restrict the conditions in which youth are able to get access to tobacco. Age restriction is a notable, effective form of these policies, as well limiting any promotion of tobacco-based products to those under legal age. Sources of tobacco should also be scrutinized and studied, especially in a community-centric context. Sources include retail outlets, vending machines, promotional campaigns, and even family members. Internationally, policies that restrict access to tobacco are achieved at the community rather than the national level. Therefore, some measure of activism is required to galvanize the community into advocating for these policies.

Smoke-Free Indoor and Outdoor Regulations

large-scale programs consist of efforts at the state and city levels. These programs create a synergistic, collaborative strategy that taps readily available resources, bolstering them with funds and a coordinated effort to gather input across a broad demographic.

Large-scale programs to create smoke-free indoor and outdoor areas of regulation at the organization, community, and city levels aim to encompass the greater part of the community's attempts to assemble a diverse set of sectors. The goal is to create a synergistic, collaborative strategy that would tap readily available resources, bolstering them with funds and a coordinated effort to gather input from several citizen participants.

At a slightly larger scale, statewide programs also share many of the goals that the aforementioned programs set out to achieve. Even though they are often difficult to evaluate, lower rates of tobacco initiation in youth have been found in the states that have extensive tobacco control policies (Luke et al., 2000). Research suggests that these programs have tangible but modest effects on prevention and cessation (Bauer et al., 2000; Cummings, 1999; Soldz et al., 2000; Sowden, Arblaster & Stead 2003; Wakefield & Chaloupka, 2000).

Local smoke-free ordinances vary widely in terms of strength, rigor, and comprehensiveness. Furthermore, tobacco interests invest heavily to block such challenges to access and use. One study of local tobacco ordinances in West Virginia—a state with one of the highest smoking rates in the United States—found that the strength of local tobacco interests had a direct relationship with the ability of communities to pass local smoking ordinances (Ferketich et al., 2010). Statewide policies, supported by legislation and a penalty structure, are poised to have greater implementation success because they are harder to manipulate or evade in the communities where they count most. Furthermore, statewide initiatives are a better investment for activists; statewide policies have a farther reach than any local ordinance could and can ultimately protect more individuals (Ferketich et al., 2010).

Prior research suggests that these large-scale tobacco control measures are effective where deployed. Studies have found that tobacco control programs reduce tobacco-related heart disease and cancer as well as overall cigarette use. For example, one Arizona tobacco control program reduced cigarette consumption by $500 million and tobacco-related health care spending by $2.33 billion, which amounted to 10 times the total initial cost of the control program (Lightwood & Glantz, 2011).

Public Policy Interventions

public policy interventions include smoking bans, taxation of tobacco products and raising the price of such products, advertising bans, regulated portrayals of smoking in popular media, and FDA product regulations regarding package warnings.

Some common **public policy interventions** include smoking bans, taxation of tobacco products, public passive smoking interventions, advertising bans, regulated portrayals of smoking in popular media, and FDA product regulations over package warnings, low-tar products, nicotine designations, advertising, and new alternative products such as e-cigarettes.

The will to face this problem in many countries across the world has never been higher (Forster & Wolfson, 1998; Lantz et al., 2000; Orleans &

Cummings, 1999; Reid et al., 2005). Campaigns that employ mass media, as well as measures taken to increase prices for tobacco products, are primary examples of population-level approaches. By far the single most powerful means of reducing access to tobacco among youth has been raising prices (Corbett, 2001). If the aim is to also reduce the allure and desirability of tobacco, carefully implemented media efforts aimed at painting tobacco use in an undesirable light can be highly effective. While these campaigns would not necessarily put a strong emphasis on the negative health ramifications of tobacco and its adoption, they would reveal some of the more reprehensible, manipulative actions of the tobacco industry at large and present a positive, youth-based subculture as a viable, favorable alternative.

Tobacco Economics and Cost Politics

economic interventions are interventions that rely on economic factors as their primary tactic. These include increasing tax rates on tobacco, which can decrease sales and tobacco use, especially in areas where disposable income is limited.

Economic interventions, such as increasing tax rates on tobacco, can have a direct effect on its consumption. It can also be indirectly affected by the revenue used for researching tobacco use, as well as cessation and prevention programs. The taxation of tobacco can have a pronounced influence on cigarette purchases, especially where disposable income is limited.

Cost is a multifaceted variable. For example, Max, Sung, Tucker, and Stark (2010) conducted a study of Black smokers in California and found that racial group bore disproportionately higher health and lost productivity costs related to their tobacco use relative to the percentage of the population they comprise. Specifically, African Americans accounted for 6% of adult Californians and 19.3% of smokers in 2002. This group bore 8% of smoking-attributable expenditures and 13% of smoking-attributable mortality costs. In real dollars, smoking costs Black Californians $1.4 billion, including $626 million in smoking-related health care costs. Additionally, unnecessarily premature deaths cost $784 million in lost productivity (Max et al., 2010).

Furthermore, rather than smokers perceiving the cost of smoking supplies and related health care expenses as an incentive to make cessation attempts, financial strain was actually associated with fewer cessation attempts and less success in attaining and maintaining smoking cessation among individuals with low socioeconomic status and racial diversity. This suggests that cessation attempts may be aided by incentives that ease financial strain or mitigate the stress cessation introduces into the lives of smokers (Martire, Mattick, Doran, & Hall, 2011).

excise taxes are taxes on the sale or production of a specific good or product.

The average cost of a pack of cigarettes has sharply increased over the last 40 years, from 38 cents in 1970 to $5.33 in 2009. Average cigarette **excise taxes** have also increased, though at a slower rate, from 18 cents in 1970 to $2.19 in 2009 (CDC, 2010b). In 2006, American consumers spent $83.6 billion on cigarettes, $3.2 billion on cigars, and $2.6 billion on all types of smokeless tobacco. In addition to the $5.33-per-pack price, smokers can also expect to pay $10.47 per pack in tobacco-related health care costs and lost work productivity (CDC, 2011c). One study found that price increases have the potential to decrease smoking between 1.89% and 7.84% among individuals with low socioeconomic status (Martire et al., 2010).

Impact of Tax Increases

Prior studies have determined cigarette tax increases have some demonstrable effect on altering smoking behavior. Choi, Toomey, Chen, and Forster (2011) found that among adolescents and young adults, ignorance of cigarette tax increases had no effect on cigarette purchasing behavior, but smokers knowledgeable of the tax increases reported a 16.7% increase in cessation attempts and a 24.1% decrease in reported smoking behavior. Tax increases also resulted in decreased cigarette frequency and consumption (Carpenter & Cook, 2008). The potential benefit of cigarette tax increases is solely as a tool for smoking cessation. There is little evidence that tax increases have any preventative effect on smoking initiation (DeCicca, Kenkel, & Mathios, 2008).

However, cigarette tax increases may have counterproductive, unintended consequences. In New York City, a large tax increase prompted rapid and expansive growth in illegal black-market cigarettes in this minority community with low socioeconomic status. Intervention programs must balance the incentives of positive and negative behavior. In New York City, a black market for cigarettes has appeared that has undermined smoking cessation efforts by making it easier for youth to access cigarettes than it is for them to access smoking cessation aids (Shelley, Cantrell, Moon-Howard, Ramjohn, & VanDevanter, 2007).

Experts today cite the critical importance of increasing the price of tobacco and regard it as a primary strategy in the reduction of tobacco use at the population level (Chaloupka, 1999; Lewit, Hyland, Kerrebrock, & Cummings, 1997; Reid et al., 1995; Willemsen & De Zwart, 1999). It can be politically difficult to pass any prohibitive pricing policies on tobacco use in public places, but these price increases do have great potential at generating far-reaching, lasting effects (Lantz et al., 2000; Nicholl, 1998; Reid et al., 1995). Even though the habitual nature of tobacco use is rooted in addiction, the demand for tobacco products has made them subject to a high measure of price elasticity. The effects of increasing tobacco price have been modeled in research, and they show that only a 10% global rise in prices could result in smoking cessation by a minimum of 40 million smokers worldwide, as well as discourage many from initiating tobacco use (World Bank, 2014). Youth are particularly responsive to increases in price, and any delay in adopting tobacco may result in reducing harm and potentially prevent initiation altogether, with varying degrees of success in subpopulations of youth (Biener, Aseltine, Cohen, & Anderka, 1998).

Laws and Regulations

Indoor air regulations reduce nonsmoker exposure to tobacco smoke, daily cigarette intake by smokers, and increased cessation success. Levy and Friend (2003) found that workplace indoor air regulations reduced overall smoking prevalence by 6% and the quantity of cigarettes smoked by 2% to 8%. Further, they found that public indoor air regulations had the potential to reduce smoking prevalence among all smokers by approximately 10%.

Household bans may be encouraged by legislation mandating **smokeless zones** or otherwise regulating public tobacco smoking (IARC, 2009) or more informal

smokeless zones, also known as smoke-free spaces, are combinations of intervention levels (organizational, policy, community, etc.) that aim to ban smoking in certain areas.

community-based public education or media campaigns about the hazards of tobacco (Mills, White, Pierce, & Messer, 2011).

Local smoke-free legislation may pave the way for individuals to implement wider-reaching smokeless legislation, especially in states where more comprehensive legislation may be difficult to pass (USDHHS, 2006). Several government agencies agree that well-designed, well-executed community public education campaigns have the potential to transform public attitudes about tobacco. However, knowledge of the dangers of tobacco may not be enough to motivate smokers to attempt cessation.

The greatest benefit of smoke-free public spaces has been to nonsmokers, who have been shown to benefit from marked decreases in exposure to the noxious chemicals associated with secondhand smoke.

SPOTLIGHT

Public smoke-free spaces laws in Scotland reduced the concentration of chemicals associated with secondhand smoke detected in schools children by nearly 40%, with similar decreases in adults. The greatest declines were reported in children and adults from smoke-free households (Hahn, 2010). Similar declines have been corroborated by studies conducted in Spain, Italy, Norway, Ireland, New Zealand, Australia, and Massachusetts (Chapman et al., 1999; Hahn, 2010; Richiardi, Vizzini, Merletti, & Barone-Adesi, 2009; Room, 2005).

Specific health benefits of smoke-free public spaces have been reported. An Italian study found that disallowing smoking in public spaces may result in an immediate 5% to 15% reduction in the risk of acute myocardial infarctions (Richiardi, Vizzini, Merletti, & Barone-Adesi, 2009).

Multilevel Tobacco Control Interventions

multilevel interventions address all levels of the Social Ecological Framework. When tackling small, specific aspects of a larger problem, it is important to consider multiple levels of influence that complement already existing approaches to postponing uptake and dependency, if not prevent them altogether.

Multilevel interventions use a mix of programs, interventions, and other efforts designed to address more than one level of the Social Ecological Framework. When tackling small, specific aspects of a larger problem, it is important that multiple levels of influence complement already existing approaches to addressing tobacco initiation to postpone uptake and dependency, if not prevent them altogether.

Employing tobacco prevention in a social ecologic manner requires multiple-level, collaborative interventions that simultaneously open up several channels and modalities. Large-scale programs, such as ASSIST, and state programs like those in California, Massachusetts, and Florida, have shown that an approach that utilizes multiple-system interventions is not only feasible but has great potential (Corbett et al., 2001; Stillman et al., 2003). Deriving experiences from other intervention initiatives should be exhaustively tailored and subjected to an uncompromising, qualitative study.

The interplay among multiple influences on health-related behaviors has been investigated, and research shows that the overall effect these influences have on smoking cessation is consistent with their emphasis within the Social Ecological Framework. The chances of a given intervention's success at the individual level are not as decidedly influenced by the specific form of treatment but rather by the combination of a number of several different forms of treatment employed (USDHHS, 2008). The importance of combining different intervention strategies has been demonstrated to have many benefits. For example, health organizations can educate health care workers about tobacco cessation while simultaneously employing measures to remind them to counsel potential patients about quitting. They can also couple telephone counseling with mass media to amplify its effects (Task Force on Community Preventive Services, 2005).

public education campaigns are efforts to educate the public about the health effects of smoking and increase awareness of cessation resources.

Certain **public education campaigns** have had a demonstrable impact on reducing home-based smoking around babies and very young children. For example, Mills, White, Pierce, and Messer (2011) identified that the National Institute of Child Health & Human Development Back to Sleep Public Education Campaign, which promotes home smoking bans as a tool to reduce Sudden Infant Death Syndrome (SIDS), has had a positive influence on increasing smoking bans in households with infants.

Comprehensive, multilayered state programs have also significantly reduced smoking at the state level. The multifaceted nature of these programs is often co-ordinated by the community and includes counter-tobacco marketing through television and billboards, public education, support services for smoking cessation, and smoking prevention programs for youth. The importance of combining these multiple components to form a comprehensive campaign has been shown through evaluations (Ferketich et al., 2010; Siegel, 2002).

A **health behavior** is what people do or how they act in relation to their health, including what they eat and drink, whether they exercise, and whether they go to the doctor. Understanding and influencing health behaviors are key ways of improving health.

Employing multilevel interventions to aid tobacco prevention has led to a de-cline in smoking rates among adults in the United States, from 42% in 1965 to nearly 21% in 2005 (CDC, 2006). This has been made possible through a systemat-ic, multilayered range of population-based interventions directed toward **health behavior**. Some of the best examples at the individual level include a broad dis-tribution of custom, individualized smoking prevention and cessation programs, nicotine dependency therapy, and counseling provided by health care professionals. At the cultural and organizational levels, a good example includes custom-tailored programs intended to reach different cultural subgroups, as well as community-based initiatives. Population-level interventions include antismoking campaigns from health organizations. Other interventions may also include restricting indoor smoking and access to cigarettes at the policy level (Task Force on Community Preventive Services, 2005). The interaction among all of the aforementioned lev-els can have an interbolstering effect between the different intervention methods. As an example, restricting smoking at the workplace can encourage employees to seek a health care professional's help in smoking cessation, while a social-marketing campaign can help smokers seek similar help. The taxation of tobacco and its price increases can also reduce its initiation among youth and make them more accepting toward public smoking restrictions.

To summarize, a varied array of maintainable interventions is almost chiefly responsible for the significant reduction of smoking in the United States. It is now widely accepted, both socially and publicly, that tobacco use is a major health problem that goes far beyond the individual level. Understanding changes in the perception of tobacco use and its consequences relies heavily on a broad, social ecologic perspective and recognizing that population-level changes are the result of the cumulative effect that multiple interventions have on tobacco prevention, not simply one all-encompassing remedy.

Effectiveness of Tobacco Interventions

While many different interventions for tobacco treatment exist, their effectiveness can be difficult to determine. The U.S. Department of Health and Public Services, in its 2008 study *Treating Tobacco Use and Dependence: 2008 Update*, states that tobacco dependence requires "repeated intervention and multiple attempts" (p. vi) in order to influence users to quit tobacco products. They also found that including interventions for quitting tobacco in health policies and insurance plans greatly increased users' likelihood to quit and remain tobacco free.

The study separated tobacco users into three distinct groups for the purpose of clinician interventions: those willing to make an attempt to quit at the time of intervention, those unwilling to do so, and former tobacco users who had recently quit and thus could benefit from continued intervention. Different interventions are necessary and effective for different people. For those willing to quit, the study includes interventions such as therapy, drugs, and nicotine replacement options. For those unwilling to quit, the study suggests a strategy called "motivational interviewing," which has been found to be "effective in increasing future quit attempts" (USDHPS, 2008, p. 57). Motivational interviewing explores users' feelings about tobacco in order to uncover areas that may be holding them back from quitting or may be exploited or emphasized to encourage quitting. For those users who have recently quit, the study suggests following up on struggles they may be having and offering solutions for preventing potential relapses, as well as praising the individual and reminding them of the benefits of quitting.

Among the interventions studied, counseling was found to be particularly effective, especially individual, group, and telephone counseling. Practical or skills-based counseling approaches were found to be best, with an added emphasis on creating and maintaining social support for abstaining from tobacco use. Counseling was found to be effective among all demographics willing to engage in such interventions. Abstinence rates were found to increase among "contact time," or length of intervention, with counseling sessions "up to 90 minutes" found to be the most effective (p. 85). The study also found that interventions tailored to individuals' needs and situations and presented in multiple formats were most effective. The study found "self-help materials" such as pamphlets or lists of programs to be more effective than no intervention but "weak" overall (p. 89), suggesting limited effectiveness of interventions such as media ads or posters.

Combining counseling with medication was found to be more effective than using medication without counseling. Medications to quit smoking include Bupropion SR, Varenicline, and nicotine gum, inhalers, lozenges, nasal sprays, and patches. "More than eight sessions" (p. 101) of counseling combined with one of these medications was found to be the most effective, though medications are not recommended for adolescents, pregnant women, or those with medical contraindications. Varenicline, a medication that stimulates nicotine receptors, was found to be the most effective, though all of the medical interventions were found to have roughly the same smoking abstinence rates. Among nicotine replacements, a nicotine patch plus a gum or nasal spray was found to be the most effective combination.

The Department found that tobacco use treatments, ranging from brief clinician advice to specialist-delivered intensive programs, including medication, have been shown not only to be clinically effective but also to be extremely cost effective relative to other commonly used disease prevention interventions and medical treatments. (USDHPS, 2008, pp. 134–135). This finding, in addition to other findings, provides strong emphasis for health insurance companies and public assistance programs to cover nicotine interventions. The affordability of such programs can make great strides in improving access to these programs and increasing abstinence from tobacco use.

Special Considerations for Tobacco Control Interventions

The following is a list of some important factors to keep in mind when planning tobacco interventions.

- Tobacco dependence is a chronic condition that can require multiple, repeated interventions. However, certain interventions have been shown to be effective across populations and in a variety of settings and delivery formats.

- Health care providers play a crucial role in identifying tobacco users, offering them quitting options, and supporting them in their quitting efforts. Training should be given to health care providers to help them identify and appropriately counsel tobacco users.

- While counseling (both individual and group) and medication have both been shown to be effective in isolation, they work best when employed together. There are a wide range of interventions available that are appropriate for tobacco users.

- Telephone quit lines have also been shown to be effective, with the added benefit of being geographically and financially accessible.

- Tobacco interventions have been shown to be cost effective for health care organizations and thus should be prioritized. Insurance coverage for tobacco cessation programs would encourage quitting as well as save organizations money in the long term.

Summary

The Social Ecological Framework for tobacco use overlaps applications in policy, economic, and scientific approaches. Most if not all of the aforementioned intervention methods are the subject of intensive research that aims to provide insights into the many determinants that would decide the intervention strategy's efficacy. The approaches that show the most promise are those that are evidenced based, including studies aimed at multiple levels of the Social Ecological Framework and those geared toward youth. Any well-designed, comprehensive initiative or campaign must employ the use of current research in order to adequately customize interventions at either end of individual or population levels, ensuring both their feasibility and efficacy. Advancing the field requires new research in many different aspects of smoking-related matters, including the effect that tobacco price increases have on tobacco initiation among youth. This will help indicate what needs to be changed in the design of interventions, such as those that are school based, and the settings that they are meant to disseminate.

Other aspects include the ever-changing definition of tobacco use among youth and its varied subcultures. Additionally, the reasons and pressures that youth face that may lead to initiation, the different trajectories that eventually lead to habitual use and nicotine dependency, the means by which youth acquire tobacco, the various preferences for smoke-based and smokeless tobacco and their many respective forms, perceptions toward tobacco-related matters, the constantly changing promotional campaigns that are employed by the tobacco industry, the effects of fluctuating demand among youth, and what type of message is effective in reaching risk-laden youth populations must be considered.

Refining social ecologic determinants is an ongoing process, since they comprise a major component in forming a foundation for results-oriented intervention research. However, there remains a sizable gap between a proper understanding of the determinants of tobacco use and their application toward tobacco prevention and cessation-based research. A firm grasp of the underlying intricacies among these determinants will help identify effective processes for successful tobacco intervention programs. The Social Ecological Framework is needed to effectively identify important, potentially modifiable relationships between determinants, ultimately leading to tobacco research interventions that are geared toward multiple levels of the system (Tobacco Control Conference Report, 2004).

Review Questions

1. (T/F) The Social Ecological Framework is a theory that considers the environmental, political, and social factors that contribute to people's behavior.

2. Approximately how many American adults smoked cigarettes in 2010?
    a. 35.6 million
    b. 45.3 million
    c. 25.8 million
    d. 52.5 million

3. Which of the following demographics are the strongest indicators of whether someone is likely to smoke cigarettes?
    a. Sex and age
    b. Income and education
    c. Education and age
    d. Income and sex

4. (T/F) The presence of a school-based smoking ban is associated with smoking initiation in youth.

5. Which of the following is NOT a level of tobacco intervention discussed in the chapter?
    a. Organizational
    b. Community
    c. Public policy
    d. Religious
    e. Economic

6. Which of the following is a drawback to tax-based interventions for tobacco use?
    a. Tobacco industries respond by putting more effort into advertising and promotion.
    b. The rising cost of cigarettes leads to black market trade that can make cigarettes easier to access.
    c. Due to the rising cost of cigarettes, smokers turn to other forms of substance abuse.
    d. Tobacco companies lobby the government to keep the price down.

7. Indoor air regulations and smokeless zones:
    a. Lead to less exposure to secondhand smoke
    b. Reduce daily cigarette intake
    c. Lead to increased cessation success
    d. All of the above
    e. None of the above

8. (T/F) Multilevel state interventions have been found to be ineffective.

9. (T/F) A single intervention method is more effective than utilizing multiple methods.

10. (Critical thinking) How do socioeconomic factors influence tobacco use, and what are some ways to design interventions to address those factors?

11. (Critical thinking) Are there drawbacks to the Social Ecological Framework when considering tobacco interventions? If so, what can be done to address those drawbacks?

Web Resources

Visit the following websites to learn more about some of the topics presented in this chapter.

Center of Disease Control and Prevention - Smoking and Tobacco Use: http://www.cdc.gov/tobacco/

World Health Organization Health Topics - Tobacco: http://www.who.int/topics/tobacco/en/

US Food and Drug Administration - Tobacco Products: http://www.fda.gov/tobaccoproducts/default.htm

National Cancer Institute - Harms of Smoking and Health Benefits of Quitting: http://www.cancer.gov/cancertopics/factsheet/Tobacco/cessation

References

Albers, A. B., Biener, L., Siegel M, Cheng, D. M., & Rigotti, N. (2008). Household smoking bans and adolescent antismoking attitudes and smoking initiation: Findings from a longitudinal study of a Massachusetts youth cohort. *American Journal of Public Health, 98*(10), 1886–1893.

Al-Delaimy, W. K., Crane, J., & Woodward, A. (2002). Is the hair nicotine level a more accurate biomarker of environmental tobacco smoke exposure than urine cotinine? *Journal of Epidemiology and Community Health, 56*(1), 66–71.

Aguilar, J., & Pampel, F. (2006). Changing patterns of cigarette use among White and Black youth, US 1976-2003. *Social Science Research, 36*(3), 1219–1236. doi:10.1016/j.ssresearch.2006.08.002.

Bauer, U.E., Johnson, T.M., Hopkins, R.S., Brooks, R.G. JAMA: *Journal of the American Medical Association,* Issue (6).

Bauer, U., Johnson, T. A., Hopkins, R., & Brooks, R. (2000). Changes in youth cigarette use and intentions following implementation of a tobacco control program: Findings from the Florida Youth Tobacco Survey. *JAMA, 284,* 723–728.

Behan, D. F., Eriksen, M. P., & Lin, Y. (2005). *Economic effects of environmental tobacco smoke.* Schaumburg, IL: Society of Actuaries. Washington, DC. Retrieved from http://www.soa.org/research/research -projects/life-insurance/research-economic-effect.aspx.

Benowitz, N. L., Hukkanen, J., & Jacob III, P. (2009). Nicotine chemistry, metabolism, kinetics and biomarkers. *Handbook of experimental pharmacology, 192,* 29–60.

Benuck, I., Gidding, S. S., & Binns, H. J. (2001). Identification of adolescent tobacco users in a pediatric practice. *Archives of Pediatrics & Adolescent Medicine, 155*(1), 32–35. Retrieved from http://www .ncbi.nlm.nih.gov/pubmed/11177059.

Biener, L., Aseltine, R. H., Cohen, B., & Anderka, M. (1998). Reactions of adult and teenaged smokers to the Massachusetts tobacco tax. *American Journal of Public Health, 88*(9), 1389–1391. Retrieved from http://www.pubmedcentral.nih.gov/articlerender.fcgi?artid=1509075&tool=pmcentrez &rendertype=abstract.

Binns, H. J., O'Neil, J., Benuck, I., & Ariza, A. J. (2009). Influences on parents' decisions for home and automobile smoking bans in households with smokers. *Patient Education and Counseling, 74*(2), 272–276.

Borio, G. (2007). Tobacco timeline: The twentieth century. Retrieved from http://archive.tobacco.org /resources/history/tobacco_history20-1.html.

Botvin, G. J., Epstein, J. A., & Botvin. E. M. (1998). Adolescent cigarette smoking: Prevalence, causes, and intervention approaches. *Adolesc Med., 9*(2), 299–313, vi.

Brownson, R. C., Hopkins, D. P., & Wakefield, M. A. (2002). Effects of smoking restrictions in the workplace. *Annual Review of Public Health, 23,* 333–348. doi:10.1146/annurev.publhealth .23.100901.140551.

Campbell, A. B. (1993). Strategic planning in health care: Methods and applications. *Quality management in health care, 1*(4), 12–23.

Carpenter, C., & Cook, P. J. (2008). Cigarette taxes and youth smoking: New evidence from national, state, and local Youth Risk Behavior Surveys. *Journal of Health Economics, 27,* 287–299.

Centers for Disease Control and Prevention (CDC). (2000). Executive summary of the Surgeon General's report titled *Reducing Tobacco Use. MMWR recommendations and reports* (Vol. 49, No. RR-16). Atlanta, GA: National Center for Chronic Disease Prevention and Health Promotion Office on Smoking and Health.

Centers for Disease Control and Prevention (CDC). (2006). Behavioral risk factor surveillance system. Retrieved from http://apps.nccd.cdc.gov/brfss/index.asp.

Centers for Disease Control and Prevention (CDC). (2009a). *Youth and tobacco use (fact sheet).* Atlanta, GA: National Center for Chronic Disease Prevention and Health Promotion Office on Smoking and Health.

Centers for Disease Control and Prevention (CDC). (2009b). *Cigars (fact sheet).* Atlanta, GA: National Center for Chronic Disease Prevention and Health Promotion Office on Smoking and Health.

Centers for Disease Control and Prevention (CDC). (2009c). *Smokeless tobacco facts (fact sheet).* Atlanta, GA: National Center for Chronic Disease Prevention and Health Promotion Office on Smoking and Health.

Centers for Disease Control and Prevention (CDC). (2009d). *Bidis and kreteks (fact sheet).* Atlanta, GA: National Center for Chronic Disease Prevention and Health Promotion Office on Smoking and Health.

Centers for Disease Control and Prevention (CDC). (2009e). *Hookahs (fact sheet).* Atlanta, GA: National Center for Chronic Disease Prevention and Health Promotion Office on Smoking and Health.

Centers for Disease Control and Prevention (CDC). (2010). *Adult cigarette smoking in the United States: Current estimate (fact sheet).* Atlanta, GA: National Center for Chronic Disease Prevention and Health Promotion Office on Smoking and Health.

Centers for Disease Control and Prevention (CDC). (2010b). *Trends in state and federal cigarette tax and retail price—United States, 1970–2009 (data table).* Atlanta, GA: National Center for Chronic Disease Prevention and Health Promotion Office on Smoking and Health.

Centers for Disease Control and Prevention (CDC). (2011a). *Adult smoking in the US.* Atlanta, GA: National Center for Chronic Disease Prevention and Health Promotion Office on Smoking and Health.

Centers for Disease Control and Prevention (CDC). (2011b). *Smokeless tobacco facts (fact sheet).* Atlanta, GA: National Center for Chronic Disease Prevention and Health Promotion Office on Smoking and Health.

Centers for Disease Control and Prevention (CDC). (2011c). *Economic facts about U. S. tobacco production and use (fact sheet).* Atlanta, GA: National Center for Chronic Disease Prevention and Health Promotion Office on Smoking and Health.

Chaloupka, F. J. (1999). Macro-social influences: The effects of prices and tobacco-control policies on the demand for tobacco products. *Nicotine & tobacco research: Official journal of the Society for Research on Nicotine and Tobacco, 1 Suppl 1,* S105–9. Retrieved from http://www.ncbi.nlm.nih.gov/pubmed/11072413.

Chapman, S., Borland, R., Scollo, M., Brownson, R. C., Dominello, A., & Woodward, S. (1999). The impact of smoke-free workplaces on declining cigarette consumption in Australia and the United States. *American Journal of Public Health, 89*(7), 1018–1023.

Choi, T. C. K., Toomey, T. L., Chen, V., & Forster, J. L. (2011). Awareness and reported consequences of a cigarette tax increase among older adolescents and young adults. *American Journal of Health Promotion, 25*(6), 379–386.

Conley Thomson, C., Siegel, M., Winickoff, J., Biener, L., & Rigotti, N. A. (2005). Household smoking bans and adolescents' perceived prevalence of smoking and social acceptability of smoking. *Preventive Medicine, 41,* 349–356. doi:10.1016/j.ypmed.2004.12.003.

Corbett, K. (1999, May/June). *Intervention to prevent adolescents from smoking.* In Proceedings of the Asia Pacific Association for the Control of Tobacco, APACT. Tenth Anniversary Symposium, Taipei, Taiwan.

Corbett, K. K. (2001). Susceptibility of youth to tobacco: A social ecological framework for prevention. *Respiration Physiology, 128*(1), 103–118. doi:10.1016/S0034-5687(01)00269-9.

Coultas, D. B., Howard, C. A., Peake, G. T., Skipper, B. J., & Samet, J. M. (1988). Discrepancies between self-reported and validated cigarette smoking in a community survey of New Mexico Hispanics. *American Review of Respiratory Disease, 137,* 810–814.

County of Santa Clara. (n.d.) Tobacco prevention and education program. Retrieved from http://www.sccgov.org/sites/sccphd/en-us/Partners/TobaccoPrevention/Pages/default.aspx.

Cummings, K. M. (1999). Community-wide interventions for tobacco control. *Nicotine & Tobacco Research: Official Journal of the Society for Research on Nicotine and Tobacco, 1 Suppl 1,* S113–116. Retrieved from http://www.ncbi.nlm.nih.gov/pubmed/11072415.

Curry, S. J., Mermelstein, R. J., Sporer, A. K., Emery, S. L., Berbaum, M. L., Campbell, R. T., Carusi, C., Flay, B., Taylor, K., Warnecke, R. B. (2010). A national evaluation of community-based youth cessation programs: Design and implementation. *Evaluation Review, 34*(6), 487–512. doi:10.1177/0193841X10391970.

Dechanet, C., Anahory, T., Mathieu Daude, J. C., Quantin, X., Reyftmann, L., Hamamah, S., Hedon, B., Dechaud, H. (2011). Effects of cigarette smoking on reproduction. *Human Reproduction Update, 17*(1), 76–95. doi:10.1093/humupd/dmq033.

DeCicca, P., Kenkel, D., & Mathios, A. (2008). Cigarette taxes and the transition from youth to adult smoking: Smoking initiation, cessation, and participation. *Journal of Health Economics, 27*(4), 904–917. doi:10.1016/j.jhealeco.2008.02.008.

Duke, J. C., Vallone, D. M., Allen, J. A., Cullen, J., Mowery, P. D., Xiao, H., Dorrier, N., Asche, E. T., Healton, C. (2009). Increasing youths' exposure to a tobacco prevention media campaign in rural and low-population-density communities. *American Journal of Public Health, 99*(12), 2210–2216.

Eisenberg, A. (n.d.) Chicago tobacco prevention project. Retrieved from http://www.lungchicago.org /chicago-tobacco-prevention-project/.

Farkas, A. J., Gilpin, E. A., White, M. M., & Pierce, J. P. (2000). Association between household and workplace smoking restrictions and adolescent smoking. *JAMA: The Journal of the American Medical Association, 284*(6), 717–722.

Faulkner, D. L., & Thomas, K. Y. (2001). Stat bite: Race/ethnicity of young U. S. smokers counseled about tobacco use. *JNCI Journal of the National Cancer Institute, 93*(1), 12–12. doi:10.1093/jnci/93.1.12.

Ferketich, A. K., Liber, A., Pennell, M., Nealy, D., Hammer, J., & Berman, M. (2010). Clean indoor air ordinance coverage in the Appalachian region of the United States. *American Journal of Public Health, 100*(7), 1313–1318.

Fisher, E. B. , Strunk R. C., Sussman L. K., Sykes R. K., Walker M. S. (2004). Community organization to reduce the need for acute care for asthma among African American children in low-income neighborhoods: The Neighborhood Asthma Coalition. *Pediatrics, 114*(1), 116–123. doi:10.1542/peds.114.1.116.

Forster, J. L., & Wolfson, M. (1998). Youth access to tobacco: Policies and politics. *Annual Review of Public Health, 19*, 203–235. doi:10.1146/annurev.publhealth.19.1.203.

Flay, B. R., McFall, S., Burton, D., Cook, T. D., & Warnecke, R.B. (1993). Health behavior changes through television: The roles of de facto and motivated selection processes. *Journal of health and human behavior, 34*(4), 322–335.

Fromme, H., Dietrich, S., Heitmann, D., Dressel, H., Diemer, J., Schulz, T., Jorres, R. A., Berlin, K., & Völkel, W. (2009). Indoor air contamination during a waterpipe (narghile) smoking session. *Food and Chemical Toxicology: An International Journal Published for the British Industrial Biological Research Association, 47*(7), 1636–1641. doi:10.1016/j.fct.2009.04.017.

Gately & Iain. (2004). "Tobacco: A Cultural History of How an Exotic Plant Seduced Civilization", Diane, pp. 3–7, ISBN 0-80213-960-4.

Get Healthy Clark County. (2008). *2008 adult tobacco survey (ATS) report.* Clark County, NV: Southern Nevada Health District Tobacco Control Program.

Gilpin, E. A., White, M. M., Farkas, A. J., & Pierce, J. P. (1999). Home smoking restrictions: Which smokers have them and how they are associated with smoking behavior. *Nicotine Tobacco Research, 1*(2), 153–162.

Glanz, K., Brekke, M., Hoffman, E., Admire, J., McComas, K., & Mullis R. (1990). Patient reactions to nutrition education for cholesterol reduction. *American journal of preventive medicine, 6*(6), 311–317.

Goodman, J. (1993). *Tobacco in history. The cultures of dependence.* London: Routledge.

Gorber, S. C., Schofield-Hurwitz, S., Hardt, J., Levasseur, G., & Tremblay, M. (2009). The accuracy of self-reported smoking: A systematic review of the relationship between self-reported and cotinine-assessed smoking status. *Nicotine Tob Res. 2009, Jan. 11*(1), 12–24.

Green, L. W., Richard, L., & Potvin, L. (1996). Ecological foundations of health promotion. *American Journal of Health Promotion, 10,* 270–281.

Grim, R. (2009). *This is your country on drugs: The secret history of getting high in America.* Hoboken, NJ: John Wiley & Sons, Inc.

Grol, R. P., Bosch, M. C., Hulscher, M. E., Eccles, M. P., & Wensing, M. (2007). Planning and studying improvement in patient care: The use of theoretical perspectives. *The Milbank Quarterly, 85*(1), 93–138. doi:10.1111/j.1468-0009.2007.00478.x.

Hahn, E. J. (2010). Smoke-free legislation: A review of health and economic outcomes research. *American Journal of Preventive Medicine, 39*(6S1), S66–S76.

International Agency for Research on Cancer (IARC). (2009). *Evaluating the effectiveness of smoke-free policies* (Volume 13). Lyon, France: World Health Organization.

Houston, T., & Kaufman, N. J. (2000). Tobacco control in the 21st century: Searching for answers in a sea of change. *JAMA: The Journal of the American Medical Association, 284*(6), 752–753. Retrieved from http://www.ncbi.nlm.nih.gov/pubmed/10927787.

James, R., & Olstad, S. (2009). A brief history of cigarette advertising. Retrieved from http://www.time.com/time/magazine/article/0,9171,1905530,00.html.

Jones, S. E., Kann, L., & Pechacek, T. F. (2011). Cigarettes smoked per day among high school students in the U. S., 1991–2009. *American Journal of Preventative Medicine, 41*(3), 297–299.

Lantz, P. M., Jacobson, P. D., Warner, K. E., Wasserman, J., Pollack, H. A., Berson, J., & Ahlstrom, A. (2000) Investing in youth tobacco control: a review of smoking prevention and control strategies. *Tobacco Control, 9*(1), 47–63.

Levesque, L., Richard, L., & Potvin, L. (2000). The ecological approach in tobacco-control practice: Health promotion practitioner characteristics related to using the ecological approach. *American Journal of Health Promotion, 14*(4), 244–252.

Levy, D. T., & Friend, K. B. (2003). The effects of clean indoor air laws: What do we know and what do we need to know? *Health Education Research, 18*(5), 592–609.

Lewis, S. J., Cherry, N. M., McL Niven, R., Barber, P. V., Wilde, K., & Povey, A. C. (2003). Cotinine levels and self-reported smoking status in patients attending a bronchoscopy clinic. *Biomarkers, 8*(3-4), 218–228.

Lewit, E. M., Hyland, A., Kerrebrock, N., & Cummings, K. M. (1997). Price, public policy, and smoking in young people. *Tobacco Control, 6*(Suppl 2), S17–24.

Lightwood, J., & Glantz, S. (2011). Effect of the Arizona tobacco control program on cigarette consumption and healthcare expenditures. *Social Science and Medicine, 72*(2), 166–172. doi:10.1016/j.socscimed.2010.11.015.

Lu, Y., Wang, S. S., Reynolds, P., Chang, E. T., Ma, H., Sullivan-Halley, J., Clarke, C. A., & Bernstein L. (2011). Cigarette smoking, passive smoking, and non-Hodgkin lymphoma risk: Evidence from the California Teachers Study. *American Journal of Epidemiology, 174*(5), 563–573.

Luke, D. A., Ribisl, K. M., Smith, C., & Sorg, A. A. (2011). Family Smoking Prevention and Tobacco Control Act: Banning outdoor tobacco advertising near schools and playgrounds. *American Journal of Preventative Medicine, 40*(3), 295–302.

Martire, K. A., Mattick, R. P., Doran, C. M., & Hall, W. D. (2011). Cigarette tax and public health: What are the implications of financially stressed smokers for the effects of price increases on smoking prevalence? *Addiction, 106*(3), 622–630. doi:10.1111/j.1360-0443.2010.03174.x.

Max, W., Sung, H. Y., Tucker, L. Y., & Stark, B. (2010). The disproportionate cost of smoking for African-Americans in California. *American Journal of Public Health, 100*(1), 152–158.

Maziak, W. (2010). Commentary: The waterpipe—a global epidemic or a passing fad. *International Journal of Epidemiology, 39*(3), 857–859. doi:10.1093/ije/dyq054.

Maziak, W., Ward, K. D., Afifi Soweid, R. A., & Eissenberg, T. (2004). Tobacco smoking using a waterpipe: A re-emerging strain in a global epidemic. *Tobacco Control, 13*(4), 327–333. doi:10.1136/tc.2004.008169.

McGoldrick, D. E., & Boonn, A. V. (2010). Public policy to maximize tobacco cessation. *American Journal of Preventative Medicine, 38*(3S), S327–332.

Melchior, M., Chastang, J.-F., Mackinnon, D., Galera, C., & Fombonne, E. (2009). The intergenerational transmission of tobacco smoking—the role of parents' long-term smoking trajectories. *Drug and Alcohol Dependence, 107*(2-3), 257–260. doi:10.1016/j.drugalcdep.2009.10.016.

Mills, A. L., White, M. M., Pierce, J. P., & Messer, K. (2011). Home smoking bans among U. S. households with children and smokers: Opportunities for intervention. *American Journal of Preventative Medicine, 41*(6), 559–565.

Nicholl, J. (1998). Tobacco tax initiatives to prevent tobacco use: A study of eight statewide campaigns. *Cancer, 83*(12 Suppl Robert), 2666–2679.

Orleans, C. T., & Cumming, K. M. (1999). Population-based tobacco control: Progress and prospects. *American Journal of Health Promotion, 14*(2), 83–91.

Porter, R., & Teich, M. (1997). *Drugs and narcotics in history.* New York, NY: Cambridge University Press.

Poulin, C. C. (2007). School smoking bans: Do they help/do they harm? *Drug and Alcohol Review, 26*(6), 615–624.

Reid, C., McNeil, J. J., Williams, F., & Powles, J. (1995). Cardiovascular risk reduction: A randomized trial of two health promotion strategies for lowering risk in a community with low socioeconomic status. *European Journal of Cardiovascular Prevention & Rehabilitation, 2*(2), 155–163. doi:10.1177/174182679500200212.

Reid, R. J., Peterson, N. A., Lowe, J. B., & Hughey, J. (2005). Tobacco outlet density and smoking prevalence: Does racial concentration matter? *Drugs: Education, Prevention and Policy, 12*(3), 233–238. doi:10.1080/09687630500035485.

Richiardi, L., Vizzini, L., Merletti, F., & Barone-Adesi, F. (2009). Cardiovascular benefits of smoking regulations: The effect of decreased exposure to passive smoking. *Preventative Medicine, 48*(2), 167–172. doi:10.1016/j.ypmed.2008.11.013.

Richter, P., Hodge, K., Stanfill, S., Zhang, L., & Watson, C. (2008). Surveillance of moist snuff: Total nicotine, moisture, pH, un-ionized nicotine, and tobacco-specific nitrosamines. *Nicotine & Tobacco Research: Official Journal of the Society for Research on Nicotine and Tobacco, 10*(11), 1645–1652. doi:10.1080/14622200802412937.

Rigotti, N. A., Arnsten, J. H., McKool, K. M., Wood-Reid, K. M., Pasternak, R. C., Singer, D. E. (1997). Efficacy of a smoking cessation program for hospital patients. *Archives of Internal Medicine, 157*(22), 2653–2660. doi:10.1001/archinte.1997.00440430135016.

Rongey, C. (2001). Advertising and tobacco use. In R. Carson-Dewitt (Ed.), *Encyclopedia of drugs, alcohol and addictive behavior* (pp. 46–51). New York, NY: Macmillan Reference.

Room, R. (2005). Banning smoking in taverns and restaurants—a research opportunity as well as a gain for public health. *Addiction, 100*(7), 888–890.

Rose, A., Fagan, P., Lawrence, D., Hart, A., Shavers, V. L., & Gibson, J. T. (2011). The role of worksite and home smoking bans in the smoking cessation among U. S. employed adult female smokers. *American Journal of Health Promotion, 26*(1), 26–36.

Shelley, D., Cantrell, M. J., Moon-Howard, J., Ramjohn, D. Q., & VanDevanter, N. (2007). The $5 man: The underground economic response to a large cigarette tax increase in New York City. *American Journal of Public Health, 97*(8), 1483–1488.

Shelley, D., Nguyen, N., Yerneni, R., & Fahs, M. (2008). Tobacco use behaviors and household smoking bans among Chinese Americans. *American Journal of Health Promotion, 22*(3), 168–175.

Sinha, D. N., Singh, S., Jha, M., & Singh, M. (2003). *Report of tobacco cessation through community intervention in India.* Patna, India: School of Preventative Oncology.

Slade, J. (1993). Nicotine dependence: intervention strategies for the physician. *New Jersey medicine: the journal of the Medical Society of New Jersey, 90*(11), 831–834.

Sleiman, M., Gundel, L. A., Pankow, J. F., Jacob, P., Singer, B. C., & Destaillats, H. (2010). Formation of carcinogens indoors by surface-mediated reactions of nicotine with nitrous acid, leading to potential thirdhand smoke hazards. *Proceedings of the National Academy of Sciences of the United States of America, 107*(15), 6576–6581. doi:10.1073/pnas.0912820107.

Smith, J. R., Novotny, T. E., Edland, S. D., Hofstetter, C. R., Lindsay, S. P., & Al-Delaimy, W. K. (2011). Determinants of hookah use among high school students. *Nicotine & Tobacco Research: Official Journal of the Society for Research on Nicotine and Tobacco, 13*(7), 565–572. doi:10.1093/ntr/ntr041.

Snider, J., & Brewster, J. M. (2002). Chapter 6—influence of health practitioners. *2002 Youth Smoking Survey* (pp. 141–160). Technical Report.

Snowden, R. (2009). Tobacco regulation bill becomes law. Retrieved from http://www.cancer.org/cancer/news/tobacco-regulation-bill-becomes-law.

Soldz, S., Kreiner, P., Clark, T. W., & Krakow, M. (2000). Tobacco use among Massachusetts youth: Is tobacco control working? *Preventive Medicine, 31*(4), 287–295.

Sowden, A., Arblaster, L., & Stead, L.Community interventions for preventing smoking in young people. In *The Cochrane database of systematic reviews 2003*, Issue 1. Art. No.: CD001291. DOI:10.1002/14651858.CD001291.

Stanton, H. J., Martin, J., & E. Henningfield, J. E. (2005). The impact of smoking on the family. *Current Paediatrics, 15*(7), 590–598. doi:10.1016/j.cupe.2005.08.010.

Stein, R. J., Haddock, C. K., O'Byrne, K. K., Hymowitz, N., & Schwab, J. (2000). The pediatrician's role in reducing tobacco exposure in children. *Pediatrics, 106*(5), E66. Retrieved from http://www.ncbi.nlm.nih.gov/pubmed/11061803.

Stokols, D. (1996). Translating social ecological theory into guidelines for community health promotion. *American Journal of Health Promotion, 10*(4) 282–298.

Sullivan, L. (Ed.). (2009). Social ecology. In *The SAGE glossary of the social and behavioral sciences* (p. 477). Thousand Oaks, CA: Sage Reference.

Task Force on Community Preventive Services. (2005). *Preventive services: What works to promote health?.* Oxford University Press. Retrieved from http://www.thecommunityguide.org/library/book/Front-Matter.pdf.

Tranah, G. J., Holly, E. A., Wang, F., & Bracci, P. M. (2011). Cigarette, cigar, and pipe smoking, passive smoke exposure, and risk of pancreatic cancer: A population-based study in the San Francisco Bay Area. *BioMed Central Cancer, 11*, 138.

Taylor II, B. (2014). A history of the pipe: Manufacturing and marketing pyrolytic graphite pipes from development to demise. Retrieved from http://www.thepipe.info/history/index.html#Introduction.

Tynan, M., Babb, S., MacNeil, A., & Griffin, M. (2011) State smoke-free laws for worksites, restaurants, and bars—United States, 2000–2010. *Office on Smoking and Health, National Center for Chronic Disease Prevention and Health Promotion, Morbidity and Mortality Weekly Report, 60*(15), 472–475.

Tyrpien, K., Bodzek, P., & Manka, G. (2001). Application of planar chromatography to the determination of cotinine in urine of active and passive smoking pregnant women. *Biomedical Chromatography, 15*(1), 50–55.

U.S. Department of Health and Human Services (USDHHS). (1994). *Preventing tobacco use among young people: A report of the Surgeon General.* USDHHS, Atlanta, GA: U.S. Department of Health and Human Services, Centers for Disease Control and Prevention, Coordinating Center for Health Promotion, National Center for Chronic Disease Prevention and Health Promotion, Office on Smoking and Health.

U.S. Department of Health and Human Services (USDHHS). (2006). *The health consequences of involuntary exposure to tobacco smoke: A report of the Surgeon General.* Atlanta, GA: U.S. Department of Health and Human Services, Centers for Disease Control and Prevention, Coordinating Center for Health Promotion, National Center for Chronic Disease Prevention and Health Promotion, Office on Smoking and Health.

U.S. Department of Health and Human Services (USDHHS). (2010). *How tobacco smoke causes disease: The biology and behavioral basis for smoking-attributable disease: A report of the Surgeon General.* Atlanta, GA: U.S. Department of Health and Human Services, Centers for Disease Control and Prevention, National Center for Chronic Disease Prevention and Health Promotion, Office on Smoking and Health.

U.S. Department of Health and Human Services (USDHHS). (2014). *The health consequences of smoking—50 years of progress: A report of the Surgeon General.* Atlanta, GA: U.S. Department of Health and Human Services, Centers for Disease Control and Prevention, National Center for Chronic Disease Prevention and Health Promotion, Office on Smoking and Health.

U.S. Department of Health and Public Services (USDHPS). (2008). *Treating tobacco use and dependence: 2008 update.* Retrieved from http://www.ahrq.gov/professionals/clinicians-providers/guidelines-recommendations/tobacco/clinicians/treating_tobacco_use08.pdf.

U.S. Surgeon General. (2006). *The health consequences of involuntary exposure to tobacco smoke: A report of the Surgeon General.* Retrieved from http://www.surgeongeneral.gov/library/reports/secondhandsmoke/fullreport.pdf.

Vardavas, C. I., & Panagiotakos, D. B. (2009). The causal relationships between passive smoking and inflammation on the development of cardiovascular disease: A review of the evidence. *Inflammation and Allergy—Drug Targets, 8*(5), 328–333.

Wakefield, M., & Chaloupka, F. (2000). Effectiveness of comprehensive tobacco control programs in reducing teenage smoking in the USA. *Tobacco Control, 9*(2), 177–186.

Wakefield, M. A., Chaloupka, F. J., Kaufman, N. J., Orleans, C. T., Barker, D. C., & Ruel, E. E. (2000). Effect of restrictions on smoking at home, at school, and in public places on teenage smoking: cross sectional study. *British medical journal / British Medical Association, 321*(7257), 333–337.

Willemsen, M. C., & De Zwart, W. M. (1999). The effectiveness of policy and health education strategies for reducing adolescent smoking: A review of the evidence. *Journal of Adolescence, 22*(5), 587–599. doi:10.1006/jado.1999.0254.

World Bank. (2014). Economics of tobacco control. Myths and facts. Retrieved from http://web.worldbank.org/WBSITE/EXTERNAL/TOPICS/EXTHEALTHNUTRITIONANDPOPULATION/EXTETC/0,,contentMDK:20365226~menuPK:478891~pagePK:148956~piPK:216618~theSitePK:376601,00.html.

Chapter 7

Sheila F. Castañeda, PhD, Jessica T. Holscher, MPH, and
Gregory A. Talavera MD, MPH

CHRONIC DISEASE MANAGEMENT

Key Terms

access to health care
activities of daily living
basic activities of daily living
caregiver
chronic care model
chronic disease
chronic disease developmental pathway
chronic disease management
community

community health worker (lay health advisor)
comorbidity
cultural competency
food deserts
functionality
health literacy
health-related quality of life
instrumental activities of daily living

interdisciplinary/ multidisciplinary care
patient empowerment
patient-centered care
patient–provider communication
promotores/as de salud/community health worker
quality of life
self-efficacy
self-management

Learning Objectives

Upon completion of this chapter, you should be able to:

1. Identify at least four chronic diseases.
2. Describe chronic disease management.
3. Describe different intervention approaches for managing chronic disease at each socio-ecological level of influence.
4. Identify common barriers to chronic disease management programs.

Chapter Outline

INTRODUCTION

While the field of public health generally focuses on disease prevention and health promotion, there is also a need to focus on the management, control, and treatment of chronic disease. This chapter will first provide an overview of chronic disease in the United States and throughout the world, followed by a comprehensive description of disease management interventions for a variety of chronic diseases using the Social Ecological Framework as a conceptual guide (see Chapter 4 for more information). Then common barriers to implementing chronic disease management intervention programs are discussed. Finally, a summary of the information and resources available for health care providers and patients in relation to chronic disease management is provided at the end of the chapter.

OVERVIEW OF CHRONIC DISEASE

chronic diseases are long-term, noncontagious, and irreversible diseases that are often related to unhealthy behaviors such as physical inactivity, poor eating habits, and cigarette smoking, as well as other factors such as family history and age.

As the name suggests, **chronic diseases** are long-term, noncontagious, and irreversible conditions that are often related to unhealthy behaviors such as tobacco use, physical inactivity, poor diet, and alcohol abuse or other factors such as family history and age. Chronic diseases are sometimes referred to as noncommunicable diseases, chronic illnesses, or chronic conditions. They cannot be prevented by a vaccination, nor can they be cured. This usually means that once an individual is diagnosed with a chronic disease, they must deal with the effects and cope with symptoms of the disease for the remainder of their lifetime. The presence of chronic disease in the United States and throughout much of the world has reached epidemic proportions. In fact, chronic diseases account for more than 70% of deaths annually in the United States, translating to more than 1.7 million deaths per year (Kung, Hoyert, Xu, & Murphy, 2008). An estimated 145 million individuals—more than half of all U.S. adults—currently live with a diagnosed chronic disease. Of these, 75 million have two or more simultaneously diagnosed chronic conditions (Parekh & Barton, 2010). There is a large impact to the economy because of the recurrent management needed to control most chronic conditions.

The management needs resulting from chronic illness diagnoses, such as regular medical appointments, prescription medications, and treatment-related complications, currently contribute to more than 75% of all annual health care expenditures in the United States (Anderson & Horvath, 2004).

Individuals with chronic illness must manage, control, or treat their disease through a variety of methods. Common strategies include (1) adherence to strict medical treatment regimens, (2) significant dietary modifications, (3) increased physical activity, and (4) other behavioral changes specific to certain conditions, such as daily glucose monitoring for diabetics. Not all chronic conditions carry the same level of management burden, because the amount of care required to control symptoms varies among conditions and the severity of the condition. For most chronic diseases, the patient is required to perform the majority of activities needed to control the condition between medical visits. However, certain diseases may require additional assistance from caregivers, such as in the case of Alzheimer's disease, where affected individuals may be unable to properly care for themselves. To better understand why management of chronic disease is important, it is necessary to first understand the historical context of disease patterns in the United States within the past century.

Historical Context of Disease Patterns

Throughout the 19th century and into the early 20th century, infectious diseases (which are also sometimes referred to as acute illnesses or communicable diseases; see Chapter 9 for more information) were highly prevalent due to improper sanitary conditions, poor hygiene practices, and a lack of immunological defense against disease. Because preventive vaccines had not yet been developed, illnesses such as cholera, polio, dengue fever, and tuberculosis were widespread during this time. In fact, in 1900, it is estimated that more than one third of all causes of mortality were due to the effects of pneumonia, tuberculosis, and diarrhea alone (Centers for Disease Control and Prevention [CDC], 1999). These infectious disease outbreaks were so commonly reported throughout the United States and Europe that life expectancy in 1900 averaged only 49.2 years.

With the advent of modern sanitation systems (e.g., clean drinking water and working toilets) and better hygienic practices (e.g., hand washing and regular bathing) after the turn of the 20th century, the incidence of infectious disease steadily began declining, especially in densely populated urban areas. It was not until the discovery of penicillin and vaccines against common childhood illnesses such as polio and measles that communicable diseases were virtually eradicated or greatly reduced in the United States. With these developments, life expectancy quickly climbed from 49.2 years in 1900 to 68.1 by 1951 and to 78.7 by 2011.

The decrease in infectious disease incidence and increased life expectancy throughout the 20th century occurred alongside economic improvement and technological advances in the United States. Where the U.S. economy of the 19th and early 20th centuries was dominated by agricultural and industrial work that often required difficult manual labor, the current economy that has emerged as a result of economic development and technology advancements includes office- and service-based labor, as well as the widespread use of the automobile for commuting and the television for recreation. These changes increased sedentary behavior in work and home environments, thereby paving the way for decreases in physical activity and increases in poor dietary behaviors. The era of chronic disease emerged as a direct result of these factors. This rapid change from infectious disease to primarily chronic disease is referred to as an epidemiological transition, in which patterns of health and disease shift from infection and nutritional deficits to long-term illnesses brought on largely by behavioral-based consequences (see Chapter 9 for a detailed discussion of the epidemiological transition).

Common Chronic Diseases

A variety of chronic illnesses affect individuals from all walks of life. These diseases often present at various stages or degrees of severity, which often determines the course of treatment for the individual. This can make chronic disease management and treatment difficult, as there is no "one-size-fits-all" approach; instead, management strategies must be tailored to the individual's unique needs in context of their social, personal, and family environment. While an exhaustive list of chronic illnesses and their associated symptomology and effects is beyond the scope of this chapter, the following is a list of the more common chronic illnesses with which one should be familiar.

Alzheimer's Disease

Alzheimer's disease is the most common form of dementia, a set of overall symptoms related to memory loss and decline in cognitive functioning. An inability or difficulty remembering newly learned information is often the most telling early symptom of the illness, while confusion, behavior changes, and impaired judgment are often present as the disease progresses (Alzheimer's Association, 2013). Age, family history, and genetics are the most apparent risk factors of the disease. So severe are the effects of the disease that it has now become the sixth leading cause of mortality in the United States (Hoyert & Xu, 2012).

Arthritis

Arthritis is thought to affect more than 50 million of the U.S. population, 21 million of whom have some level of disability as a result of the condition (CDC, 2011a). The term "arthritis" encapsulates different forms of the illness (including osteoarthritis, rheumatoid arthritis, and juvenile arthritis). Although more specific symptoms may be present in certain subtypes of arthritis, all of these diseases are characterized by joint inflammation and pain related to joints and the associated surrounding tissue. Moreover, while dependent on the type of arthritis with which an individual is diagnosed, treatment includes a combination of medication to reduce pain and inflammation, tailored physical activity to maintain joint mobility, healthy eating to reduce weight, and stress management.

Asthma

Characterized by shortness of breath, chest tightness, and wheezing, asthma is thought to affect nearly 19 million U.S. adults and 7 million U.S. children annually

(National Center for Environmental Health, 2012). When an asthmatic individual has an asthma attack, the airways will contract and narrow, causing difficulty with breathing. Various triggers can instigate an attack: tobacco smoke, air pollution, and common allergens such as pet dander and pollen. However, there are effective treatment options that, when taken as prescribed by a medical provider, can provide relief of many asthmatic symptoms. The most common treatment for asthma is the regular use of an inhaler, which dilates the airways in the lungs, and oral medications that reduce inflammation, thereby expanding the airway to the lungs.

Cancer

Characterized by the presence of abnormal cell growth leading to malignant tumors, there are more than 100 types of diagnosable cancers. The most commonly diagnosed cancers among U.S. men include prostate (28% of new cases), lung (14%), and colon (9%). Among U.S. women, the most common cases include breast (29%), lung (14%), and colon (9%) cancer (American Cancer Society, 2013). While certain risk factors such as age and genetic predisposition are out of an individual's hands, an estimated one third of all cancer deaths are due to the effects of tobacco smoking, and another one third of deaths are due to physical inactivity, poor dietary choices, and excessive weight (American Cancer Society, 2013). Although it is the second leading cause of death in the United States (Hoyert & Xu, 2012), a variety of cancer types have relatively high survival rates due to advances in cancer research and care; as a result, many cancer patients and their medical providers are able to monitor and control their condition better.

Cardiovascular Diseases

The leading cause of mortality in the United States (Hoyert & Xu, 2012), cardiovascular diseases are characterized by the presence of artery-clogging plaque, mainly in the heart and brain, which can reduce oxygen flow over time and cause a heart attack or stroke. Risk factors for cardiovascular diseases can include preexisting conditions such as diabetes, obesity, hypertension, and high cholesterol, as well as behavioral and lifestyle choices such as physical inactivity, poor diet, cigarette smoking, and excessive alcohol consumption (CDC, 2013a). Treatment will include targeting behaviors, such as quitting smoking, increasing daily exercise, and improving diet, as well as taking prescribed medications as needed and receiving regular monitoring by a medical team.

Chronic Obstructive Pulmonary Disease (COPD)

As the name suggests, COPD is an obstruction or blockage of air in the lungs that leads to breathing issues. It is diagnosed by a simple pulmonary function test called spirometry, which measures lung capacity. Largely due to the effects of smoking and environmental triggers such as air pollution, COPD is characterized by any combination of wheezing, cough, and fatigue. While these symptoms can often be controlled with medications, the best and most effective treatment option for patients with COPD is smoking cessation and limiting exposure to air pollutants. With an estimated 15 million people diagnosed with the condition, COPD is currently the third leading cause of death in the United States (Hoyert & Xu, 2012).

Diabetes Mellitus (Diabetes Type 1 and Type 2)

Diabetes develops when the body is unable to properly use or produce insulin, causing sugar to accumulate in the bloodstream and produce high blood glucose levels. While type 1 diabetes is largely due to genetic predisposition, development of type 2 diabetes is often the result of harmful health behaviors such as obesity, physical inactivity, and poor eating habits. Combined, the two types affect an estimated 26 million U.S. adults; of those, approximately 95% have type 2 diabetes (CDC, 2011b). Treatment for type 2 diabetes will often involve a combination of regular glucose monitoring, prescribed medications, increases in physical activity, and healthier eating. If not properly treated, diabetes can lead to major complications such as vision problems (including blindness), kidney damage, and foot problems due to nerve damage and poor circulation that can lead to amputations; moreover, diabetes is a contributor to heart disease and stroke.

Hypertension (High Blood Pressure)

Often referred to as hypertension, high blood pressure prevalence in the United States is at roughly 33% (for those 50 or older, hypertension is estimated to affect more than 50%), meaning approximately 68 million U.S. adults must learn to control their blood pressure as part of daily living, which includes use of both medicine and diet modification (CDC, 2013b). If not properly treated, high blood pressure can lead to a variety of serious problems, including stroke and heart disease. In fact, roughly 50% of all heart disease and stroke incidents are related to hypertension (World Health Organization, 2013). Risks for the condition include behavior-related factors (smoking cigarettes, poor dietary choices, and lack of exercise) as well as factors out of an individual's control, such as genetics or age; however, it is of note that hypertension often occurs without any noticeable symptoms (and thus is sometimes called "the silent disease"). Routine blood pressure checks from a medical professional are important for the early diagnosis of hypertension.

   The remainder of this chapter discusses management strategies for some of the aforementioned chronic conditions from a social ecological framework. Following is a discussion of underlying components that increase risk of chronic disease development, with a focus on behavioral, genetic, environmental, and social factors.

Chronic Disease Risk Factors

Research suggests that chronic diseases, such as those listed earlier, are related to certain changes in behavior. The mechanisms that are linked with chronic diseases are complex and also require consideration of the social environment in which individuals live. Certain causal factors (called modifiable risk factors) can be addressed by changing behaviors and the local environment, while others are due to factors out of one's control that cannot be changed, such as genetic predisposition and aging (referred to as non-modifiable risk factors). Examples of modifiable and nonmodifiable chronic disease risk factors are described in the following "Spotlight" box.

SPOTLIGHT

Behavioral (Modifiable) Risk Factors

1. The combined effects of *poor dietary choices* from processed foods and increased consumption of foods high in saturated fats and refined sugars and low in essential nutrients have aided in the extreme increase in obesity rates and are linked to chronic conditions such as hypertension and diabetes.

2. A higher degree of *sedentary lifestyle* due in large part to the advances in technology and computers has led to a general decrease in physical activity throughout much of the world. These more sedentary behaviors have contributed to rapid increases in obesity, which is directly related to increases in cardiovascular diseases and other chronic conditions.

3. Continued high rates of *tobacco smoking*, despite the overwhelming evidence of the harmful health effects to the smoker and individuals in close proximity, as well as to the environment, is considered to be related to at least one third of all cancer diagnoses (American Cancer Society, 2014) and is considered one of the main causes of increases in stroke and chronic respiratory diseases such as asthma and COPD.

Nonmodifiable Risk Factors

1. The *aging* of the Baby Boomer generation has meant there are now more individuals over the age of 65 than ever before. Most chronic diseases manifest at a later age, so with increased life expectancy, older individuals are more likely to develop a chronic illness and—more importantly—multiple chronic conditions.

2. *Genetic predisposition/heredity* may contribute to increased risk of developing certain chronic conditions in specific populations. This is especially true for certain ethnic minority groups, who are more likely to be diagnosed with certain chronic illnesses. For instance, the Pima Native American tribe has been extensively studied by the National Institute of Diabetes and Digestive and Kidney Diseases (NIDDK) for the past 50 years. Within this span of time, researchers have determined a strong genetic predisposition for diabetes among Pima tribe members that has shed light on the contribution of genetics among certain ethnic groups may have for certain chronic illness.

The health consequences of certain social and environmental factors—commonly referred to as **social determinants of health**—are directly linked to modifiable chronic disease risk factors. This is especially true of low-income areas, which are more likely to be located in **food deserts**, areas with little to no access to quality healthy foods and supermarkets, and thus have increased exposure to fast food restaurants, liquor stores, and convenience stores. These areas are also more likely to have higher rates of crime and less access to safe recreational spaces, factors contributing to higher rates of physical inactivity. The U.S. Community Preventive

food deserts are areas with little to no access to healthy foods and supermarkets and thus have increased exposure to fast food restaurants, liquor stores, and convenience stores.

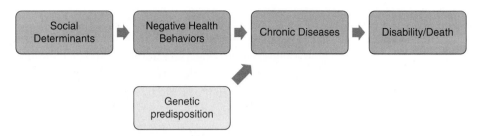

FIGURE 7-1 The Chronic Disease Developmental Pathway

Services Task Force (Anderson, Scrimshaw, Fullilove, & Fielding, 2003) categorizes social determinants of health into three areas of influence:

1. Social institutions

2. Surroundings

3. Social relationships

The **chronic disease developmental pathway** is a hypothesized theoretical that explains the link among social determinants such as income, education, access to resources, air pollution, and health outcomes such as morbidity and mortality.

These three categories form most all of the underlying causes of chronic disease in the United States and throughout the world. As Figure 7-1 highlights, a **chronic disease developmental pathway** is hypothesized to explain the link among social determinants such as income, education, access to resources, air pollution, and morbidity or mortality. A deeper societal root is hypothesized to be a major cause of many of these harmful health behaviors, where the social determinants affect access to health insurance and health-promoting resources, which then can increase the likelihood of an individual participating in certain negative behaviors such as smoking cigarettes or eating fast food regularly. Increased exposure to these unhealthy behaviors then leads to increased prevalence of chronic diseases. Additionally, genetic factors may play a role in the increased likelihood of developing chronic diseases among certain groups, so genetic predisposition is a factor that medical providers will assess as appropriate when evaluating an individual's likelihood of developing specific chronic conditions. When these diseases are not managed or controlled properly, multiple chronic conditions, increased disability, or even death may result. Needless to say, there are many components at play that can affect the occurrence of chronic disease, and as such, interventions and control efforts must seek to intervene at a number of levels.

Genetics

As mentioned previously, genetic predisposition can play a role in the development of certain chronic conditions, as is the case for various types of cancer in which genetic predisposition accounts for approximately 5% to 10% of new cases (National Cancer Institute, 2013). Advances in genetic research have made it possible to test for certain genetic mutations that are linked to specific diseases. If an individual receives a positive genetic result, an opportunity may arise to assess possible prevention or treatment and control of the disease in a proactive manner. Possibly the most well-known genetic testing application for chronic illness is for the breast cancer susceptibility gene 1 (BRCA1) and the breast cancer susceptibility gene 2 (BRCA2) genes. Individuals (both female and male) with high family risk due to presence of harmful BRCA1 or BRCA2 mutations have a much greater likelihood of developing cancer (breast and ovarian cancer among females and breast, pancreatic, and testicular cancer among males) over their lifetime than those without the inherited gene mutations (National Cancer Institute, 2009). To possibly prevent or detect early the presence of cancer, genetic tests that can detect the presence of BRCA1 and BRCA2 genes can be used to provide individuals with the best treatment options for an individual with this increased cancer risk. Because this genetic predisposition cannot be intervened with in the same way a medical provider could intervene with harmful health behaviors, it is important to identify populations at high risk for certain illnesses, as highlighted with increased diabetes diagnoses in the Pima Native American tribe discussed previously.

comorbidity is the presence and interaction of two or more chronic conditions.

SPOTLIGHT

Special Considerations: Comorbidity of Chronic Conditions

Many chronic conditions share several of the same risk factors that have been previously described: older age, smoking status, and increased weight. This makes multiple disease diagnoses—referred to as **comorbidity**—common in chronic care management. In fact, recent estimates indicate approximately 75 million U.S. adults are living with two or more chronic diseases (Parekh & Barton, 2010). Of those, nearly 11 million have five or more chronic conditions. The interaction among risk factors for each separate illness can speed up disease complications when they are not treated properly or not treated at early onset of the disease. This can then lead to increased disability or early mortality. As a result of increased rates of complication, care for individuals with comorbid conditions must be properly coordinated and managed on a routine basis.

Because of the increasing occurrence of comorbidity in chronic disease care, more research is needed to study the interactions of treating multiple diseases. An increasing number of programs are being developed that are critically examining the effects of comorbidity on health outcomes and quality of life of patients with multiple conditions. From a healthcare perspective, comorbid chronic conditions require collaboration of multiple clinicians who work in tandem to ensure treatment options are effectively carried out for the patient. When one of these conditions is depression, proper care can be even more complex, as the addition of depression requires integration of both primary and behavioral care to properly treat all conditions. An example of a successful approach to managing and caring for multiple conditions is the TEAMcare study, which focuses on care for individuals with chronic illnesses such as diabetes and/or cardiovascular disease and co-occurring depression using a collaborative, team-based approach in which the patient becomes an active member of his or her treatment (Katon et al., 2010). This study is especially relevant given the high prevalence of comorbid depression found in those with chronic illnesses such as diabetes. If left untreated or not treated properly, depression can become a barrier to self-management of the co-occurring chronic illness such as diabetes. However, treating the depression by itself does not ensure that self-care practices of the co-occurring chronic illness will be successful. As a result, it is important to treat the conditions simultaneously and in ways that are likely to be long term.

CHRONIC DISEASE MANAGEMENT

chronic disease management (CDM) includes the actions and behaviors taken by health providers, caregivers, and patients to reduce the complications and impact of a chronic disease.

quality of life (QOL) is the subjective measurement of categorical factors such as income and socioeconomic status, environmental quality, or educational attainment.

health-related quality of life (HRQOL) includes an individual's perceived mental and physical health, as well as the perceived experience the individual has of his or her illness and activity limitations.

functionality describes an individual's mental and physical ability to perform activities of daily living.

activities of daily living (ADL) are activities that are performed or completed throughout an individual's day.

basic activities of daily living (BADL) are self-care responsibilities, including bathing, dressing, feeding, toileting, and walking, that are performed by individuals themselves or with the aid of a caregiver.

instrumental activities of daily living (IADL) include tasks that are not considered self-care responsibilities and are thus supplemental activities, including personal financial management, preparing and cooking meals, shopping, and using communication devices.

Strategies of care for chronically ill individuals vary, but most focus on increasing quality of life and functionality, as well as decreased mortality. Chronic disease management is an important way to ensure and address positive outcomes for the patient such as decreased morbidity and increased quality of life and functionality. As there is yet no cure for chronic illnesses, chronic disease management strategies and interventions seek to provide optimal quality of life and functionality to patients in place of the immediate curability frequently seen in acute-care situations. **Chronic disease management (CDM)** comprises the actions and behaviors taken by health providers, caregivers, and patients to reduce the complications and impact of the chronic disease. Stemming from the Social Ecological Framework (defined in Chapter 4), chronic disease management is accomplished through collaboration among the individual, interpersonal relationships such as family and caregivers, and health care providers.

Quality of life (QOL) can be a subjective measurement, largely dependent on the context in which it is used. Different occupational industries use it to describe a variety of categories, including income and socioeconomic status, environmental quality, and educational attainment (Haas, 1999). To better understand QOL specifically in terms of health and well-being, health practitioners often refer to **health-related quality of life (HRQOL)** to denote a patient's perceived mental and physical health over time (Ôunpuu, Chambers, Patterson, Chan, & Yusuf, 2001), as well as a patient's perception of their illness experience and activity limitations (Haas, 1999). **Functionality** refers to the patient's ability to perform normal daily functions and activities, usually categorized as **activities of daily living (ADL)**. These ADLs can be further grouped into basic functions and instrumental functions. **Basic activities of daily living (BADL)** are self-care responsibilities such as bathing, dressing, feeding, toileting, and walking, while **instrumental activities of daily living (IADL)** are tasks that fall outside the realm of self-care, such as personal finance management, cooking meals, shopping, and using communication devices. Individuals requiring assistance with BADL are said to have low functionality and therefore usually rely on caregivers to complete daily activities.

While health care systems have recognized the importance of management as a long-term solution to the chronic disease epidemic, delivery of successful disease-management practices can be considerably difficult for a variety of reasons, a few of which stem from societal and economic barriers. For management to be most effective, a system of organized and insightful education and skills must be passed down to the patient; likewise, the health provider must be equipped to provide appropriate care and advice to the patient and the caregiver and work collaboratively with a team of care providers.

Frameworks for Chronic Disease Management

With the continued rise of chronic disease diagnoses in the United States, the need for standardized but tailored care is essential. The current U.S. health care system has struggled to keep pace with the epidemiological disease shift that has taken place within the last century. Historically, acute and infectious diseases were treated using a reactive approach, meaning treatment was provided only once an individual became sick or showed symptoms. Treatment methods such as antibiotics or surgery were then used to fix or cure the health problem.

This health care delivery system based around treating and curing acute symptoms does not translate well to chronic illness care, mainly because of the long-term nature of care needed to manage most chronic conditions. Chronic diseases cannot generally be cured, which means tangible financial resources are necessary to ensure that treatment is successful in the long term. In fact, treatment and care for chronic disease currently contributes to more than 75% of all annual health care expenditures in the United States (Anderson & Horvath, 2004). Moreover, according to the CDC's National Center for Health Statistics (NCHS), the United States currently spends more money per capita on medical needs than any other developed country, largely because the current health system is incentivized to deliver care that fixes acute problems, not to manage recurrent symptoms on a long-term, continual basis (CDC, 2009). If these care practices are not drastically improved, a strain will remain on the U.S. economy. Fortunately, public health researchers and health care professionals have begun to recognize the importance of providing proactive chronic disease managed care in order to limit further strain on both the patient and the economy. The following sections provide an overview of existing chronic disease management models at each level of the Social Ecological Framework.

Chronic Disease Management at the Individual Level

self-management includes the actions and behaviors taken by patients to successfully manage and control the effects and symptoms of their illness on a routine basis.

Due to the long-term, often irreversible nature of chronic illness, the majority of the burden of treatment and care involves patients themselves successfully managing the effects and symptoms of their illness on a routine basis. This is referred to as **self-management**. Self-management strategies vary according to illness, as does the amount of time and resources needed for each patient to successfully manage and control their symptoms. Self-management is widely recognized as an essential component of effective chronic disease management. These strategies must be learned and practiced; as such, the health care system has acknowledged the importance of helping patients develop the proper skills needed to accomplish these management tasks. For management and control of disease symptoms to be effective, patients must be confident in their ability to perform self-care and monitoring activities with or without assistance, a notion referred to as **self-efficacy**.

self-efficacy is an individual's confidence in her or his own ability to perform certain actions or behaviors.

The first of its kind, the Stanford University Patient Education Research Center has established a series of self-management patient education programs for an array of chronic illnesses, all with the goal of increasing the self-efficacy of the patients enrolled to perform self-management tasks and, by doing so, lowering the burden of disease (Lorig, Mazonson, & Holman, 1993). With patients more confident in their ability to manage their illness, less money is spent on preventable hospitalizations and trips to the emergency room, thereby decreasing the overall economic burden placed on the health system. The Stanford programs have become the evidence-based standard around which most self-management programs are modeled.

Model for Understanding

Arthritis Self-Management Program (ASMP)

The Arthritis Self-Management Program (ASMP) is the original chronic disease management program at Stanford University—thought to be the first of its kind in the United States—and has served as the model for additional disease-specific education programs. In addition, Stanford has evidence-based self-management programs focusing on other chronic diseases, such as diabetes. Chronic arthritis is often painful, requiring medication and pain-management techniques; if not properly treated, the condition can lead to a level of disability and low functionality. In fact, an estimated 50 million U.S. adults have been diagnosed with arthritis, with nearly half reporting activity limitations of some kind due to the effects of the disease (CDC, 2012). Through the use of peer leaders/educators, the Stanford ASMP teaches participants beneficial exercises and techniques for maintaining strength and coping with the effects of pain and fatigue associated with their condition. Additional topics include medication management, communication with family, friends, and health professionals, and making informed decisions about treatment (Holman & Lorig, 2004). Participants who complete the program regularly report decreased pain episodes and fewer visits to physicians. Perhaps more importantly, patients have markedly increased self-efficacy after participating in the program. This increased confidence in treating and controlling their condition is a positive sign for long-term successful management of the disease.

In the "Model for Understanding" box, one of the many successful applications of these programs is highlighted: the Arthritis Self-Management Program.

As discussed earlier, chronic disease management strategies will vary by disease and will be dependent on an individual's health status. This can prove to be a challenge for those diagnosed with multiple chronic conditions in which symptom management and control differ for each disease. Recent studies suggest that self-management programs originally developed for single chronic diseases may not be appropriate for those with comorbid conditions (Bayliss, Steiner, Fernald, Crane, & Main, 2003), causing difficulties when simultaneously treating all conditions. For instance, an individual with both hypertension and type 2 diabetes mellitus may have to coordinate with a registered dietician to follow the Dietary Approaches to Stop Hypertension (DASH) diet to aid in lowering salt intake (thereby lowering blood pressure) but might also need to take a self-management course on proper insulin usage to control diabetes. Another example may find asthmatic individuals experiencing trouble breathing when following recommended physical activity plans as treatment for osteoarthritis. **Adherence to medications**, generally defined as the degree to which prescribed medications are taken by patients, can also be affected by the presence of multiple conditions, especially if side effects from one medication exacerbate the symptoms of another condition. In each of the described situations, the competing demands of self-management required for each chronic disease may leave the patient feeling overwhelmed and unsure how to balance treatment for each illness. Perhaps this individual is then afraid to ask for help in managing these issues or loses confidence in his or her ability to successfully control his or her health (see "Spotlight" box on Patient Empowerment).

SPOTLIGHT

Patient Empowerment

To better ensure successful self-management practices, the process of patient empowerment is often employed between provider and patient. **Patient empowerment** is a method to help individuals increase their self-efficacy and take control of their health by obtaining the necessary skills and knowledge to make informed and educated behavioral decisions, with the ultimate goal for patients to better manage their disease. Patients are given the power to make informed decisions regarding their day-to-day management of symptoms without solely relying on the health care professional to provide detailed instructions on management tasks (Anderson & Funnell, 2010). In this way, the patient assumes responsibility and works in partnership with the health care provider. By putting the responsibility and power in the hands of the patient rather than the physician, proponents of empowerment argue that management of the disease will be most effective in the long run. This also has implications for health expenditures, as patient self-management is more cost effective than the traditional medical model in place where individuals may have multiple medical appointments.

patient empowerment is a method to help individuals to increase their self-efficacy and take control of their health by obtaining skills and knowledge necessary to make informed and educated behavioral decisions.

Barriers to Individual-Level Chronic Disease-Management Programs

Despite the importance of self-management to the overall success of many chronic disease treatment plans, the burden of care can be quite high for chronically ill individuals. This can be especially true of individuals with low health literacy. **Health literacy** refers to an individual's ability to find, process, and understand information and services relevant to their medical and health needs (U.S. Department of Health and Human Services, 2012). This includes an individual's ability to perform essential health functions such as reading prescription labels, appointment slips, and health brochures and communicating with—and understanding instructions from—their health care provider. Health literacy is often dependent on an individual's level of comfort in negotiating the U.S. health care system, with the elderly, poor, new immigrants, and non-English speakers most negatively affected (Nielsen-Bohlman, Panzer, & Kindig, 2004). If an individual does not feel comfortable discussing health issues with their provider— or perhaps even going to see a provider—that individual might not receive optimal care, which may translate to undiagnosed conditions or increased risk for illness complications. With increased emphasis placed on managing chronic conditions, individuals need to be more attentive to their health needs, requiring high health literacy to ensure optimal disease management. Unfortunately, research estimates nearly half of the U.S. population has low health literacy, with the average reading

health literacy is an individual's ability to find, process, and understand information and services relevant to medical and health needs and to perform essential health functions such as reading and comprehending health information and communicating with health care providers.

ability among adults only at a seventh-grade level. As a consequence, many in the United States are lacking the skills needed to make informed health decisions and potentially manage their chronic conditions (Nielsen-Bohlman et al., 2004).

Chronic Disease Management at the Interpersonal Level

A **caregiver** is an individual, often a friend or family member, who assists and supports another individual through management and treatment of an illness.

Support from family, friends, and social networks can be a powerful tool for both one's physical and emotional well-being. These support systems can be a particularly valuable resource for the management of chronic conditions, especially as a historically acute-centered health system continues to struggle with providing appropriate care to a growing number of chronically ill patients. **Caregivers** are family members, friends, and other individuals who assist and support patients through management and treatment on a day-to-day basis. It is estimated that 29% of U.S. adults are caregivers in some form (National Alliance for Caregiving, 2009). Research has found that proactive social support and disease management assistance from caregivers generally leads to more positive health outcomes across the chronic disease spectrum (Rosland & Piette, 2010). This can be especially true of self-management programs geared toward young people, which will be the focus of this section.

Social Support Techniques for Children

It is estimated that roughly 7% to 15% of children under the age of 18 are diagnosed with a chronic condition every year in the United States (see Eiser, 1997, for instance), more than three times the annual number of children diagnosed 50 years ago. The self-management needed for these specific illnesses is often intensive, calling on individuals to practice self-care and monitoring on a routine basis. Children are generally not equipped to handle these management practices on their own, thus relying on parental figures to ensure illness symptoms are kept under control. While different chronic illnesses require different supportive measures, the most common forms of support caregivers provide to children include emotional support and helping with self-care practices (Rosland & Piette, 2010). This can mean anything from a parental figure encouraging their child to engage in physical activity every day to assisting in glucose monitoring for diabetic children or measuring peak air-flow outputs for asthmatic children. Interventions targeting the adult caregiver as a means of increasing the quality of life and long-term functionality of chronically ill children are becoming increasingly relevant. These interventions are usually mutually beneficial to the caregiver, as the caregiver must frequently deal with their own coping and stress-management techniques as they help their child. One area that has seen a rise in caregiver interventions in recent years is pediatric asthma.

Rising rates of obesity, secondhand smoke exposure from tobacco, and poor indoor and outdoor air quality have led to a record number of children aged 18 and younger being diagnosed with asthma, with estimates of more than 7 million children living with asthma in the United States alone (CDC, 2012). As a result, asthma is now the most commonly diagnosed chronic condition among children. Even still, leading asthma researchers believe pediatric asthma to be underdiagnosed and undertreated compared to adult-onset asthma (Szefler, 2001).

Model for Understanding

One of the first comprehensive asthma education programs directed specifically at parents and caregivers of young asthmatic children is the Wee Wheezers Asthma Education Program, developed and validated in both Spanish and English, and used throughout the United States in clinical and home-based settings (CDC, 2009b). The primary goal of the program is to increase the knowledge, skills, and motivation of caregivers to better manage exacerbations of asthma symptoms in children under the age of 7. This goal is obtained through several small-group sessions focusing on practical changes caregivers can make for young children with asthma: identifying asthmatic triggers and using preventive medications, among others (Wilson, Fish, Page, & Starr-Schneidkraut, 1994). Loosely based on Albert Bandura's social cognitive theory, group sessions target caregiver self-efficacy through the use of such constructs as feedback, modeling of behaviors and mastery experiences with children, information sharing among group members, and reinforcement of positive behaviors displayed by the caregivers. As a result of these efforts, parents and caregivers often report becoming more effective and confident managers of their child's asthma, as well as more consistent symptom-free days for the child.

When left uncontrolled and untreated, chronic asthma can lead to a loss of pulmonary (lung) function or increases in wheezing attacks after basic activity, among other challenges. These consequences of poor asthma control can then lead to a decreased quality of life, sleepless nights, missed school days for the child, missed work days for the adult caregiver, increased emergency room visits, hospitalization, and occasionally even death. With more than 145,000 children 15 and under hospitalized annually for asthma-related reasons (Buie, Owings, DeFrances, & Golosinsky, 2010), interventions targeting management techniques and education for pediatric asthma are greatly needed for both child and adult caregiver alike.

Barriers to Interpersonal Chronic Disease Programs

While social support is an important component of successful chronic disease self-management, there are certain barriers to effective care at the interpersonal level. In order for an intervention targeting caregivers to be most effective, caregivers must be open to receiving educational messages and feedback on supportive methods. However, due to social, environmental, and economic factors, a number of challenges might hinder this process, including a lack of time or transportation, both of which might make it difficult for a family to dedicate attention to such matters.

Additional barriers may arise for caregivers. For example, research studies have shown that, especially among adolescents, social support from parental figures is not always well received (Roseland & Piette, 2010). For young adults with chronic conditions but few functional limitations, a sense of independence is often important to emotional and physical well-being. Parental figures, while well intentioned, may inadvertently pose a threat to this independence by overstepping boundaries or interrupting self-care schedules.

Along with caregiver support for children, the aging trends among the U.S. population—as well as the growing number of older adults diagnosed with Alzheimer's disease—has led to a rising number of middle-aged U.S. adults caring for chronically ill adult parents who require closely monitored care. This can especially place a strain on individuals who themselves have full-time jobs or are raising their own children. Providing skills and training on effectively facilitating care for others is one way for the health system to decrease the burden on caregivers. Participation in support groups and interventions such as the one described previously are successful methods used previously.

Chronic Disease Management at the Organizational Level

Another way chronic disease management is supported and disseminated is through organizations such as schools, job sites, and health care settings. These settings can provide a platform for change on a large scale, especially considering the significant amount of time many individuals spend within these institutions and organizations on a regular basis (Whittemore, Melkus, & Grey, 2004). In fact, schools and worksites have shown substantial success with chronic disease prevention interventions such as physical activity and antismoking policies. Health care settings, however, may prove more appropriate avenues for chronic disease-management interventions, compared to other organizational settings such as schools and workplaces. As the health care system shifts focus toward chronic care, the impact of its influence over management and control of chronic illness cannot be underestimated. The following sections highlight organizational-level chronic disease-management strategies occurring through implementation of the Chronic Care Model in primary care settings.

The Chronic Care Model

Depending on conditions, an individual with a chronic disease may require multiple health advisors, with the number of providers increasing with each additional chronic condition diagnosis. Unsurprisingly, the need for collaboration among all necessary health providers is essential to satisfactory care. This collaboration among health care specialists is known as **interdisciplinary** or **multidisciplinary care**. Previous research suggests that, in fact, the most successful treatment of chronic disease is achieved through a system of collaboration in which the patient is the recipient of tailored care from a team of health care professionals, commonly including a general practitioner, nurses, dieticians, pharmacists, and other specialists. Money, resources, and time are all needed to successfully produce this system change but are often hard to obtain and even harder to delegate among the vast network of health care services available in the United States. To address this care shift challenge, Wagner and colleagues developed the **Chronic Care Model (CCM)**, the first theoretical framework of its kind designed to answer the increasing need for medical care targeting long-term management of heart disease, diabetes, asthma, and other chronic conditions.

The CCM was born out of the idea that positive health outcomes are obtainable if a patient is informed and confident in his or her ability to communicate with

interdisciplinary or **multidisciplinary care** is the collaboration of health care specialists from various fields who come together to effectively and efficiently treat a patient.

The **chronic care model (CCM)** is a framework designed to increase positive health outcomes among chronically ill individuals by ensuring the patient and the health provider work in partnership and utilize a series of community and health system elements, including self-management support, resources and policies, delivery system design, organization of health care, decision support, and clinical information systems.

providers who themselves are accessible and prepared to offer assistance. Conversely, this partnership between patient and provider can only succeed when supported by a set of community and health system elements, including self-management support, resources and policies, delivery system redesign (transforming care from reactive to proactive), organization of health care, decision support (evidence-based guidelines), and clinical information systems (electronic patient registries; Wagner et al., & Bonomi, 2001). When all these elements are used together, optimal chronic care can be achieved for the patient. By improving the delivery of chronic care, the health system as a whole becomes more efficient and streamlined, translating to more effective quality care to chronically ill patients and more effective use of health care expenditure over the long term (Coleman, Austin, Brach, & Wagner, 2009). To date, the CCM has been implemented across a variety of settings both in the United States and throughout the world, with the World Health Organization (WHO) recommending its use in health systems worldwide (Oprea, Braunack-Mayer, Rogers, & Stocks, 2009). The framework has now been adapted for a range of chronic conditions and has been tailored to specific cultural groups. Many of the most successful examples of CCM utilization involve primary care settings, where health professionals change the underlying process for care delivery to chronically ill patients through a system of collaboration. Originally used in diabetes care management, the CCM has been implemented across a variety of chronic illnesses, including depression. One such example is highlighted in the "Spotlight" box on depression.

SPOTLIGHT

Depression

Depression affects many individuals in the United States and throughout much of the world. Consequences of depression can range from a persistent sense of sadness to more extreme functional impairment such as disturbed sleep and appetite changes, making the completion of daily tasks especially difficult; severe cases of depression can lead to self-harm and suicide (WHO, 2012). A growing concern in the literature is the rise of major depressive disorder (MDD) diagnoses in older adults. Estimates place more than 7 million U.S. adults aged 65 or older suffering from the effects of depression (Steinman et al., 2007). Moreover, depression is more likely to occur in those with chronic diseases, with up to 50% of older individuals with diagnosed chronic conditions such hypertension and diabetes believed to have comorbid depression (McEvoy & Barnes, 2007). Grounded on evidence-based reviews, the U.S. Community Preventive Services Task Force (thecommunityguide.org) recommends a collaborative approach to management of depressive disorders. This recommendation has been supported by other research teams (see Katon & Guico-Pabia, 2011, for example). The CCM aligns with collaborative care approaches, as these models are highly structured and utilize decision support, information systems, and community resources to elicit positive patient outcomes (McEvoy & Barnes, 2007).

Intervention Focus at the Organizational Level

The Improving Mood Promoting Access to Collaborative Care Treatment (IMPACT) randomized control trial was implemented in a series of primary care settings in the United States, utilizing approximately 1,800 study participants aged 60 and older over a 12-month period (Unützer, Katon, Callahan et al., 2002). A collaborative team approach was employed, with nurses and psychologists functioning as depression care managers and working alongside participants' primary physicians to disseminate treatment and care. IMPACT participants received tailored education, medication management, problem-solving treatment, and relapse-prevention training (McEvoy & Barnes, 2007). Results indicate study participants who were assigned to this collaborative team of providers had higher antidepressant medication adherence, mental functioning, and quality of life than those receiving usual care (Hunkeler et al., 2006). The IMPACT program has since been implemented in a variety of settings both in the United States and abroad, with a comprehensive online resource available to mental health providers looking to implement the program in various care settings. These subsequent versions of the program have found similar results across settings, highlighting the effectiveness of implementation of a collaborative care approach. Further information on the IMPACT program may be found at the end of this chapter.

SPOTLIGHT

Where Does Technology Fit in the Equation?

As society becomes more reliant on technology for the completion of daily tasks, the health care system must adapt to this growing dependency, using technology to its benefit. In fact, technology can play a vital role in many areas of chronic disease management, including the facilitation of self-care practices and assisting in effective communication between patient and provider. Cell phones and the Internet can be powerful tools for managing symptoms and providing pertinent information to patients, caregivers, providers, and the general public. Health care systems and nonprofit organizations dedicated to specific chronic diseases are able to provide tailored information to a wide audience through comprehensive websites. Specific to diabetes care, the National Diabetes Education Program (ndep.nih.gov) provides resources such as fact sheets, risk test assessments, and print public service announcements (PSAs) for patients, clinicians, and caregivers. Similar resources are available for other chronic conditions, such as asthma, cancer, and depression. More information can be found at the end of the chapter.

These technological resources can be used alone or with more comprehensive patient-centered primary care to provide support and increased knowledge. The use of technology as a means to increase effectiveness of patient education and long-term care can play an important role in primary care health delivery and can enhance care through all of the elements within the CCM. For example, the clinical information systems component of the CCM calls on the health system to utilize electronic-based patient registries that are able to provide proactive

Continues

automated reminders to physicians and patients, medication reviews, and performance monitoring of provider staff (Wagner et al., 2001). An increasing number of programs are exploring the use of communication devices to enhance care to patients and their caregivers, as well as to support the primary care provider in collaborating with other providers and disseminating health information. For example, many chronic disease management programs offer interactive web-based intervention components that allow patients and their caregivers to interact with other patients and receive tailored care to address barriers to management (see Meischke, Lozano, Zhou, Garrison, & Christakis, 2011, for information on "My Child's Asthma," a web-based pediatric asthma management intervention).

Barriers to Organizational Chronic Disease Management Programs

cultural competency
describes an individual's or organization's level of awareness, familiarity, and comfort with the values, traditions, and behaviors of a specific cultural, ethnic, or racial group.

There is evidence that cultural competence among health care professionals may aid in positive patient outcomes, including increased satisfaction, adherence to medication, and better self-management of symptoms (California Endowment, 2003). **Cultural competency** refers to an individual's or organization's level of awareness, familiarity, and comfort with the values, traditions, and behaviors of a specific cultural, ethnic, or racial group (U.S. Office of Minority Health, 2002). Additionally, cultural competence as a whole includes learned skills and knowledge that must be acquired and practiced (California Endowment, 2005). While helpful, a health care professional does not necessarily need to be of the same cultural background as a patient; basic familiarity with the customs and traditions of ethnic and racial groups is a small token of cultural sensitivity and may be the difference needed to ensure a patient receives proper care. Just for this reason, an increasing number of health professionals are required or at the very least encouraged to take continuing education courses in cultural competence, especially those in areas rich with diversity.

Chronic Disease Management at the Community Level

A **community** is a group of individuals who share common values and beliefs and provide a sense of belonging to the members of the group.

community health worker or **lay health advisors**
is an individual selected by his or her community who provides culturally tailored health information to community members and who often shares similar health struggles to the population of interest.

A **community** is a group of individuals who share common values and beliefs and provide a sense of belonging to the members of its group. Community-level interventions focus on the needs of a specific population of people. Interventions at this level involve techniques and strategies that focus on the most appropriate care for certain communities. For instance, an intervention targeting young mothers with gestational diabetes in an urban area with a large Somali refugee population will employ different strategies than a hypertension intervention targeting older Asian American adults in a suburban area.

One way public health professionals are better able to implement community-based chronic disease programs is through the use of **community health workers** or **lay health advisors**. Community health workers are usually of similar cultural and linguistic background to the community of interest and often share similar health struggles. For example, in predominately Hispanic/Latino communities, particularly those along the U.S./Mexico border, these individuals providing outreach and support are referred to as **promotores/as de salud** (health promoters). Interventions utilizing promotores/as in Hispanic/Latino community settings have shown considerable long-term success with chronic disease management (Ayala, Vaz, Earp, Elder, & Cherrington, 2010). Consequently, the Hispanic/Latino population of the United States has been particularly affected by rising rates of chronic disease, especially diabetes and obesity, and yet often has limited access to health care and important health-promoting resources. Because of their strong ties to the community and their personal experiences with health concerns, the use of promotores/as is a successful method for providing culturally appropriate and effective chronic disease management within Latino communities. Promotores/as are able to train members of the community by teaching and modeling practical skills for improving health-related behaviors in familiar, trusted, and nonthreatening environments such as community centers and churches (Thompson, Horton, & Flores, 2007).

Engaging the community in effecting change strategies is a successful method of involving chronically ill individuals in long-term management of their disease. Likewise, particularly effective promotore/a-led management interventions often utilize resources available in a primary care setting. This collaborative approach allows for proper communication between patient and provider, which then allows for more operational treatment and control of the chronic condition. These promotores/as also can provide health professionals with valuable insights into the community of interest, acting as a liaison between patient and provider. In this sense, the promotore/a may serve as a "patient navigator," facilitating navigation through the health care system by assisting patients with scheduling and keeping medical appointments, adhering to medication treatments, and communicating with health providers.

Promotora interventions have been widely used in diabetes management among Latino communities. As it is, Latinos are 1.7 times more likely to be diagnosed with diabetes compared to non-Hispanic Whites; nearly 12% of Latinos are diabetic, higher than the national average (CDC, 2011b). The following "Model for Understanding" box reviews a community-based intervention targeting Latinos living with diabetes.

Barriers to Chronic Disease Management at the Community Level

While the impact that management efforts can have at the community level is extensive, creating a successful infrastructure with resources and available personnel can be quite the undertaking. Needless to say, barriers can emerge in these endeavors. For example, a complex infrastructure composed of appropriate resources to both train community workers and provide education and skills for patients is necessary for sustained success. However, many of the community-based organizations that assist in implementing these interventions are largely funded through grants and other public and private endowments; for those organizations funded by governmental entities, any budgetary concerns may translate into a reduction in funding or the complete withdrawal of assistance.

> Similar to a community health worker or lay health advisor, **promotores/as de salud** are individuals who are part of the Hispanic/Latino community and who provide outreach, education, and support to individuals of similar background.

Model for Understanding

Community-Level Intervention Focus

One such example of a successful randomized control trial that tested a community-based, promotore/a-led intervention model found positive effects on glycemic control (measured by hemoglobin A1c levels) and increased diabetes management knowledge (Lujan, Ostwald, & Ortiz, 2007). Before the intervention began, the promotores were first trained to motivate behavior change. At the start of the intervention, group educational meetings were scheduled and were supplemented by follow-up calls by the promotores to the diabetic patients. The motivational messages used were tailored to focus on religion and faith so as to acknowledge the high prevalence of fatalistic beliefs among participants (i.e., "only God can decide if I will suffer complications of diabetes"; Lujan et al., 2007). This intervention was successful because promotores delivered diabetes education in a family-like and mutually supportive environment between the participants and the health educators. This partnership fostered trust, belonging, and greater receptivity to educational messages, thus influencing effective behavior change: in this case, glycemic control. Similar positive results have been found in other chronic disease management and prevention interventions that have successfully utilized a promotore/a model to deliver intervention components (see Ayala, Vaz, Earp, Elder, & Cherrington, 2010, for a comprehensive overview of existing promotore/a-led interventions in chronic disease).

Chronic Disease Management at the Policy Level

This chapter thus far has discussed strategies for managing and controlling chronic disease at the first four levels of the Social Ecological Framework. In order for each of these levels of influence to be effective channels for change, the policies guiding them must be sustainable and reliable and able to affect change at a larger, population level. Considerable attention has been given to public policies targeting health behaviors and the prevention of disease, such as additional taxes on cigarettes that directly decrease smoking rates. In addition, public health advocates have focused on laws requiring fast food chains to disclose nutritional and caloric information to customers to allow for informed decision making. Many of these strategies aimed at the prevention of disease are applicable to the management and control of chronic illness (Institute of Medicine, 2012). For instance, improving dietary choices, becoming more physically active, and quitting smoking are cornerstones of chronic disease management, just as they are prevention efforts. These behavior modifications are not a substitute for proper management of chronic illness but are instead supplementary well-being support. By adopting these positive health behaviors, improved quality of life and optimal functioning are more obtainable for the chronically ill patient.

While the prevention of disease is an important component of public health, policies focused on the management and control of chronic disease also have implications for society. Next, a discussion of recent policy advances in chronic disease management is described, followed by an overview of current chronic disease policy guidelines from the Institute of Medicine.

Recent Chronic Disease Management Policy Advances

In 2001, the Institute of Medicine (IOM) released a report ("Crossing the Quality Chasm: A New Health System for the 21st Century") outlining the state of health care in the United States. The report brought attention to the looming health disparities and inefficiency plaguing the current health system and opened the eyes of many previously unaware of the difficulties with care delivery in the United States and around the world. Within the 2001 report, the IOM outlined six aims that, when closely followed by providers and organizations, would lead to better, more sustainable care for patients, especially those chronically ill; these aims have since become the basis by which quality care in the United States is now framed. Positive health outcomes and better use of health expenditures can be obtained when health professionals and organizations provide quality health care that is:

1. *Safe*: Care should intend to help the patient and avoid harm

2. *Effective*: Providing services based on scientific knowledge to all who may benefit and avoid providing services to those who will not to benefit

3. *Patient centered*: Providing care that corresponds to patient preferences, needs, and values

4. *Timely*: Reducing wait time and delays in seeking care and care delivery

5. *Efficient*: Avoiding waste of equipment, supplies, and resources

6. *Equitable*: Providing quality care that does not vary by personal gender, ethnicity, geographic location, and socioeconomic status (Committee on Quality of Health Care in America, Institute of Medicine, 2001).

Since the IOM (2001) report was first published, efforts at bridging the quality gap in care delivery and increasing collaboration among providers have drastically increased, likely due in part to greater exposure to the components of the Chronic Care Model and other integrated care models. As part of the 2001 IOM report, the Agency for Healthcare Research and Quality (AHRQ) was charged with determining the most effective and efficient health care policies for the U.S. population, given the substantial increases in chronic care needs. As a result, the AHRQ has determined that patient–provider communication must be improved for any health policy to have lasting effect (Agency for Healthcare Research and Quality, 2008), a sentiment echoed in the CCM. **Patient–provider communication** relates to a patient's satisfaction, level of disclosure, and adherence with treatment regimens and physician recommendations. Effective communication between patient and provider can lead to more positive health behaviors, including increased adherence to treatment, and improved patient outcomes (DeVoe, Wallace, & Fryer, 2009). Even so, research suggests a gap exists in communication efforts among providers and those of lower educational attainment and certain ethnic minorities, where certain socioeconomic factors are correlated with more fragmented communication

patient–provider communication affects a patient's satisfaction, level of disclosure, and adherence to treatment regimens and physician recommendations, which all increase as patients feel communication levels with providers are improved.

patterns between provider and patient (Siminoff, Graham, & Gordon, 2006). Efforts are currently underway to provide more comprehensive training and education to health care professionals to bridge this gap. A growing number of medical schools are recognizing this concern; seeking to establish a more patient-centered medical preparation, these educational programs are providing semester- or year-long courses on appropriate communication styles.

SPOTLIGHT

Healthy People 2020

Healthy People, a broad, national initiative that uses evidence-based and evaluated research to inform social, environmental, and economic policies on prevention, intervention, and management of disease, is a success story of collaboration among various organizations at the federal, state and local levels. Started in 1980 and maintained via the U.S. Department of Health and Human Services, the initiative tracks and monitors progress in a variety of areas as chosen by key stakeholders over a 10-year timespan (Green & Fielding, 2011). As each new iteration of Healthy People is launched at the start of a new decade, the findings and developments of the previous Healthy People program are used to inform the direction and goals of the current initiative, which then inform public health policy. These data are then made available to organizations, community leaders, and the general public through the Healthy People 2020 website. In this way, the goals and objectives of Healthy People can be implemented in smaller, more localized efforts to reach greater results.

Due to the shifting landscape of disease in the United States, the majority of the topic areas and objectives of the newest version, Healthy People 2020, target chronic illness and the most appropriate and successful ways in which to prevent and manage these diseases. Healthy People 2020 focuses on and monitors progress in four areas relevant to current public health needs:

1. General health status
2. Health-related quality of life and well-being
3. Determinants of health
4. Health disparities

Within these four measures, there are more than 40 topic areas that have their own unique objectives that are used to track, evaluate, and monitor progress over the decade. In total, there are almost 600 objectives that will be monitored throughout the decade. Special consideration is paid to what Healthy People 2020 refers to as "Leading Health Indicators," areas that are of high priority given current public health needs: access to health services; clinical preventive services; environmental quality; injury and violence; maternal, infant, and child health; mental health; nutrition, physical activity, and obesity; oral health; reproductive and sexual health; and social determinants (U.S. Department of Health and Human Services, 2013).

Transforming Primary Care

As referenced previously in this chapter, the traditional medical model of treating acute illness is no longer an appropriate method of care, as the disease landscape has shifted to chronic conditions. A result of this fragmented care system, sky-rocketing health care costs and inefficient use of personnel and resources all have negative consequences for the patient. A full paradigm shift that makes efficient chronic care possible is greatly needed. Before this shift can take place, a few key issues must be addressed at a systemwide level. First, the way in which health providers are reimbursed for their services does not often support the ways in which chronic conditions are most effectively treated. For example, the widely used fee-for-service reimbursement schedule pays providers based on the volume (number) of patients treated and not the quality of care provided. This system is set up to reward quantity over quality and does not align with the long-term, in-depth care needed for most chronic conditions. Another issue present is the reimbursement system in place with the traditional system of care; currently, this traditional system does not reward health providers for better coordination of chronic care services. Despite the coordination and collaboration needed to successfully treat chronically ill individuals (especially those patients living with multiple chronic conditions), there is currently no system of financial incentives set up for providers who share in the responsibility of care and treatment in a collaborative, multidisciplinary fashion.

The recent passage of the Patient Protection and Affordable Care Act (ACA) alleviates some of these primary-care reimbursement issues. Certain provisions within the ACA are designed to reward medical professionals who do engage in collaboration to better treat and deliver care for individuals with chronic illness. The idea behind these provisions is twofold: to provide adequate and appropriate **patient-centered care**, care that is based on the patient's preferences, needs, and values, for those chronically ill and to save costs across the health care spectrum by utilizing a proactive approach to care delivery and treatment. So important is the need for chronic illness health care reform that 2 of the 10 main titles (or major chapters) of the ACA, Title III: Improving the Quality and Efficiency of Health Care and Title IV: The Prevention of Chronic Disease and Improving Public Health, focus on the issues discussed throughout this chapter and how these issues can be ameliorated (Senate Bill 2702, 2010).

> **patient-centered care** is health care that is respectful and delivered in a way that is responsive to the patient's preferences, needs, and values.

Barriers to Chronic Disease Management at the Policy Level

Due to the shift from acute to chronic disease in the past century, the health care system in the United States has not yet expanded to include policy directed at improvements to patient care and treatment of chronic illness. With this current lack of evidence-based policy interventions geared at management and control of chronic illness, it is difficult to secure funding for programs and studies that seek to narrow this gap. As a result, barriers to disease management at the policy level are significant. Policy is often influenced and affected by politics (where certain issues are given priority due to financial, economic, and political reasons) and agenda setting, making substantial change a slow process. Other barriers present at the policy level include the sheer number of individuals lacking insurance or proper health care; this concept—known as access to health care—has implications for individuals' quality of life and functionality.

access to health care is used to describe the degree to which individuals are able to obtain health care services when needed, measured by the presence of resources that facilitate health care use, such as insurance coverage, having had a recent physician's visit, and adequate economic resources.

According to a 1993 Institute of Medicine (IOM) report, **access to health care** describes the degree to which individuals are able to obtain health care services when needed (Millman, 1993). Access to health care is measured by the presence of resources that facilitate health care use like insurance coverage, having a recent physician's visit, and adequate economic resources (Millman, 1993). Health insurance plays a powerful role in the process of using health services, in that certain state and federal legislation exists to ensure that insurance companies cover certain chronic disease screening and treatment procedures. Because U.S. health care costs per capita are the highest in the world, having health insurance can potentially protect individuals from paying high medical costs associated with managing their disease (Hoffman & Paradise, 2008). Yet a significant portion of the U.S. population remains uninsured. For example, in 2004, 45.8 million Americans were without health insurance, equating to 15.7% of the total population (DeNavas-Walt, Proctor, & Lee 2005). This number increased to 49.9 million in 2010, with an estimated 16.3% of the total U.S. population uninsured as of 2010 (DeNavas-Walt, Proctor, & Smith, 2011). Most recent data have shown that uninsured rates are decreasing as a result of the ACA. For example, data from 2014 show the uninsured rate has dropped to approximately 14% (Levy, 2014). Receiving insurance is often difficult for those with preexisting chronic conditions, and as a result, many individuals with comorbid chronic conditions do not receive adequate treatment. Given the importance of access to health care in the prevention and control of disease, one provision of the ACA limits the ability of insurance companies to deny medical coverage to individuals with preexisting conditions—including chronic conditions (Senate Bill 2702, 2010). This will mean that more individuals with chronic conditions—especially those with multiple conditions—will have access to more comprehensive treatment, including extensive self-management plans, thus increasing patient–provider communication.

Summary

While it is imperative for public health departments and health care providers to take steps to ensure individuals are given adequate and accurate information on the prevention of chronic disease, it is also necessary to focus on the large percentage of individuals already diagnosed with long-term health conditions. By doing so, one can help ensure further disability—and even death—do not occur. This chapter highlights the many ways by which chronic disease management is achieved, ultimately demonstrating that optimal care is achieved when all levels of the Social Ecological Framework work together to provide increased functionality and greatest quality of life for patients and their caregivers.

This chapter has highlighted successes at each level, learning about self-management strategies and programs at the individual level; the importance of social support from caregivers at the interpersonal level; the perennial theoretical framework guiding chronic care in the 21st century, the Chronic Care Model, at the organizational level; the use of promotores/as and community health workers to effect change at the community level; and the various policies that have the ability to affect management of chronic disease at each level of the Social Ecological Framework. As chronic illness becomes more of an issue in the United States and throughout the world, the health system must be prepared to manage, treat, and control the symptoms and consequences of these chronic conditions.

Review Questions

1. What is the difference between a modifiable and nonmodifiable risk factor for chronic disease?

2. What is the definition of chronic disease management?

3. (T/F) Health literacy refers to the degree to which prescribed medication is correctly taken by a patient.

4. What does the Chronic Care Model component of delivery system design entail?
   a. The use of electronic medical records
   b. Transforming care from a reactive approach to a proactive approach
   c. Community support
   d. Effective use of health expenditure

5. What are some of the benefits to using a community health worker/lay health advisor/promotore/a de salud model in chronic disease self-care management?

6. What are the components used to measure an individual's access to health care?
   a. Presence of disease
   b. Health insurance coverage
   c. Economic resources
   d. Only B and C
   e. All of the above

7. (T/F) An example of culturally competent care is when a provider speaks the same language as the patient.

8. Self-efficacy is important in chronic disease management interventions because:
    a. It prevents one from being depressed.
    b. It is one's own perceived confidence in managing their disease.
    c. It is one's perceived confident in their spouse's ability to manage their disease.
    d. It promotes social support for chronic disease management.

9. Which of the following chronic diseases were not discussed in this chapter?
    a. Diabetes
    b. Arthritis
    c. Obesity
    d. Asthma

Web Resources

Visit the following websites to learn more about some of the topics presented in this chapter.

The following websites offer information applicable to health practitioners, patients and caregivers alike:

The Community Guide (http://www.thecommunityguide.org). From the Community Services Preventive Task Force, this resource provides evidence-based research and systematic reviews of health promotion–related programs for use in the community.

Healthy People 2020 (www.healthypeople.gov). Detailed information on U.S. national health objectives guided by evidence-based research in the areas of chronic illness and communicable/acute diseases.

Healthcare.gov (www.healthcare.gov). Comprehensive resource on the Patient Protection and Affordable Care Act, including information on the most important provisions of the law and the health insurance marketplace.

The Cochrane Reviews (www.cochrane.org/cochrane-reviews). Systematic reviews that provide evidence-based evaluation of health policies and intervention efforts (including for treatment and prevention).

The National Alliance for Caregiving (www.caregiving.org). Provides support for caregivers of chronically and acutely ill individuals.

IMPACT Program (impact-uw.org). Comprehensive resource page with information and program materials for the preeminent depression-care program targeting older adults. The resources available are primarily for clinicians and other health providers.

The Institute of Medicine (www.iom.edu). Information on research and policy related to health issues in the United States.

Stanford Self-Management Courses and Resources (patienteducation.stanford.edu/programs/). Further information on the preeminent chronic disease self-management programs available.

Chronic Disease–Specific Resources

National Heart, Lung, and Blood Institute (www.nhlbi.nih.gov) and ***American Heart Association*** (www.heart.org) for more information on cardiovascular diseases, including hypertension and heart attack.

National Heart, Lung, and Blood Institute (www.nhlbi.nih.gov) and ***American Lung Association*** (www.lung.org) for more information on pulmonary diseases, including asthma and COPD.

National Diabetes Education Program (ndep.nih.gov) and ***American Diabetes Association*** (www.diabetes.org) for more information on diabetes mellitus type 1 and type 2.

National Cancer Institute (www.cancer.gov) and ***American Cancer Society*** (www.cancer.org) for more information on cancer.

National Institute of Arthritis and Musculoskeletal and Skin Diseases (www.niams.nih.gov) and ***Arthritis Foundation*** (www.arthritis.org) for more information on arthritis.

Alzheimer's Disease Education and Referral Center (www.nia.nih.gov/alzheimers) and ***Alzheimer's Association*** (www.alz.org) for more information on Alzheimer's disease.

National Institute of Mental Health (www.nimh.nih.gov) and ***National Alliance on Mental Illness*** (www.nami.org) for more information on mental illness, including depression.

References

Agency for Healthcare Research and Quality. (2008). *2007 National Healthcare Disparities Report* (AHRQ Pub. No. 08-0041). Rockville, MD: U.S. Department of Health and Human Services, Agency for Healthcare Research and Quality.

Alzheimer's Association. (2013). *What is Alzheimer's?* Retrieved on May 20, 2013, from http://www.alz.org/alzheimers_disease_what_is_alzheimers.asp

American Cancer Society. (2013). *Cancer facts & figures 2013.* Atlanta, GA: Author.

American Cancer Society. (2014). *Cancer facts & figures 2014.* Atlanta, GA: Author.

Anderson, R. M., & Funnell, M. M. (2010). Patient empowerment: Myths and misconceptions. *Patient Education and Counseling, 79*(3), 277–282.

Anderson, G., & Horvath, J. (2004). The growing burden of chronic disease in America. *Public Health Reports, 119*(3), 263–270.

Anderson, L. M., Scrimshaw, S. C., Fullilove, M. T., & Fielding, J. E. (2003). The Community Guide's model for linking the social environment to health. *American Journal of Preventive Medicine, 24* (3S), 12–20.

Ayala, G. X., Vaz, L., Earp, J. A., Elder, J. P., & Cherrington, A. (2010). Outcome effectiveness of the lay health advisor model among Latinos in the United States: An examination by role. *Health Education Research, 25* (5), 815–840.

Bayliss, E. A., Steiner, J. F., Fernald, D. H., Crane, L. A., & Main, D. S. (2003). Description of barriers to self-care by persons with comorbid chronic diseases. *Annals of Family Medicine, 1* (1), 15–21.

Buie, V. C., Owings, M. F., DeFrances, C. J., & Golosinky, A. (2010). National Hospital Discharge Survey: 2006 Summary. *Vital Health Statistics, 13* (168), 1–79.

California Endowment, The. (2003). *Principles and recommended standards for cultural competence education of health care professionals.* Woodland Hills, CA: Author.

Centers for Disease Control and Prevention (CDC). (1999). *Leading causes of death, 1900–1998.* National Center for Health Statistics, Atlanta, GA.

Centers for Disease Control and Prevention (CDC). (2009a). *The power of prevention: Chronic disease . . . the public health challenge of the 21st century.* Retrieved February 22, 2012, from http://www.cdc .gov/chronicdisease/pdf/2009-power-of-prevention.pdf

Centers for Disease Control and Prevention (CDC). (2009b). *Wee Wheezers asthma education program.* Retrieved February 22, 2012, from http://www.cdc.gov/asthma/interventions/wee_wheezers _programcomponents.htm.

Centers for Disease Control and Prevention (CDC). (2011a). *Arthritis—data and statistics.* Retrieved on May 20, 2013, from http://www.cdc.gov/arthritis/data_statistics.htm

Centers for Disease Control and Prevention (CDC). (2011b). *National diabetes fact sheet: National estimates and general information on diabetes and prediabetes in the United States, 2011.* Atlanta, GA: United States Department of Health and Human Services Centers for Disease Control and Prevention.

Centers for Disease Control and Prevention (CDC). (2013a). *Heart disease fact sheet.* Atlanta, GA: United States Department of Health and Human Services Centers for Disease Control and Prevention.

Centers for Disease Control and Prevention (CDC). (2013b). *High blood pressure fact sheet.* Atlanta, GA: United States Department of Health and Human Services Centers for Disease Control and Prevention.

Coleman, K., Austin, B. T., Brach, C., & Wagner, E. H. (2009). Evidence on the chronic care model in the new millennium. *Health Affairs, 28* (1), 75–85.

Committee on Quality of Health Care in America, Institute of Medicine (IOM). (2001). *Crossing the quality chasm: A new health system for the 21st century.* Washington, DC: National Academies Press.

Eiser, C. (1997). Effects of chronic illness on children and their families. *Advances in Psychiatric Treatment: Journal of Continuing Professional Development, 3,* 204–210.

DeNavas-Walt, C. Proctor, B. D., & Lee, C. H. (2005). *Income, poverty, and health insurance coverage in the United States: 2004* (U.S. Census Bureau, Current Population Reports, P60-229). Washington, DC: U.S. Government Printing Office.

DeNavas-Walt, C., Proctor, B. D., & Smith, J. C. (2011). *Income, poverty, and health insurance coverage in the United States: 2010* (U.S. Census Bureau, Current Population Reports, P60-239). Washington, DC: U.S. Government Printing Office.

DeVoe, J. E., Wallace, L. S., & Fryer, Jr., G. E. (2009). Measuring patients' perceptions of communication with healthcare providers: Do differences in demographic and sociodemographic characteristics matter? *Health Expectations, 12* (1), 70–80.

Green, L. W., & Fielding, J. (2011). The U.S. Healthy People initiative: Its genesis and its sustainability. *Annual Review of Public Health, 32,* 451–470.

Haas, B. (1999). A multidisciplinary concept analysis of quality of life. *Western Journal of Nursing Research, 21* (6), 728–742.

Hoffman, C. B., & Paradise, J. (2008). Health insurance and access to health care in the United States. *Annals of the New York Academy of Sciences, 1136,* 149—160.

Holman, H., & Lorig, K. (2004). Patient self-management: A key to effectiveness and efficiency in care of chronic disease. *Public Health Reports, 119*(3), 239–243.

Hoyert, D. L., & Xu, J. (2012). *Deaths: Preliminary data for 2011. National vital statistics report,* Vol. 61, no. 6. Hyattsville, MD: National Center for Health Statistics.

Hunkeler, E. M., Katon, W., Tang, L., Williams, Jr., J. W., Kroenke, K., Lin, E. H. Harpole, L. H., Arean, P., Levine, S. Grypma, L. M., Hargreaves, W. A., & Unützer, J. (2006). Long-term outcomes from the IMPACT randomized trial for depressed elderly patients in primary care. *British Medical Journal, 332*(7536), 1–5.

Institute of Medicine. (2012). *Living well with chronic illness: A call for public health action.* Washington, DC: National Academies Press.

Katon, W., & Guico-Pabia, C. J. (2011). Improving quality of depression care using organized systems of care: A review of the literature. *Primary Care Companion to CNS disorders, 13* (1). doi: 10.4088 /PCC.10r01019blu

Katon, W., Lin, E. H., Von Korff, M., Ciechanowski, P., Ludman, E., Young, B., Rutter, C., Oliver, M., & McGregor, M. (2010). Integrating depression and chronic disease care among patients with diabetes and/or coronary heart disease: The design of the TEAMcare study. *Contemporary Clinic Trials, 31* (4). 312–322.

Kung, H. C., Hoyert, D. L., Xu, J. Q., & Murphy, S. L. (2008). Deaths: Final data for 2005. *National Vital Statistics Report 2008,* 56(10), 1–121.

Levy, J. (2014). *U.S. uninsured rate drops to 13.4%: Uninsured rate down nearly four percentage points since late 2013.* Retrieved August 30, 2014 from http://www.gallup.com/poll/168821/uninsured-rate -drops.aspx

Lorig, K. R., Mazonson, P. D., & Holman, H. R. (1993). Evidence suggesting that health education for self-management in patients with chronic arthritis has sustained health benefits while reducing health care costs. *Arthritis and Rheumatism, 36* (4), 439–446.

Lujan, J., Ostwald, S. K., & Ortiz, M. (2007). Promotora diabetes intervention for Mexican Americans. *The Diabetes Educator, 33* (4), 660–670.

McEvoy, P., & Barnes, P. (2007). Using the chronic care model to tackle depression among older adults who have long-term physical conditions. *Journal of Psychiatric and Mental Health Nursing, 14*(3), 233–238.

Meischke, H., Lozano, P., Zhou, C., Garrison, M. M., & Christakis, D. (2011). Engagement in "My Child's Asthma,' an interactive web-based pediatric asthma management intervention. *Int J Med Inform, 80* (11), 765–774.

Millman, M. (Ed.). (1993). *Access to health care in America.* Washington, DC: National Academies Press.

National Alliance for Caregiving. (2009). *Caregiving in the U.S.: Executive summary.* Retrieved on March 1, 2012, from http://www.caregiving.org/research/caregiving-research/general-caregiving.

National Cancer Institute. (2009). *FactSheet: BRCA1 and BRCA2: Cancer risk and genetic testing.* Retrieved on May 17, 2013 from http://www.cancer.gov/cancertopics/factsheet/Risk/BRCA.

National Cancer Institute. (2013). *FactSheet: Genetic testing hereditary cancer syndromes.* Retrieved on June 17, 2013 from http://www.cancer.gov/cancertopics/factsheet/Risk/genetic-testing.

National Center for Environmental Health. Division of Environmental Hazards and Health Effects. (2012). *Asthma's impact on the nation.* Retrieved on August 7, 2014, from http://www.cdc.gov/asthma/impacts_nation/

Nielsen-Bohlman, L., Panzer, A. M., & Kindig, D. A. (Eds.). (2004). *Health literacy: A prescription to end confusion.* Washington, DC: National Academies Press.

Oprea, L., Braunack-Mayer, A., Rogers, W. A., & Stocks, N. (2010). An ethical justification for the Chronic Care Model (CCM). *Health Expectations, 13* (1), 55–64.

Ôunpuu, S., Chambers, L. W., Patterson, C., Chan, D., & Yusuf, S. (2001). Validity of the United States Behavioral Risk Factor Surveillance System's health-related quality of life survey tool in a group of older Canadians. *Chronic Diseases in Canada, 22* (3–4), 93–101.

Parekh, A. K., & Barton, M. B. (2010). The challenge of multiple comorbidity for the US health care system. *Journal of the American Medical Association, 303* (13), 1303–1304.

Rosland, A., & Piette, J. D. (2010). Emerging models for mobilizing family support for chronic disease management: A structured review. *Chronic Illness, 6* (1), 7–21.

Siminoff, L. A., Graham, G. C., & Gordon, N. H. (2006). Cancer communication patterns and the influence of patient characteristics: Disparities in information-giving and affective behaviors. *Patient Education and Counseling, 62* (3), 355–360.

Steinman, L. E., Frederick, J. T., Prohaska, T., Satariano, W. A., Dornberg-Lee, S., Fisher, R., Graub P. B., Leith K., Presby K., Sharkey J., Snyder S., Turner D., Wilson N., Yagoda L., Unutzer J. & Snowden, M. (2007). Recommendations for treating depression in community-based older adults. *American Journal of Preventive Medicine, 33* (3), 175–181.

Szefler, S. J. (2001). Challenges in assessing outcomes for pediatric asthma. *Journal of Allergy and Clinical Immunology, 107* (S5), S456–S464.

Thompson, J. R., Horton, C., & Flores, C. (2007). Advancing diabetes self-management in the Mexican American population: A community health worker model in a primary care setting. *The Diabetes Educator, 33* (S6), 159S–165S.

Unützer, J., Katon, W., Callahan, C. M., Williams, J. W., Jr., Hunkeler, E., Harpole, Hoffing, M., Della Penna, R. D., Noel, P. H., Lin, E. H., Arean, P. A., Hegel, M. T., Tang, L., Belin, T. R., Qishi, S., & Langston, C. (2002). Impact investigators. Improving mood-promoting access to collaborative treatment. Collaborative care management of late-life depression in the primary care setting: A randomized controlled trial. *Journal of the American Medical Association, 288* (22), 2836–2845.

U.S. Department of Health and Human Services Office of Disease Prevention and Health Promotion. (2012). *What is health literacy?* Retrieved on March 14, 2012, from http://www.health.gov/communication/literacy/quickguide/.

U.S. Department of Health and Human Services Office of Disease Prevention and Health Promotion. (2013). *Healthy People 2020.* Retrieved on May 22, 2013, from http://www.healthypeople.gov/2020.

U.S. Department of Health and Human Services Office of Minority Health. (2002). Teaching cultural competency in health care: A review of current concepts, policies and practices. Retrieved on August 5, 2014, from http://minorityhealth.hhs.gov/assets/pdf/checked/1/em01garcia1.pdf

Wagner, E. H., Austin, B. T., Davis, C., Hindmarsh, M., Schaefer, J., Bonomi, A. (2001). Improving chronic illness care: Translating evidence into action. *Health Affairs, 20* (6), 64–78.

Whittemore, R., Melkus, G. D., & Grey, M. (2004). Applying the social ecological theory to type 2 diabetes prevention and management. *Journal of Community Health Nursing, 21* (2), 87–99.

Wilson, S. R., Fish, L., Page, A., & Starr-Schneidkraut, N. (1994). *Wee Wheezers: An educational program for parents of children with asthma under the age of seven.* Palo Alto, CA: American Institutes for Research.

World Health Organization. (2012). *Depression: What is depression?* Retrieved March 21, 2014, from: http://www.who.int/topics/depression/en/

World Health Organization. (2013). *A global brief on hypertension: Silent killer, global public health crisis.* Geneva, Switzerland: Author.

Chapter 8

Maria Luisa Zúñiga, PhD and Isela Martinez, BA

HUMAN IMMUNODEFICIENCY VIRUS AND SEXUALLY TRANSMITTED INFECTIONS

Key Terms

acquired immune deficiency syndrome (AIDS)

CD4 cells

comorbidities

drug addiction

drug resistance

health behavior model

health disparity

HIV–related stigma

human immunodeficiency virus (HIV)

medication adherence

migration

post-exposure prophylaxis

pre-exposure prophylaxis (PrEP)

risk behaviors

structural intervention

vulnerable populations

Learning Objectives

Upon completion of this chapter, you should be able to:

1. Describe basic characteristics and global health impact of the Human Immunodeficiency Virus (HIV) and sexually transmitted infections (STIs).
2. Identify risk behaviors associated with HIV and STI transmission and acquisition.
3. Recognize basic elements of health behavior models used to guide HIV/STI prevention programs and research.

4. Distinguish behavioral and structural interventions to prevent HIV/STI transmission.

5. Explain the role of HIV and STI testing in stemming transmission.

6. Describe how HIV– and STI–related risk behaviors are measured and monitored.

7. Indicate which populations are disproportionately impacted by HIV and STIs and why they are disproportionately impacted.

8. Identify policy-level approaches to reduce HIV/STI transmission.

9. Discuss global health challenges to eliminating HIV and STIs.

Chapter Outline

HIV, AIDS, and STIs
> *Other Routes of Exposure to HIV*
> *The Global Health Impact of HIV and STIs*

Health Behavior Theories and Models Used to Guide HIV/STI Prevention Programs and Research
> *Characteristics of Effective HIV–Prevention Interventions*
> *Applying the Social Ecological Framework to HIV–Prevention Interventions*
> *Improving Patient Antiretroviral Medication Adherence*
> *Prevention of HIV and STI Transmission*
> *Health Disparities in HIV and STIs*
> *HIV and STI Global Health Policies*
> *Global Health Challenges to Eliminating HIV and STIs*

INTRODUCTION

human immunodeficiency virus (HIV) is the virus that impacts an individual's immune system by destroying specific blood cells (see *CD4 cells* definition below) that are crucial to helping the body fight disease.

acquired immune deficiency syndrome (AIDS) is a term used to indicate when HIV has impacted an individual's immune system to the extent that their CD4+T-cell count falls below a certain threshold. It is an advanced stage of HIV infection when a person's immune system is damaged and has difficulty fighting diseases and certain cancers.

Diseases transmitted through sexual contact date back thousands of years. These sexually transmitted infections (STIs) such as chlamydia, gonorrhea, and syphilis are acquired by more than 4.3 million people in the United States each year. You are most likely to hear news about **Human Immunodeficiency Virus (HIV)** infections (with about 48,100 new cases diagnosed in the United States every year; Centers for Disease Control and Prevention, HIV in the United States: At a glance, 2013a). Unlike most STIs, HIV and the advanced form of infection, **Acquired Immune Deficiency Syndrome (AIDS)**, can be managed but not cured. Over the last 20 years, HIV has had a devastating impact on millions of persons, both in the United States and throughout the world. HIV has been termed an "exceptional disease" because it has proven a particularly elusive and adaptable bug that destroys an individual's immune response system and, consequently, his or her ability to fight off disease. HIV shares some similarities with other STIs in terms of the risk-transmitting behaviors, but unlike other STIs, it can also spread through sharing needles used to inject drugs or vitamins and through transfusions using blood that has not been properly treated to kill microorganisms such as HIV. This chapter will discuss HIV and common STIs with the broader goal of considering the types of behaviors that put individuals at risk for acquiring HIV and STIs. Protective behaviors and interventions that prevent transmission will also be discussed, and three **health behavior models** (i.e., frameworks) will be introduced that can help us understand how to approach behavior change to reduce likelihood of transmitting infections. The chapter closes with thoughts on why HIV/STIs impact some communities more than others (i.e., HIV–related health disparities) and a brief review of HIV–global health policies.

health behavior models or theories are frameworks that help us explain and predict human behavior and are especially helpful when planning health promotion programs

HIV, AIDS, AND STIs

AIDS was first identified in the mid-1980s when physicians started to report AIDS symptoms in homosexual patients. HIV, the virus that causes AIDS, was not identified until 1983 (CDC, 2014a). "HIV/AIDS" are often written together, but it is important to understand the distinction. HIV refers to the actual infection with the virus and includes individuals at any stage of illness. An AIDS diagnosis means that someone living with HIV shows specific signs associated with advanced stages of illness. AIDS or AIDS–defining illness is designated for individuals whose blood shows a very low number of specific white cells (the T4 lymphocyte) that are much higher in noninfected persons and/or those who have specific illnesses that are a direct result of having low white blood cell counts. Examples of AIDS–defining illnesses include Kaposi's sarcoma (KS; a specific type of cancer that causes abnormal tissue to grow under the skin, the lining of the mouth, nose, and throat, and other organs), tuberculosis, and wasting (extreme loss of body weight), among others. With the availability of new HIV therapies and opportunities to connect people to HIV treatment once they are diagnosed with HIV, many individuals are able to maintain their immune systems and lead healthy, productive lives.

A person is diagnosed as HIV positive after getting tested for HIV and the result indicates that the virus is present in the blood. There are specific indicators of how the body responds to infection and how sensitive HIV tests are to detecting the virus that are beyond the scope of this chapter. For detailed information about getting tested for HIV and what the testing process involves, please visit the Centers for Disease Control and Prevention (CDC) website at http://www.cdc.gov/actagainstaids.

STIs refer to infections transmitted by sexual contact. This is why HIV can be considered a sexually transmitted infection. HIV can also be transmitted in nonsexual ways such as from mother to child (described later in this chapter). However, unlike other STIs, HIV has a devastating impact on an individual's immune system. It is important to remember that all types of STIs, including HIV, can be stigmatizing and make people feel embarrassed or ashamed to seek medical care or obtain support from others.

The most common STIs are chlamydia, gonorrhea, and syphilis. These three diseases are responsible for about 4.3 million infections per year in the United States. Each of these STIs is very different in terms of the type of agent and type of infection that it causes. Chlamydia is the most commonly reported STI in the United States. Caused by the bacterium *Chlamydia trachomatis*, chlamydia is known as a "silent" disease because the majority of infected people exhibit no symptoms. Chlamydia can damage a woman's reproductive organs and, if untreated, can cause infertility (CDC, 2014b). Gonorrhea is almost as common as chlamydia and is also caused by bacteria that can grow easily in a woman's reproductive tract, both men and women's urethras, as well as a person's mouth, throat, eyes, and anus. The symptoms for gonorrhea may be mild and can be mistaken for urinary tract infections, although most women do not experience any symptoms. In men, symptoms can include a burning sensation when urinating or white, yellow, or green discharge from the penis. Anyone having sex is at risk for acquiring an infection, and an untreated pregnant woman can spread it to her baby during childbirth (CDC, 2014c). Chlamydia and gonorrhea are particularly common among adolescents and young adults because these individuals may have less access to accurate information and testing resources (CDC, 2014c). Syphilis is another STI caused by a bacterium, but it can cause long-term complications or death if left untreated or if treated inadequately. Although less common than chlamydia and gonorrhea, syphilis is a public health concern. Syphilis is contracted through direct contact with sores and through sexual contact with an infected person, as well as from mother to child during childbirth. Syphilis is particularly worrisome because of its prevalence among men who have sex with men (MSM), who comprise 67% of all cases (CDC, 2014d). The end of this chapter includes a list of references that provide more information on HIV and STIs.

> **risk behaviors** are behaviors that place a person at risk for poor health. For HIV, this includes activities in which people engage that place them at risk for acquiring HIV (e.g., using drugs and/or alcohol before having sex, having unprotected sex, and using contaminated syringes).

Because HIV/STIs are included in most health curricula, you are likely familiar with the types of **risk behaviors** that are associated with HIV/STI transmission. Most common are unprotected (i.e., without using a condom) vaginal, anal, and oral sex. The CDC's website on HIV/AIDS has an extensive number of web-based resources that contain complete information about HIV, chlamydia, gonorrhea, and syphilis, including individuals at highest risk for infection due to unprotected sexual and drug-using behavior. For example, HIV infection among persons who use methamphetamine is very common because use of this drug increases sexual appetite while severely impairing judgment that may otherwise foster use of condoms. Because of such high HIV risk among individuals who use methamphetamine, substantial research has been devoted to determining how to work with this population to reduce their risk for HIV acquisition (i.e., getting infected) and, if they are positive, engaging the persons into HIV care and drug addiction treatment to reduce the risk that they transmit the virus to an uninfected person.

Other Routes of Exposure to HIV

Throughout the world, mother-to-child transmission is the most common way that children become infected with HIV. In the absence of any health interventions (e.g., access to antiretroviral medication), the likelihood that transmission of HIV from an HIV–positive pregnant woman to the fetus or infant can be anywhere from 25% to 48% (De Cock et al., 2000). Transmission of HIV from mother to child can occur under three different conditions: during the pregnancy (in utero), during birth, and during breastfeeding. If an HIV–positive woman is able to receive the antiretroviral medication she needs while pregnant, have a caesarean section before she is in labor, receive infant formula and the family support needed to avoid breastfeeding, then the likelihood of passing the virus to the infant becomes very small (1%–2%; Sturt et al., 2010).

Other HIV transmission routes include transmission through use of contaminated syringes (i.e., needles) or drug paraphernalia among injection drug users or through use of contaminated syringes used for injectable medications or vitamins. Health workers may be exposed to HIV through needle-stick injuries in the workplace.

The Global Health Impact of HIV and STIs

As mentioned in the introduction, the global health impact of HIV has been profound, especially in Sub-Saharan Africa, where 68% of the world's HIV–infected individuals live (Joint United Nations Programme on HIV/AIDS [UNAIDS], 2010). In order to better understand the impact of HIV in the United States and around the world, it is critical to understand how primary transmission routes (i.e., infection routes) vary by country and region. Remember that HIV can be transmitted among men who have sex with men, heterosexual contact, mother-to-child transmission, through sharing contaminated needles, and through blood transfusion. In the United States, most individuals living with HIV were infected by male-to-male sexual contact (CDC, 2013b); however, the most common transmission routes differ by community. For example, among Latinos of Puerto Rican background, the predominant transmission category is through sharing infected syringes, but among African-American women, the exposure is predominantly through unprotected heterosexual sex. The primary transmission route in Sub-Saharan Africa is through heterosexual contact, but infected persons in Sub-Saharan Africa include children, women, and men.

HEALTH BEHAVIOR THEORIES AND MODELS USED TO GUIDE HIV/STI PREVENTION PROGRAMS AND RESEARCH

Drawing from a combination of the theories and models summarized in Zúñiga, Strathdee, Blanco, and Patterson (2010), we learn that an effective behavior-change intervention requires the following key components:

1. A clearly defined target behavior (e.g., consistent condom use for vaginal sex with a new sex partner)

2. Knowledge on the individual's part about the behavior (e.g., What can a condom prevent? How is a condom properly used?)

3. Sufficient importance to the individual or community to warrant adoption of the behavior (this incorporates elements of perceived risk and motivation to change).

4. Adequate skill and confidence on the individual's part to carry out the behavior on his or her own (e.g., self-efficacy).

5. Individual belief in the value of the anticipated outcome (i.e., outcome expectancy).

6. Adequate access to materials (e.g., condoms, sterile needles for injection drug users, or IDUs) or environments (e.g., HIV testing centers) needed to carry out or adopt the behavior.

7. Ability to anticipate barriers beyond the individual's control that could inhibit change in behavior and to formulate plans to overcome those barriers (e.g., prohibitive cost, laws or regulations, cultural beliefs or taboos, and stigma).

Characteristics of Effective HIV–Prevention Interventions

Evaluation of HIV–prevention interventions in target populations (e.g., youth; IDUs; persons with high-risk sexual behavior) has helped to identify several key characteristics of successful interventions (Kirby, Laris, & Rolleri, 2007; Lyles et al., 2007a, 2007b; Nation et al., 2003). A variety of factors can make it challenging to identify effective intervention characteristics, including differences in intervention design, data reporting methods, and evaluation methods (Lyles et al., 2007a). It is important that intervention results be clearly defined and measurable (e.g., a person's viral load, how frequently she takes the HIV medications as prescribed, etc.) and must match the intended outcome (Lyles et al., 2007b). For example, an intervention to improve antiretroviral (ARV) therapy adherence should consider biological markers such as the number of specialized infection-fighting white blood cells (CD4 cells) in a person's immune system, viral load, or viral resistance, whereas an intervention to reduce syringe sharing among IDUs should consider whether the outcome of interest is receptive sharing (i.e., using a borrowed or rented syringe that someone else has already used), distributive needle sharing (i.e., passing on a used syringe to others), or both. Clearly, receptive sharing poses a risk to self, whereas distributive sharing poses a risk to others.

CD4 cells or T-cells are specialized white blood cells in the human immune system that help fight infections. These cells send signals to activate the body's immune response when they detect a virus (like HIV).

Health promotion programs to prevent HIV transmission should include a variety of approaches that engage the target community. For example, since knowledge alone does not necessarily translate into sustained behavioral change, rather than provide only educational information (e.g., how to use a condom), successful programs should include skill-building activities (e.g., participants use a model to practice correct condom placement). Second, programs should include different types of approaches to learning depending on the audience to be reached. For example, when working with a youth population, you might consider using social networking or Internet-based interventions that are more relevant to this population in order maintain the target population's interest. Effective group-level programs may have a single facilitator, but this facilitator may need to adapt his message and encourage different types of learning depending on the participants' needs (e.g., using videos, games, role playing, and scenarios for practicing risk-reduction negotiations). Third, any prevention program needs to provide enough instruction (also known as the "intervention dose") to produce the desired effect. How much instruction is needed should be based on knowledge of and relevant experience with the target population. For example, it would be unrealistic to expect children of elementary school age to stay interested in a lecture about HIV/AIDS that lasted several hours. Fourth, effective programs should optimally match the target population's needs. Administering an intervention at the time of highest possible impact (e.g., education about sexual health and HIV risk behaviors prior to sexual debut in youth) would be such an example.

Applying the Social Ecological Framework Model to HIV–Prevention Interventions

When thinking about who is at higher risk for acquiring HIV or an STI, it is helpful to use the Social Ecological Framework as a reference. The Social Ecological Framework (SEF) has to do with understanding health and health behavior from individual, interpersonal, community, and environmental/structural/policy levels. This model helps us to understand that people do not live or make decisions about HIV prevention or HIV care in isolation but that they will be influenced by how they feel, their relationships (e.g., family and sexual partners), community/societal norms (e.g., stigmatizing attitudes toward people living with HIV), and public health systems or policies (e.g., availability of HIV/STI testing centers).

Figure 8-1 applies the Social Ecological Framework to HIV testing behavior in order to illustrate examples of influential factors at each level of the model that could determine whether an individual is tested for HIV. At the *individual level*, a person may avoid HIV testing because he does not have enough information about HIV (i.e., limited knowledge) or may not know that HIV can be effectively treated and HIV–positive individuals can lead healthy, productive lives. At the *interpersonal level*, HIV–testing behavior may be influenced by family or sexual partner perceptions about HIV that could promote or inhibit testing behaviors. For example, if a person's sexual partner was recently tested for HIV, she may encourage the individual to also get tested. At the *community/societal level*, we may see the influence of social norms and perceptions about HIV, including stigmatizing attitudes that may inhibit HIV testing. In this case, individuals may be reluctant to get tested for fear that their community will judge or reject them if they learn that the individual is HIV positive. In the broadest sphere, we consider *environmental/policy-level* influences on HIV testing. Environmental/policy-level influences on behavior includes factors that are structural (e.g., location of testing centers is far away), organizational (e.g., testing location hours are not convenient), or policy driven (e.g., adolescents need parent permission to get tested). For example, in order for an individual to get an HIV or STI test, there must be HIV/STI testing centers to which the person has access. Federal, state, or local health policies can promote HIV testing and influence testing norms.

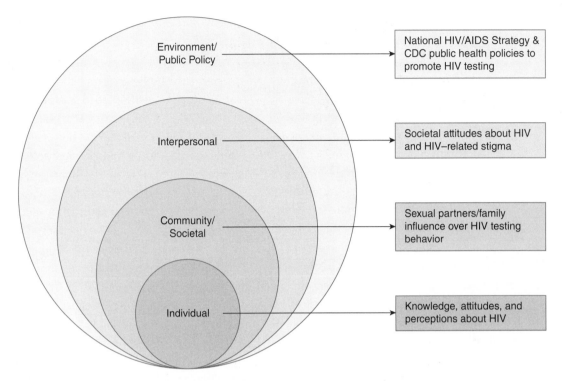

FIGURE 8–1 Social Ecological Framework Applied to HIV Testing Behavior

In 2006, the CDC revised HIV testing guidelines to recommend HIV testing of individuals during all routine health visits and in settings such as drug treatment centers (Branson et al., 2006).

Improving Patient Antiretroviral Medication Adherence

In general, there are several factors that enter into the equation of whether a person is able to take his medications as prescribed. The ability of an HIV–positive person to take his medications at the correct time and dose each day (at least 95% of the time) is very important in order to reduce the amount of HIV circulating in the person's blood (i.e., viral load). A low or very low level of virus in the blood (e.g., where standard laboratory tests are unable to detect the virus in the blood) leads to improved health and well-being of the individual and makes it far less likely that the individual could transmit HIV through unprotected sex or sharing syringes with someone who is not HIV positive. The following example uses levels of the SEF to highlight important factors that favor high medication adherence to antiretroviral therapy.

Prevention of HIV and STI Transmission

What makes HIV so difficult to control? About 20% of the 1.2 million people in the United States who are living with HIV infection do not know that they are

Model for Understanding

Because cell phone access and use are very common, especially among young persons, researchers have been studying the application of cell phone technology to help HIV–positive individuals adhere better to their medications. To this effect, Dowshen and colleagues (2012) pilot tested a cell phone text messaging intervention to improve adherence to antiretroviral therapy among a small sample ($N = 25$) of HIV–positive youth in a U.S. clinic. Eligible youth were HIV positive, age 14 to 29 years, used a personal cell phone, were English speaking, and reported having problems adhering to their HIV medications. Youth who enrolled in the study worked with the study coordinator to create their own personalized Short Message Service (SMS) text reminder messages, which were programmed through the study's website to be delivered daily at specified times for the patient. Participants also created a personalized reminder message for 1 hour later to determine whether they took the medication. Participants were asked to respond via text message whether they took their medications. The pilot study showed that the personalized, interactive, daily text reminders were acceptable to the youth and that they significantly improved self-reported adherence. Importantly, participants who completed the study said they wanted to continue to receive text messages, as almost all said that the text messages were very helpful for them to miss fewer doses of their medication (Dowshen et al., 2012). This pilot study illustrates the potential effect that interventions can have at the individual level to make a difference in adherence. Although cell phone–mediated interventions to promote adherence are still being developed and tested, it is important to see how researchers are focusing on the technology we use in our daily lives to help us take better care of ourselves.

HIV–related stigma is a socially driven negative attitude toward or response to individuals living with HIV. This type of attitude may build upon and reinforce other negative attitudes about marginalized behaviors, such as sex work, drug use, and homosexual and transgender sexual practice. Stigma can have negative repercussions on the health and well-being of individuals who are stigmatized.

infected (CDC, 2013a). As with many diseases that are spread person to person, individuals may carry and transmit HIV without realizing it. One reason is that when people do not know that they are infected, they continue to engage in unprotected sex or share contaminated syringes, which increases the opportunity for transmitting the virus to an uninfected person. Frequently the problem is more complicated. There are many reasons some individuals who have received an HIV–positive test result do not go for care. One of the most important reasons is **HIV–related stigma**; individuals may feel socially excluded and ashamed to be HIV positive, feel stigmatized about having HIV, or fear that others may find out that they are HIV positive. These individuals have been known to delay care (Pollini et al., 2011). HIV–related stigma comes from deeply rooted negative feelings that many societies have against particular groups or behaviors. For example, homosexual men and injection drug users are communities that are frequently ostracized, blamed, and associated with HIV transmission. HIV–positive women may also feel stigmatized because of the perception that their sexual behavior exposed them to the virus; women may feel judged and delay getting the health care that they need. In what follows, we discuss why women represent a group with particular vulnerabilities to HIV.

Other issues that complicate stopping HIV transmission include denial about being HIV positive and concern that one may not be able to afford treatment. Although HIV–related stigma and concerns about being able to afford care are very real, most countries, including the United States, have made enormous strides in making health care and treatment available to those who need it. Importantly, one of the most critical times to get an HIV–positive person into care is at the time she is diagnosed. Research shows that when you offer to help a newly positive person make an appointment for care or are able to go with her to her appointment, she will be more likely to engage in her HIV care (Gilman et al., 2012). The problem is that offering this level of support to newly diagnosed HIV–positive persons is not always feasible due to staffing shortages. In the United States, routine HIV testing (also called routine screening) is part of the National HIV/AIDS Strategy to stop HIV transmission. The CDC recommends that individuals who are seen for any type of health care should get tested for HIV.

Once a person has started to receive HIV care and is able to obtain her HIV medications (i.e., antiretroviral therapy), the next critical step is to make sure that she has access to her medications and is able to take her pills as prescribed. The connection between the behavior of taking one's antiretroviral medicine as prescribed (i.e., **medication adherence**) and HIV transmission is important. Over time, when a person is able to take her HIV medicine as prescribed, this usually reduces the amount of circulating HIV in the person's blood to a very, very small amount. When the amount of virus in a person's blood is so small that it cannot be measured by laboratory test, the person's HIV is said to be "undetectable," which means that the likelihood of transmitting HIV to others, even if she has sex without a condom, is low. Offering HIV medication as soon as possible to newly diagnosed people is known as a **structural intervention** to reduce HIV transmission in a population. Achieving and sustaining high antiretroviral adherence, however, is not an easy battle for persons living with HIV.

If you have ever had to take antibiotics over several days, even when you feel better, you may appreciate how hard medication adherence can be. Now try to imagine yourself having to take medications every day for the rest of your life. Although many living with HIV have successfully figured out how to take their medications with very high adherence, many face barriers to taking their medications as they would like to. Some of the challenges include HIV–related stigma—having to hide the fact that he is taking pills for fear that someone may find out he is HIV positive. Some individuals lose access to their pills if their health care insurance gets cancelled. These are a few of the many reasons that make it difficult (but not impossible) to stop HIV transmission.

Stopping HIV transmission is a complicated matter. First and foremost, people need to know their HIV status. They also need adequate support to get HIV care, to keep taking their medications as prescribed, and to continue using condoms and clean syringes if they use injected drugs. Public health policies are needed that promote the type of testing and health care environment that help HIV–positive people succeed in caring for themselves, but this can be very costly, and in many countries, HIV is one of several important diseases that compete for public resources, which makes stopping HIV transmission a challenging public health

medication adherence involves following a recommended medication regimen closely every day: taking the correct dose of a medication and at the correct time as prescribed by a clinician. High medication adherence to HIV treatment is critical to the health of the individual and can contribute to decreased HIV transmission at the community level.

structural intervention is an action or a series of actions designed to reduce or remove barriers to health or health behavior. In terms of HIV prevention, structural interventions may address physical, social, cultural, organizational, community, economic, legal, or policy barriers that contribute to HIV transmission.

endeavor. The following section discusses the difference between primary and secondary prevention, behavioral strategies that have been used to prevent transmission, and clinical strategies to combat HIV, such as treatment as prevention.

HIV–prevention interventions (programs designed to stop the transmission of HIV) include strategies to keep uninfected persons from becoming infected (this could be at any of the four levels of the Social Ecological Framework). Prevention efforts can include promoting HIV testing so that uninfected persons are aware of their HIV status and can take precautions to reduce risk of future infection. Prevention could also be in the form of individual behavioral counseling for HIV–negative persons who engage in behaviors that place them at risk for HIV infection (individual level of the Social Ecological Framework).

Prevention among individuals who are already living with HIV is designed to provide a timely HIV–positive test result so that they know they are infected with HIV and engage them into HIV care as soon as possible. Because getting people into care and on antiretroviral treatment is very effective at reducing HIV transmission, getting individuals linked to care and on treatment is a critical part of HIV prevention. Among populations of persons living with HIV, other prevention strategies may include reducing risk behaviors (e.g., increasing consistent condom use). When newly HIV–positive persons obtain timely access to antiretroviral medications and are able to lower the amount of virus in their bodies to undetectable levels, transmission of HIV can be avoided. This approach is called "treatment as prevention" because by *treating* recently diagnosed HIV–positive individuals with antiretroviral therapy as soon as possible and promoting widespread coverage of ARVs among HIV–infected populations, one can *prevent* HIV transmission and substantially reduce the number of individuals infected with HIV at the community level (Wood, 2012).

Health Disparities in HIV and STIs

health disparity is a difference in the incidence, prevalence, mortality, or burden of disease that is observed in specific subgroups when compared to the health status of the general population.

vulnerable populations are populations who may be at increased risk for HIV acquisition by virtue of conditions such as their socio-economic status, gender, age, disability status, and risk status related to low access to condoms or other effective prevention of HIV.

A **health disparity** is when there is a disproportionate disease burden on one group versus another group or when a group is overrepresented in a disease in comparison to their proportion of the population. This may be an observable difference in health conditions (e.g., greater disease), health outcomes, or access to care in a population subgroup when compared to a larger group. Health disparities (also known as inequities in health) are unfortunately very common in HIV. From our discussion so far, you can see that there are **vulnerable populations** that are at higher risk for HIV or STIs than others. For example, if we look to see which populations in the United States are most impacted by HIV infection, we would see that risk groups are gay, bisexual, and other men who have sex with men (individuals who may not identify as gay) and individuals who use injection drugs. There may also be some at-risk groups you have not considered. HIV transmission among heterosexual women is also a consideration. For some women, their only risk factor is being married or being in a monogamous sexual relationship—that is, they may have a partner who is an injection drug user or who has been exposed to HIV through sexual contact, and the female partner is then exposed to the virus.

HIV has disproportionately affected U.S. minority populations, especially African Americans. African Americans represent 14% of the U.S. population; however, they account for about 44% of new HIV infections (CDC, 2013c).

Factors that contribute to vulnerability to becoming HIV infected are very complex. For individuals who are injection drug users, it may seem obvious that if a person is going to inject a drug, she should use a clean syringe. Using our Social Ecological Framework as a framework, we might see that at the individual level, the person is facing an addiction to drugs and may not know where to get clean syringes. She may also not have money to purchase them. At the interpersonal level, her social and sexual network may include other injection drug users or individuals with high-risk sexual behavior, some of whom are infected with HIV and may not know it. If there is sharing of contaminated syringes, the likelihood of transmitting the virus is higher. If an individual lives in an environment that does not provide access to clean syringes or does not have easily accessible, effective, and affordable drug treatment programs, these factors may limit the individual's opportunities to use clean syringes and receive treatment for her addiction, which can lead to HIV–transmitting behavior. You can see from this example the role that socioeconomic factors can play in HIV transmission. Individuals who live in impoverished conditions do not have access to many protective factors that would help reduce their risk of acquiring HIV or STIs. Poverty is one of the main underlying contributors to transmission of HIV and STIs in the United States and worldwide.

Critical Thinking

Think about the steps you would take to promote access to clean syringes and promote uptake of substance use treatment in an underserved community in which addiction to heroin or other injectable drugs is problematic. What key questions would need to address at the individual, community, and environmental/structural/policy levels in order to provide access to clean syringes and addiction treatment? With which agencies would you work to accomplish your health promotion goals?

HIV and STI Global Health Policies

As research provides new insights into effective programs and interventions to help uninfected persons stay disease free (primary prevention) and help individuals who are infected achieve and maintain the best health possible (secondary prevention), this allows for improved federal and global policy-level efforts to reduce HIV/STI transmission and the burden of HIV.

In the last few years, new HIV–prevention strategies have focused on getting people tested for HIV on a routine basis and promoting testing as soon as possible

SPOTLIGHT

Special Considerations for Interventions that Prevent Transmission of HIV

Purpose

- Interventions should include **clearly defined and measurable outcomes** (e.g., frequency of unprotected sex, frequency of using a clean syringe to inject drugs, how often HIV–positive individuals are able to take their HIV medications as prescribed, etc.).

Health Disparities and Target Populations

- Health disparities are common among individuals at risk for and living with HIV.
- Populations most impacted by HIV may vary by country and region and often include vulnerable populations such as people living in extreme poverty, children of HIV–positive mothers, and injection drug users.
- Effective interventions should be tailored to specific subpopulations, include a variety of approaches, and match the target population's needs.

Social Ecological Framework

- It is important to understand HIV at different levels, including individual, interpersonal, community, and environmental/structural/policy levels.
- Effective interventions should recognize that people do not live or make decisions about HIV prevention or HIV care in isolation; individuals are influenced by how they feel, their relationships, community/societal norms, and public health systems or policies.

HIV–Related Stigma

- Individuals may feel ashamed to be HIV positive or fear that others may find out that they are HIV positive and discriminate against them.
- HIV–related stigma comes from deeply rooted negative feelings that many societies have against particular groups or behaviors.
- When engaging HIV–positive populations in HIV interventions, showing respect, sensitivity, confidentiality, and privacy are of utmost importance.

Global Health Challenges

- Effective interventions should consider that mobile populations, such as migrants, may live in high-risk environments (e.g., easy and inexpensive access to drugs or alcohol) and lack social support and access to health care and information that place them at very high risk for acquiring and or transmitting HIV or STIs.

pre-exposure prophylaxis (PrEP) is an HIV–prevention strategy for individuals who are at high risk for acquiring HIV. PrEP involves taking one combination antiretroviral pill every day to reduce the risk of becoming infected with HIV.

post-exposure prophylaxis involves taking antiretroviral medication as soon as possible after exposure to HIV to decrease the chance that a newly exposed person will become infected.

migration is the movement of a person or a group of persons, either across an international border or within a country. This population mobility could encompass any kind of movement of people, regardless of the length of time they move, the composition of mobile groups, and causes of mobility. Migration includes refugees, victims of natural disasters, economic migrants, and persons moving for other purposes such as for family reunification.

comorbidities are the presence of more than one disease or condition in the same person at the same time. Conditions described as comorbidities are often chronic or long-term conditions. Other names to describe comorbid conditions are coexisting or co-occurring conditions. For example, tuberculosis could be a comorbid condition among individuals living with HIV.

when someone suspects she may have been exposed to HIV. The newest strategy is called "test and treat," which involves starting HIV treatment as soon as possible (versus waiting until the person has lower immune function or health problems due to HIV). This strategy was developed based on research that shows that by getting as many HIV–positive persons as possible on treatment as soon as possible, you are lowering the amount of circulating virus in the population (Hull, Wu, & Montaner, 2012). There is evidence that this approach could be very effective as a national policy to reduce disease transmission, and it is currently recommended by the CDC as a comprehensive policy to prevent HIV through testing, getting HIV–positive persons into HIV care, and helping them start antiretroviral treatment as soon as possible.

Promising prevention avenues to stem HIV transmission include **pre-exposure prophylaxis** and **post-exposure prophylaxis**. Pre-exposure prophylaxis (PrEP) is a relatively new HIV–prevention strategy used with HIV–uninfected individuals who are at high risk for acquiring HIV. PrEP involves taking antiretroviral medication (a combination medication currently available in one pill) every day to reduce their risk of becoming infected with HIV. PrEP requires high medication adherence to work properly; research has shown that when the medication is taken consistently, it reduces risk of HIV infection among adults with sexual or injection-drug use behavioral risk. Post-exposure prophylaxis is an HIV–prevention strategy for individuals who believe they may have been exposed to HIV through sexual, injection drug use, or other nonoccupational exposure. Also referred to as "nonoccupational post-exposure prophylaxis" (nPEP), current CDC guidelines indicate that this prevention strategy must be initiated within 72 hours after the individual believes he was exposed to HIV (e.g., had unprotected sex with someone who is HIV positive). Individuals with potential exposure are given antiretroviral medication to prevent them from acquiring HIV. Research is still needed to understand how PrEP and nPEP can work at a population level, but these strategies offer a promising avenue of research.

Global Health Challenges to Eliminating HIV and STI

drug addiction is a chronic disease characterized by the compulsive use of a substance (e.g., alcohol or drug) despite negative or dangerous personal or societal impact.

In considering some of the global health challenges to managing HIV and reducing transmission, countries with high unemployment may also have high **migration** of their population to other countries. Migration is a well-documented risk factor for high-risk sexual behavior (Sanchez et al., 2012). Migrants may live in high-risk environments (e.g., easy and inexpensive access to drugs or alcohol) and lack social support and access to care and information and have other factors that place them at very high risk for acquiring HIV or STIs. Because HIV lowers your immune system's capacity to fight off infection, individuals who are HIV positive may also be at very high risk for other diseases such as tuberculosis. When you have diseases that are highly linked, this is known as **comorbidities** or co-occurring diseases. **Drug addiction** is another co-occurring disease that exposes individuals to higher-risk behavior and HIV or STI infection (e.g., less likelihood of using a condom when under the influence of alcohol or a drug). Addictions also complicate the health of individuals who are living with HIV. For example, someone with a drug or alcohol addiction may not remember to take his medications on time and may suffer from poorer health than another HIV–positive person who does not have an addiction. Individuals who do not take their medications as prescribed may also have problems with the medication not effectively working on the HIV; this is called drug resistance. **Drug resistance** is a global health problem because there are only certain drugs that work on HIV, so if a person has a drug-resistant strain of HIV, he may have more limited options about which drugs will work for him. Infections can be even harder to treat if they are drug resistant. This is the case for HIV, STIs, and many other infections.

> **drug resistance** occurs when microorganisms such as bacteria, viruses, fungi, and parasites change in ways that reduce the medication's effectiveness to cure or treat the health problem. HIV drug resistance may occur if antiretroviral treatment is not taken as prescribed (e.g., when medication doses are missed).

Summary

HIV and STIs present an enormous health challenge and burden to the United States as well as to the global community. Primary and secondary prevention play a major role in stopping transmission of HIV and STIs, and there are significant behavioral as well as environmental factors that influence how well an intervention may work. Treatment as prevention is a promising avenue to reducing HIV transmission among people who test HIV positive; however, this will require effective engagement of at-risk populations into testing, making sure that individuals have timely access to HIV treatment and care, and seeing that they are supported to take their medications as prescribed. As HIV is treatable, it is considered a chronic condition. Paying for lifelong treatment of HIV represents a large economic burden on many countries. As research progresses and availability of lower-cost drugs increases, however, better and more accessible treatments are on the horizon. Public health practitioners will also be in a better position to help individuals avoid infection and help keep infected persons healthy and support them in their efforts to not transmit the virus.

CASE STUDY 8-1

Interpersonal Level of the SEF: Couples Voluntary Counseling and Testing (CVCT) in Africa (Allen et al., 2003)

Supporting heterosexual couples to reduce HIV transmission from the infected to the uninfected partner is crucial, especially in regions where heterosexual contact continues to be the main mode of HIV transmission (e.g., Sub-Saharan Africa; El-Bassel & Wechsberg, 2012). There is convincing evidence that couples voluntary counseling and testing (CVCT) interventions have the potential to prevent more than two thirds of new HIV infections. Testing centers that are sensitive to couples can provide a supportive environment in which testing and disclosure can be privately discussed, where a couple can learn safe-sex negotiation skills and discuss gender differences, imbalances, and expectations. These sites may be particularly useful for women who are fearful, uncomfortable, or unable to negotiate safer sexual practices with their partner (El-Bassel & Wechsberg, 2012). Allen and colleagues (2003) conducted a study of 818 couples in Lusaka, the capital of Zambia, where one in five cohabiting couples is serodiscordant (i.e., one partner is HIV positive and the other is negative). This research team found that sexual behavior changed after couples participated in CVCT. Before receiving their HIV test results, less than 3% of discordant couples had reported condom use with each other, whereas after CVCT, condom use increased to more than 80% among couples. More importantly, this percentage remained stable throughout more than 1 year of follow-up. Among couples in which the man was HIV positive, the couple had less frequent intercourse but were more likely to use a condom 100% of the time. This is significant because in areas where women may have a more difficult time negotiating condom use, the CVCT may be promoting greater willingness to use condoms among men who know they are HIV positive. Although the study also found that unprotected intercourse was frequently underreported, after the intervention, discordant couples complied with condom use fairly well. Couple-based voluntary counseling and testing has worked so well to decrease HIV–transmission rates among heterosexual couples in Africa that it has become a reduction strategy in the Unites States and is being modified for interventions with couples who are men who have sex with men.

Thought Questions

1. Even when individuals understand that their behavior places them at risk for acquiring or transmitting HIV/STI, what factors make it difficult for many to reduce their risk behaviors and adopt behaviors that favor prevention? What considerations should a public health professional make when trying to work with individuals with high-risk behaviors?

2. What modifications must take place in order to foster success of an intervention such as CVCT in a different country?

8-2

CASE STUDY

Community/Societal Level of the SEF: Reducing HIV Transmission Among Injection Drug Users in Vancouver, Canada (Tyndall et al., 2006)

In 2003, Canada was the first North American country to pilot test a medically supported safer injection facility (SIF) in response to high rates of HIV and hepatitis C among injection drug users (IDUs) in Vancouver. The goal of the SIF was to reduce syringe sharing and use of contaminated injection equipment that might transmit HIV or hepatitis C to other IDUs, their sexual partners, and their families (e.g., mother-to-child transmission). The SIF was implemented as a harm-reduction strategy that provided IDUs with sterile syringes and clean injection equipment in a controlled environment (e.g., staffed by public health professionals and counselors trained to work with IDUs). Because the SIF provided services that were culturally relevant to IDU populations in the region, the SIF attracted a large number of Aboriginal people, a group disproportionately affected by HIV in Canada. The SIF then became a point of service for this community and other marginalized groups, creating an important public health opportunity to engage populations at very high risk for HIV with health and social services, including HIV–prevention education and referrals to other services such as counseling and detoxification.

Thought Questions

1. What are some of the challenges to implementing structural-level interventions?

2. Can you think of any local policies that would aid/hinder the implementation of a structural-level intervention such as a safer injection facility?

CASE STUDY 8-3

Environment/Public Policy Level of the SEF: HIV/AIDS National Health Policy in Brazil: "From the bottom up" (Berkman et al., 2005; World Health Organization [WHO], 2004)

Brazil's National AIDS Program (NAP) is a leading example of a country-level, integrated HIV/AIDS prevention, care, and treatment program. Although efforts to stem HIV transmission and increase access to HIV care among Brazil's most vulnerable communities were initiated in the late 1980s, it was changes in Brazil's political landscape in the 1990s that fostered government collaboration with communities and health and social service practitioners. The NAP has successfully reduced transmission of HIV and, in the last decade, decreased HIV mortality rates by 50% (Berkman et al., 2005). As democracy reemerged in the 1990s, there was a rebirth of societal involvement with the government. This process led to involvement of many different sectors of society (e.g., persons living with HIV, gay persons, health professionals, etc.) that together set the priorities for the National Unitary Health System (SUS [Portuguese acronym]). Pressure from nongovernmental organizations and local governments on the federal government was vital in the creation of an AIDS program that would reflect the view of health care as a human right, which is recognized in the Brazilian constitution. The Brazilian government acknowledged that health care is a central responsibility of the government and refused to comply with international agencies such as the International Monetary Fund and the World Bank for loans that would require them to slash public spending expenditures as part of their economic policies. Brazil was the first developing country to implement a large-scale universal antiretroviral access program, which started in the early 1990s and became federal law in 1996 (WHO, 2004).

By targeting HIV-related stigma and discrimination and strengthening sexual rights and expression, the Brazilian NAP was able to make HIV–prevention programs more effective by virtue of being culturally appropriate and relevant. In this way, HIV–prevention programs could address sexuality more openly than in other countries and be much more impactful. Additionally, local initiatives at the municipal and state levels included harm-reduction strategies such as SIFs and viewing drug use as a public health issue rather than a criminal justice one, which led to better control of the HIV epidemic. The Brazilian initiative successfully reduced HIV transmission and substantially improved care; however, in order to implement this program in other countries, it will need to be adapted to the countries' cultural, social, political, and resource contexts.

Thought Questions

1. What cultural-, social-, political-, and resource-context adaptations would be necessary for the Brazilian initiative to succeed in a country such as the United States?

2. Why don't more countries that are affected by HIV at a similar level adopt initiatives such as Brazil's?

Review Questions

1. Which of the following is/are associated with HIV transmission?

    a. Crowded living conditions
    b. Lack of access to clean syringes among injection drug users
    c. Having active tuberculosis
    d. Having an STI
    e. a, b, and c
    f. b, c, and d
    g. All of the above

2. Which of the following should be supported as a primary prevention strategy among people already living with HIV to prevent HIV transmission to others?

    a. Consistent condom use
    b. Seeking drug treatment if addicted
    c. Promoting high antiretroviral medication adherence
    d. Disclosure of HIV status to new partners
    e. All of the above are important strategies to prevent transmission.

3. Which of the following responses is a critical component of the HIV testing process?

    a. Offer HIV–negative persons a brochure on how to prevent contracting HIV.
    b. Promote frequent HIV testing among persons who test HIV negative.
    c. Provide persons who test HIV positive with a brochure about clinics in the area.
    d. Offer to make a clinic appointment for persons who test HIV positive.

4. Which of the following is NOT generally considered primary prevention?

    a. Condom use

    b. Syringe exchange programs

    c. HIV testing

    d. Prevention education with high-risk populations

5. Which of the following health conditions is considered a common comorbidity with HIV?

    a. Drug addiction

    b. Tuberculosis

    c. Hepatitis C

    d. STIs

    e. All of the above

6. An effective HIV–prevention intervention program should include which of the following?

    a. Skill-building activities

    b. Diverse learning approaches tailored to the learner

    c. Adequate "intervention dose"

    d. All of the above

7. _____ refers to the legislative, regulatory actions taken by local, state, or federal governments that are meant to influence behavior by promoting specific behaviors or inhibiting others.

    a. Environmental support

    b. Policy

    c. Community support

    d. None of the above

8. Prevention of mother-to-child HIV transmission should include:

    a. Timely access to antiretroviral medication for the mother

    b. Infant-care classes that teach the mother how to breastfeed

    c. Performing a cesarean section to deliver the child

    d. Both a and b

    e. Both a and c

9. Current efforts to stop HIV transmission include:

    a. Pre-exposure prophylaxis

    b. Early HIV testing

    c. Early HIV treatment for people who have been recently diagnosed with HIV

    d. Promoting high adherence to antiretroviral medications

    e. All of the above

10. Treatment as prevention is a promising avenue to reducing HIV transmission among people who test HIV positive and will require which of the following?

    a. Effective engagement of at-risk populations into HIV testing
    b. Making sure that individuals have timely access to HIV treatment and care
    c. Providing social support for individuals to take their medications as prescribed
    d. All of the above

Web Resources

Visit the following websites to learn more about some of the topics presented in this chapter.

Centers for Disease Control and Prevention: HIV Fact Sheets http://www.cdc.gov/hiv/resources/factsheets/

Centers for Disease Control and Prevention: Chlamydia Fact Sheet http://www.cdc.gov/std/chlamydia/STDFact-Chlamydia.htm

Centers for Disease Control and Prevention: Gonorrhea Fact Sheet http://www.cdc.gov/std/gonorrhea/STDFact-gonorrhea.htm

Centers for Disease Control and Prevention: Syphilis Fact Sheet http://www.cdc.gov/std/syphilis/STDFact-Syphilis.htm

Centers for Disease Control and Prevention: Pre-Exposure Prophylaxis (PrEP) http://www.cdc.gov/hiv/prevention/research/prep/

References

Allen, S., Meinzen-Derr, J., Kautzman, M., Zulu, I., Trask, S., Fideli, U., Musonda, R., Kasolo, F., Gao, F., & Haworth, A. (2003). Sexual behavior of HIV discordant couples after HIV counseling and testing. *AIDS, 17*(5), 733–740.

Berkman, A., Garcia, J., Muñoz-Laboy, M., Paiva, V., & Parker, R. (2005). A critical analysis of the Brazilian response to HIV/AIDS: lessons learned for controlling and mitigating the epidemic in developing countries. *Am J Public Health, 95*(7), 1162–1172. Epub 2005 Jun 2.

Branson, B. M, Handsfield, H. H., Lampe, M. A., Janssen, R. S., Taylor, A. W., Lyss, S. B., Clark, J. E., & Centers for Disease Control and Prevention (CDC). (2006). Revised recommendations for HIV testing of adults, adolescents, and pregnant women in health-care settings. *MMWR Recomm Rep., 55*(RR-14), 1–17; quiz CE1-4.

Bronfenbrenner, U. (1994). Ecological models of human development. *International Encyclopedia of Education* (Vol. 3, 2nd ed.). Oxford: Elsevier.

Centers for Disease Control and Prevention. (2008). HIV Surveillance Report, 2008; vol. 20. http://www.cdc.gov/hiv/topics/surveillance/resources/reports/.

Centers for Disease Control and Prevention. (2013a). HIV in the United States: At a glance. http://www.cdc.gov/hiv/statistics/basics/ataglance.html. Accessed August 2014.

Centers for Disease Control and Prevention. (2013b). HIV Incidence. http://www.cdc.gov/hiv/statistics/surveillance/incidence/. Accessed August 2014.

Centers for Disease Control and Prevention. (2014a). HIV basics. http://www.cdc.gov/hiv/basics/index.html. Accessed August 2014.

Centers for Disease Control and Prevention. (2014b). Sexually transmitted diseases. Fact sheet: Chlamydia. http://www.cdc.gov/std/chlamydia/stdfact-chlamydia.htm. Accessed August 2014.

Centers for Disease Control and Prevention. (2014c). Sexually transmitted diseases. Fact sheet: Gonorrhea. http://www.cdc.gov/std/gonorrhea/STDFact-gonorrhea-detailed.htm. Accessed August 2014.

Centers for Disease Control and Prevention. (2014d). Sexually transmitted diseases. Fact sheet: Syphilis. http://www.cdc.gov/std/syphilis/stdfact-syphilis.htm. Accessed August 2014.

De Cock, K. M., Fowler, M. G., Mercier, E., de Vincenzi, I., Saba, J., Hoff, E., Alnwick, D. J., Rogers, M., & Shaffer, N. (2000). Prevention of mother-to-child HIV transmission in resource-poor countries: translating research into policy and practice. *JAMA : the journal of the American Medical Association, 283*(9), 1175–82. [PUBMED: 10703780]

Dowshen, N., Kuhns L. M., Johnson, A., Holoyda, B. J., & Garofalo, R. (2012). Improving adherence to antiretroviral therapy for youth living with HIV/AIDS: a pilot study using personalized, interactive, daily text message reminders. *J Med Internet Res., 14*(2), e51.

El-Bassel, N., & Wechsberg, W. M. (2012). Couple-based behavioral HIV interventions: Placing HIV risk-reduction responsibility and agency on the female and male dyad. *Couple and Family Psychology: Research and Practice, 1*(2), 94–105.

Gilman, B., Hidalgo, J., Thomas, C., Au, M., & Hargreaves, M. (2012). Linkages to care for newly diagnosed individuals who test HIV positive in nonprimary care settings. *AIDS Patient Care STDS, 26*(3),132–140.

Hull, M. W., Wu, Z. & Montaner, J. S. (2012). Optimizing the engagement of care cascade: A critical step to maximize the impact of HIV treatment as prevention. *Curr Opin HIV AIDS*, 7(6):579-86. doi: 10.1097/COH.0b013e3283590617.

Joint United Nations Programme on HIV/AIDS (UNAIDS). (2010). *Global report: UNAIDS report on the global AIDS epidemic 2010*. ISBN 978-92-9173-871-7 Retrieved from http://www.unaids.org/globalreport/documents/20101123_GlobalReport_full_en.pdf.

Kirby, D. B., Laris, B. A., & Rolleri, L. A. (2007). Sex and HIV education programs: Their impact on sexual behaviors of young people throughout the world. *Journal of Adolescent Health, 40*, 206–217.

Lyles, C. M., Kay, L. S., Crepaz, N., Herbst, J. H., Passin, W. F., Kim, A. S., Rama, S. M., Thadiparthi, S., DeLuca, J. B., & Mullins, M. M. (2007a). Best-evidence interventions: Findings from a systematic review of HIV behavioral interventions for US populations at high risk, 2000-2004. *American Journal of Public Health, 97*, 133–143.

Lyles, C. M., Crepaz, N., Herbst, J. H., Kay, L. S., & The HIV/AIDS Prevention Research Synthesis Team. (2007b). Evidence-based behavioral prevention from the perspective of the CDC's HIV/AIDS Prevention Research Synthesis Team. *AIDS Education and Prevention, 18*(4SSA), 21–31.

Nation, M., Crusto, C., Wandersman, A., Kumpfer, K. L., Seybolt, D., Morrissey-Kane, E., & Davino, K. (2003). What works in prevention: Principles of effective prevention programs. *American Psychologist, 58*, 449–456.

Pollini, R. A., Blanco, E. B., Crump, C., Zúñiga, M. L. (2011). A community-based study of barriers to HIV care initiation. *AIDS Patient Care and STDs, 25*(10), 601–609.

Sanchez, M. A. L., Hernández, M. T., Hanson, J. E., Vera, A., Magis-Rodríguez, C., Ruiz, J. D., Garza, A. H., Castañeda, X., Aoki, B. K., & Lemp, G. F. (2012). The effect of migration on HIV high-risk behaviors among Mexican migrants. *J Acquir Immune Defic Syndr, 61*(5), 610–607. doi: 10.1097/QAI.0b013e318273b651.

Sturt, A. S., Dokubo, E. K., & Sint, T. T. (2010). Antiretroviral therapy (ART) for treating HIV infection in ART-eligible pregnant women. *Cochrane Database Syst Rev.* (3): CD008440.

Tyndall, M. W., Wood, E., Zhang, R., Lai, C., Montaner, J. S. G., & Kerr, T. (2006). HIV seroprevalence among participants at a supervised injection facility in Vancouver, Canada: Implications for prevention, care and treatment. *Harm Reduction Journal, 3*(36). Accessed November 2012 at http://www.harmreductionjournal.com/content/pdf/1477-7517-3-36.pdf.

Wood, E., Milloy, M. J., & Montaner, J. S. (2012). HIV treatment as prevention among injection drug users. *Curr Opin HIV AIDS, 7*(2), 151–156.

World Health Organization. (2004). *The world health report 2004: Changing history.* Available at: http://www.who.int/whr/2004/en/.

Zúñiga, M. L., Strathdee, S. A., Blanco, E., & Patterson, T. L. (2010). Community HIV preventive interventions. In Suls, J., Kaplan, R. M., & Davidson, K. W. (eds.), *Handbook of health psychology.* New York: Guilford Press.

Chapter 9

Joe Smyser, PhD, MSPH and John P. Elder, PhD, MPH

TROPICAL INFECTIOUS DISEASE

Key Terms

agent	host	vector
asymptomatic	hydrocele	vector-borne diseases
bacteria	infectious diseases	
bacterial infections	ITNs	vertical control programs
chronic diseases	lesions	
elephantiasis	Lymphedema	viral infections
endemic	ministries of health	virus
entomological surveillance	tropical infectious diseases	World Health Organization (WHO)

Learning Objectives

Upon completion of this chapter, you should be able to:

1. List at least six of the diseases in the World Health Organization's Special Programme for Research and Training in Tropical Diseases disease portfolio (TDR).

2. Describe "epidemiological transition."

3. Describe the treatment of diarrheal diseases and the main age group they affect.

4. Identify at least three of the six challenges in public health disease control.

Chapter Outline

INTRODUCTION

infectious diseases are illnesses that are caused by an organism such as a virus, bacteria, parasite, or fungus (otherwise known as pathogens).

A **virus** is an infectious pathogen many times smaller than bacteria that replicates inside an organism's cells.

bacteria are one-celled (unicellular) microorganisms, some of which are harmful to humans.

tropical infectious diseases are diseases that occur solely or principally in the tropics.

WHO stands for the World Health Organization, the United Nations public health arm.

Infectious diseases are illnesses caused by an organism such as a **virus, bacteria,** parasite, or fungus. Infectious diseases can occur anywhere and cause illness in any population, though some are more common in certain parts of the world and among certain groups of people. This chapter focuses on those infectious diseases common to the Global South, or developing countries in tropical or subtropical regions. These countries receive a disproportionate burden of infectious disease when compared to wealthier nations, or those commonly referred to as "developed," or "more developed countries (MDC)." For this reason, the diseases covered in this chapter fall under the category of "**tropical infectious diseases**." According to the **World Health Organization (WHO)**, tropical diseases are "diseases that occur solely, or principally, in the tropics" (World Health Organization, 2011a). This definition is often extended to subtropical regions, or regions which are hot and humid.

A list of diseases classified as tropical infectious diseases is provided at the end of this chapter, along with descriptions provided by TDR. However, prior to examining the details of any of these particular diseases, it is important to understand the global environment in which they operate and current efforts by public health authorities to control and eradicate them.

THE EPIDEMIOLOGICAL TRANSITION

The concept of the *epidemiological transition* has been with us for more than three decades. Most of the age of human existence has been characterized by high fertility and high mortality rates, the latter spiking during times of famine, plague, and war. As Hobbes famously put it in *Leviathan*, human life was "solitary, poor, nasty, brutish and short" (Ch. 13, Para. 9). Life expectancy and population levels both remained fairly low until only two centuries ago. Orman (1971) and other seminal writers taking a historical perspective on mortality, fertility, and society noted that the West (especially northwestern Europe) witnessed a gradual reduction in mortality rates in the 18th century, largely due to a reduction in extreme poverty and improved nutrition. As fertility rate changes lagged behind mortality reduction for several decades, the West realized a major population boom in the 18th and 19th centuries, leveling off thereafter as fertility rates began to decline. This transition has been paralleled in other regions of the world over the past century, including in much of East Asia, the Middle East, and Latin America.

Orman (1971) characterizes these and other aspects of the epidemiological transition in terms of "propositions," three of which are:

1. Mortality and fertility rates explain most of the dynamics in population change;

2. Over periods of time, chronic "degenerative" diseases displace infectious disease pandemics as major causes of mortality, and the West and elsewhere have now left the "age of pestilence and famine" and entered the "age of degenerative and man-made disease"; and,

3. Improvements in mortality patterns have favored infants, children, and women.

> **chronic diseases** are incurable diseases that last a lifetime and typically advance slowly in the body.

However, some have challenged the current applicability of the epidemiological transition model. **Chronic diseases** are no longer the reserve of industrialized, prosperous, and well-fed societies, as witnessed by the globalization of cigarette smoking, obesity, and other public health challenges, reaching into the poorest nations (World Health Organization, 2012c). Socioeconomic inequality has grown alarmingly even in Western democracies, foreshadowing a possible regression to earlier and less favorable illness and mortality patterns even in the world's healthiest regions. Habitat destruction may lessen the planet's "carrying capacity," both in terms of reduced food production and global climate change, which alter the livability of large parts of the earth's surfaces. Infectious diseases, once considered "diseases of poverty," are not only expanding in terms of incidence but are increasingly demonstrating chronic disease aspects in that many are never truly cured (e.g., tuberculosis, HIV). At the same time, cancer and other chronic diseases may be caused by viral or bacterial infections. Thus, "infectious diseases" in general comprise a very heterogeneous category. This chapter presents some of the complexities in approaching these and other problems common to many tropical, developing countries.

INFECTIOUS DISEASE CONTROL

In 1974, the WHO announced the global eradication of smallpox, one of the great scourges of humankind into the 20th century. Polio and other killers seemed nearly ready to be consigned to public health history as well. However, the past 30 years have witnessed the advent of "emerging and reemerging infectious diseases," largely **bacterial** and **viral infections** that were initially thought to have been largely under control or that were considered almost completely the province of underdeveloped countries. With the explosion of the HIV/AIDS epidemic 30 years ago, which rapidly spread throughout Africa then East Asia, as well as the United States and other industrialized countries, public health experts became increasingly aware that diseases know few boundaries. Other infectious diseases such as malaria and dengue fever, spread by different types of mosquitoes, spread into urban and semirural areas as forests and other natural habitats have increasingly been destroyed and the human population has grown rapidly.

> **bacterial infection** is the invasion of bacteria into the body and subsequent growth/multiplication of the bacteria.
>
> **viral infection** is the invasion of a virus into the body and subsequent replication of the virus.

Perhaps forgotten in current "Western models" is that the profession of public health was largely developed to combat and control such diseases. The discipline of epidemiology had its roots in determining the causes of disease, such as in John Snow's determination of the drinking water source of a cholera epidemic in 18th-century London. Increasing military and economic expansion of the Imperial powers in the 19th century, such as colonization by Europeans of Africa and southern Asia and the building of the Panama Canal, required at least a modicum of "tropical hygiene." Over the past two centuries, infectious disease control has witnessed much progress plus a range of outcomes, including the following categories (Dowdle & Hopkins, 1998):

1. *Control.* Reduction of the incidence and prevalence of illness and death as a result of public health interventions.

2. *Elimination.* Reduction of disease incidence to a zero level, at least within defined geographic areas.

3. *Infection elimination.* Reduction of infection due to a specific agent to zero as a result of the elimination of that agent.

4. *Eradication.* The permanent reduction of disease incidence worldwide caused by the reduction of a specific agent to a zero level.

5. *Extinction.* The elimination of a specific agent both in a laboratory and in nature.

> An **agent** is an organic or nonorganic factor that causes disease, otherwise known as a pathogen.
>
> The **host** is the organism a parasite attaches itself to or lives within.

Infectious diseases involve the **agent** (bacterium or virus), the **host** (for our purposes, the human who becomes ill), and the mode of transmission. The latter includes human-to-human contact (e.g., sexual transmission of HIV), vector-borne transmission (e.g., through insects, animals, or birds), and vehicle-borne transmission (through air, water, food, etc.). The control of these diseases depends on the ability of public health to combat them through either early treatment or prophylactic services for the individual or prevention of the contact between the host and the agent or vector. This section reviews some of the previous efforts and challenges related to control of waterborne and **vector-borne diseases**. Although historically thought to be the province of clinical and public health experts, the emphasis of this next section is on the central role of health promotion and behavior change in reducing remerging diseases and diseases of poverty. Three examples of tropical diseases will be presented for purposes of comparison: infant and childhood diarrhea, malaria, and dengue.

> A **vector-borne disease** is a disease that is transmitted to humans via a carrier of a different species.

Diarrheal Diseases

Diarrhea is a symptom of numerous types of intestinal diseases among which the agent may be viral, bacterial, or parasitic. All children are likely to get diarrhea, as are most adults, at various points in their lives. Usually in well-nourished populations with access to clean water, the diarrheal episode is short lived and may not require special attention. In some cases however, especially in malnourished communities with limited access to clean water and medical services, responses to diarrhea should be immediate. This is especially the case in children under 5; diarrhea and resulting dehydration kill approximately 2 million children every year.

Most children who die from diarrhea actually die from dehydration and loss of nutrients associated with the infection. Dehydration, in turn, can be treated at home through a combination of liquids, salt, energy, and potassium. The form that these ingredients take may be found in some home-based remedies (even chicken soup). It may be especially effective if the parents use oral rehydration salts solutions (ORS), which are premixed powders available through pharmacies, clinics, and public health offices.

The concept of oral rehydration is a fairly simple one: mixing water with a powdered solution and feeding it to a baby or young child. However, the parent or caretaker using and feeding the solution must generally be well skilled with respect to how best to mix the solution, why and how to use clean water, determining correct proportions of powder and water to use, and how much to feed the child. Mastery of each of these techniques can mean the difference between recovery or prolonged illness or worse for the child. Most countries have found that it is necessary to educate a large number of community health workers or volunteers to spread the message about oral rehydration solution, as poor parents may have limited access to or may be unable to afford health services. Thus, the community health workers themselves must also be able to master the oral rehydration intervention. "Counseling cards" comprise one technique for improving both community health worker and caregiver skills among even semiliterate populations (Figure 9-1). These cards, typically large and laminated, afford the community health worker the possibility of visiting homes with a sick child to review with the caretaker step-by-step procedures for keeping a child healthy during bouts of diarrhea. Counseling cards have been shown to significantly improve both community health workers' and mothers' skills in Indonesia and elsewhere (Elder et al., 1992).

Malaria and Dengue: A Tale of Two Mosquitoes

A **Vector** is any living thing that carries an infectious agent.

Vector control typically comprises vertical programs to reduce the source of transmission. For example, yellow fever and malarial eradication programs primarily rely on the eradication of the mosquitoes implicated in these diseases. Specifically, larval production sites and house spraying with systemic insecticides can be successful if substantial administrative and political support is provided. However, for many vectors, such eradication is simply short-term control, as areas

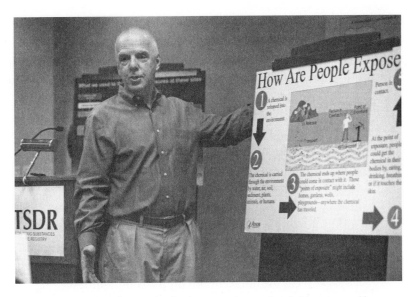

FIGURE 9–1 Counseling cards, also known as instructional aides, are used by health educators all over the world.

Source: Courtesy of Centers for Disease Control and Prevention/Dawn Arlotta

vertical control programs are focused on a specific disease, health issue, or population.

will become reinfested in a fairly short period of time. Thus, **vertical control programs** may be ineffective because individuals, families, and communities are not active partners in the control but rather passive participants in or recipients of the eradication effort (Gubler, 1988). Therefore, the true issue for vector control is not whether source reduction is effective but whether and how individual and community participation can be a part of that source-reduction effort (Winch et al., 1991). Public health's work is not performed "on" communities. Effective programs do not "parachute in," achieve short-term objectives, and then disappear. The heart of any public health program is the community it operates in, because health cannot be imposed by a small group of individuals, however well intentioned. Health is a human right and is therefore the collective responsibility of all.

The most prominent among vector-borne infectious diseases is malaria, which represents the greatest vector-borne disease threat in the world. Transmitted by the *Anopheles* mosquito, a nighttime biter, malaria causes more than one million deaths annually in Africa alone. Approximately one fourth of these cases comprise children under the age of 5 years old.

An **ITN** is an insecticide-treated bed net.

The two primary approaches to malaria control are transmission reduction and chemotherapy. Based on strong evidence that they reduce malaria transmission and related morbidity and child mortality, local and international organizations in Africa have been promoting and distributing insecticide-treated nets (ITNs) for more than two decades. Although this has resulted in greater ITN availability in sub-Saharan African countries, getting people to use ITNs correctly and consistently is difficult. Given the recognized gap between ITN ownership and use, designing effective strategies to promote use is critical, especially among children under 5 and pregnant women. In a recent attempt to inform the development of such strategies, Eisele and colleagues (2009) conducted an extensive review of standardized national surveys across 15 countries to document the factors associated with ITN use among these vulnerable groups. They concluded that there is increasing support for involving community health workers to go house to house to provide accurate information on malaria transmission, to explain how ITNs protect against malaria, and to help households hang their nets properly.

Not only is additional research needed to develop effective strategies for promoting ITN use, but such research should have sufficient internal and external validity for policy makers and consumers to make appropriate and informed decisions. The purpose of the Net Use Intervention (NUI) community trial, therefore, was (a) to identify how to bridge the gap between ITN ownership and use, (b) to identify the best mix of communication tools to affect the behavior of ITN owners to become consistent ITN users, and (c) to do so with optimal internal and external validity. The following presents the results of a multichannel, multisector intervention process conducted between June and August 2009 in southern Ghana and the impact of the interventions on the communities.

Insecticide-treated nets (ITNs) reduce malaria transmission and related morbidity and child mortality; however, incorrect and inconsistent use limits their protective factors. An experiment was used to evaluate a multichannel, multisector program over the course of 8 weeks. Health and education personnel used mobile vans to broadcast net use messages, involved drama groups who role played the need for and correct use of nets (Figure 9-2), and engaged volunteers, who went door to door to encourage their neighbors to correctly use nets and protect themselves (especially pregnant women and babies) every evening. The program resulted in an overall increase in ITN

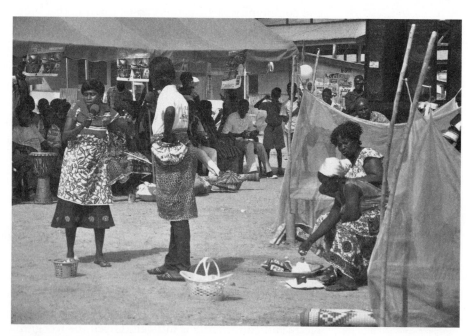

FIGURE 9-2 Community members in Ghana perform a scene to educate others on how and why to use bednets.

Source: Courtesy of USAID/Kasia McCormick

coverage of approximately one person per night per every two households. The promotion efforts succeeded well beyond the planners' expectations, not only promoting usage but also dramatically increasing demand for new ITNs (Elder et al., 2011).

Although also a disease borne by the mosquito vector, dengue fever prevention and control presents a very different and arguably more complex challenge than malaria. The *Aedes aegypti* mosquito is a daytime biter; thus, encouraging individuals to sleep under nets would have no impact on the disease. Instead, programs have typically involved complete vector control rather than individual protection, including **entomological surveillance**, breeding site reduction, and selective killing of adult mosquitoes, supported by health education. Such programs must be done throughout entire communities; however, as individuals or households that take up the challenge themselves will still be exposed to mosquitoes breeding nearby where no control measures have taken place. In many communities, residents often have other problems or priorities and are not interested in or able to take actions to prevent possible dengue transmission in their neighborhood. Some residents may be unaware of how dengue is transmitted, others may be unaware of the source of the vector mosquito, and still others may know where the *Ae. aegypti* mosquito is produced and how these sites can be controlled or eliminated but are not motivated to take preventive actions. And finally, even those who follow the recommended actions may still have *Ae. aegypti* or other mosquitoes in their houses and, worse yet, may suffer dengue infections since their neighbors do not participate in controlling domestic breeding sites, or they may get bitten by an infected mosquito at their place of work or study. As a result of some or all of these challenges, comprehensive community action is needed.

> **entomological surveillance** involves monitoring the location and number of disease vectors, such as mosquitoes, as well as eradication effectiveness.

Challenges in Implementing Infectious Disease Control

Childhood diarrhea and dehydration, malaria, and dengue control are three examples of common and deadly tropical diseases, resulting in millions of infections and deaths annually. However, these three illnesses present very different challenges for health promotion and public health in terms of the types of outcomes we can expect from individual and community interventions. These challenges can be summarized as follows:

- Is disease prevention feasible and effective?

- Can the disease be effectively treated?

- Can the mode of transmission be controlled or eliminated?

- Is individual action effective, or does the program need to be communitywide to have an impact?

- Can programs "go to scale," that is, can they be made to work in entire regions or populations?

- Are programs sustainable over a long period of time?

TABLE 9-1 Comparisons of Health Promotion Interventions for Tropical Disease Control per Types of Outcomes*

Dimension of Outcome	Disease		
	Diarrhea	**Dengue**	**Malaria**
Efficacy of prevention	2	3	1
Complexity of target behavior	2	3	1
Efficacy of treatment once disease is contracted	1**	3	2
Transmission/vector control	3	2	2
Possibility of protecting individual when larger groups are not protected	1	3	1
Scalability	1	3	2
Sustainability	2	2	2

**Refers to efficacy of treatment of dehydration, not diarrhea per se
*3 = least favorable rating; 1 = most favorable

The evidence for intervention outcomes varies for diarrhea, malaria and dengue, as shown in Table 9-1. In this table, the number 3 represents a least-favorable rating, with the number 1 representing most favorable. For instance, the evidence base for interventions designed to prevent malaria (rating of 1 in Table 9-1) is greater than those for diarrhea (rating of 2), which in turn is greater than those for dengue (rating of 3).

Decades of persistent efforts and commitment of resources have paid off for diarrhea and malaria, with oral rehydration, insecticide-treated nets, and other program elements making headway in reducing morbidity and mortality. Current control efforts for dengue have been relatively ineffective given the complexity of the target behavior and the questionable sustainability of efforts needed. Hopefully, progress in all three of these disease threats will continue, or at a minimum, they will not be exacerbated by overpopulation, environmental damage, and other interrelated challenges.

TDR DISEASE PORTFOLIO

As stated previously, infectious diseases are a heterogeneous group. This section provides details on a selection of tropical infectious diseases, with information taken almost exclusively from their corresponding WHO fact sheets. The WHO's Special Programme for Research and Training in Tropical Diseases, or TDR, "is a global programme of scientific collaboration that helps coordinate, support and influence global efforts to combat a portfolio of major diseases of the poor and disadvantaged" (World Health Organization, 2012e). The TDR's disease portfolio includes the following diseases:*

- African trypanosomiasis (sleeping sickness)

- Chagas

- Dengue

- Helminths

- Leishmaniasis

- Leprosy

- Lymphatic filariasis

- Malaria

- Onchocerciasis (river blindness)

- Schistosomiasis

- Tuberculosis (TB)

Sleeping Sickness

Occurring in 36 countries in sub-Saharan Africa, sleeping sickness is a vector-borne parasitic disease. This means that the disease is transmitted to humans via a carrier of a different species, or vector, while the agent of disease is a parasite. In the case of sleeping sickness, the vector is the tsetse fly, *Glossina* genus, which acquires the parasite, protozoa of the *Trypanosoma* genus, from either humans or other carrying animals (World Health Organization, 2010g; see Figure 9-3). Once bitten by the tsetse fly, a person develops flu-like symptoms within weeks. If left untreated, the parasite eventually attacks the central nervous system, resulting in neurological symptoms (brain function), loss of motor control (movement), and eventually death. There are two forms of sleeping sickness, the Gambiense and the Rhodesiense. In the Gambiense form, the disease typically takes years to fully affect the body, whereas the Rhodesiense form can result in death within months (World Health Organization, 2012f). As of 2011, the estimated number of cases of sleeping sickness was 30,000, although 2009, the most recent year of reporting, saw reported cases drop below 10,000 for the first time in 50 years (World Health Organization, 2010h). This drop was due to sustained prevention efforts by public–private partnerships including the WHO, pharmaceutical companies, nongovernmental organizations, and national organizations engaged in vector-control activities such as **ministries of health**.

ministries of health are government bodies in charge of public health nationally.

*The portfolio also includes sexually transmitted diseases and TB/HIV coinfection; however, these conditions will not be covered in this chapter. Additionally, there are many more tropical infectious diseases than are listed here.

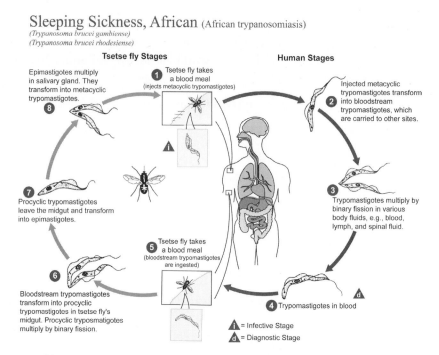

FIGURE 9–3 This illustration shows the life cycle of the parasitic agents that cause African sleeping sickness, or African trypanosomiasis.

Source: Courtesy of Centers for Disease Control and Prevention, DPDx/Alexander J. da Silva, PhD, Melanie Moser

Chagas Disease

endemic refers to a disease regularly found in a particular geographic area or population.

Chagas disease occurs mainly in Latin America, where it is **endemic** and is a vector-borne parasitic disease. Transmitted in the feces of triatomine bugs, or "kissing bugs," the protozoan parasite *Trypanosoma cruzi* currently infects an estimated 10 million people worldwide (World Health Organization, 2010f; see Figure 9-4). Triatomine bugs typically encounter humans when they emerge at night from exposed cracks in roughly constructed structures. The bugs feed on blood, biting into skin and then defecating near the wound they create while feeding. The parasites in their feces can come into contact with human blood, such as when a person rubs the area of a bite. Chagas disease can be transmitted person to person as well, in infected blood. Therefore blood transfusions, pregnancy and childbirth, organ transplants, and accidents where exposure to blood occurs can transmit Chagas disease, in addition to contact with triatomine bug feces (World Health Organization, 2010f). Chagas occurs in two stages, the first lasting from the moment a person is infected to approximately 2 months, characterized by flu-like symptoms and occasionally a skin lesion or swelling of the eyelids. The second stage is chronic, with the parasite slowly attacking the heart and digestive muscles over the course of years, which can lead to death.

Dengue and Dengue Hemorrhagic Fever

Dengue is a mosquito-borne infection caused by any of four different viruses. Dengue infects an estimated 50 million people worldwide every year, though it

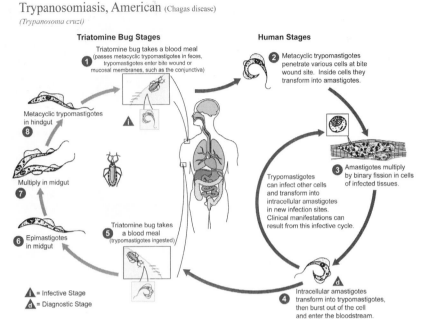

Trypanosomiasis, American (Chagas disease)
(Trypanosoma cruzi)

FIGURE 9–4 This illustration depicts the life cycle of *Trypanosoma cruzi*, the causal agent of American trypanosomiasis.

Source: Courtesy of Centers for Disease Control and Prevention, Alexander J. da Silva, PhD, Melanie Moser

is found mostly in Asian countries, where it has become a leading cause of death in children (World Health Organization, 2009a). Female *Aedes* mosquitoes circulate among human populations, mainly in urban and semi-urban areas, becoming infected with the dengue virus when they feed on a human carrier (Figure 9-5). A mosquito carrying dengue can transmit the virus for the remainder of its lifespan. Dengue manifests as a severe flu and is most often not fatal, though in some cases complications occur, leading to dengue hemorrhagic fever. In such instances, fatality rates can exceed 20% without the necessary medical attention (World Health Organization, 2009b). Dengue has seen a significant increase over the years due to growing mosquito populations in urban and semi-urban areas.

Helminths

Globally, an estimated 182 million preschool children have stunted growth when compared to well-nourished children of similar age and height, with 33% of cases occurring in the developing world (World Health Organization, 2003). Although growth stunting can occur solely due to poor nutrition intake, it is often due to a combination of malnutrition and helminth infection (see Figure 9-6). Soil-transmitted helminths resemble worms and include the intestinal parasite roundworms (*Ascaris lumbricoides*), whipworms (*Trichuris trichiura*), and hookworms (*Necator americanus* and *Ancylostoma duodenale*). Helminth infection occurs by the ingestion of eggs or larvae in contaminated food, or, in the case of hookworms, by skin penetration via contact with larvae in soil. Once inside the body, helminths reproduce and can affect the ability to absorb nutrients through

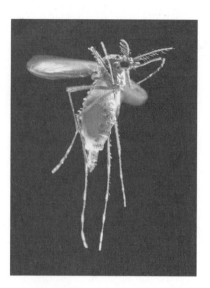

FIGURE 9–5 An *Aedes* mosquito, having just fed. The *Aedes* is responsible for the majority of dengue infections.

Source: Courtesy of Centers for Disease Control and Prevention/Prof. Frank Hadley Collins, Dir., Cntr. for Global Health and Infectious Diseases, Univ. of Notre Dame

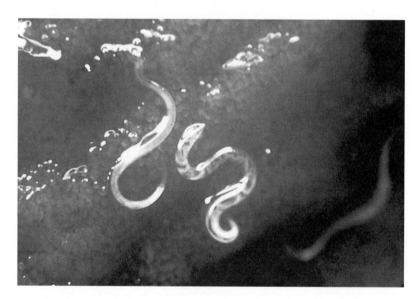

FIGURE 9–6 Hookworm attached to the intestinal mucosa.

Source: Courtesy of Centers for Disease Control and Prevention

the digestive system, as well as cause damage to brain function and tissue. This loss of digestive function due to helminth infection, coupled with general malnutrition, is referred to as malnutrition–infection complex.

Leishmaniasis

Approximately 80% of areas endemic for leishmaniasis are in the developing world (World Health Organization, 2012d). The phlebotomine sandflies that transmit the parasitic protozoa that cause the disease (genus *Leishmania*) live in forested and

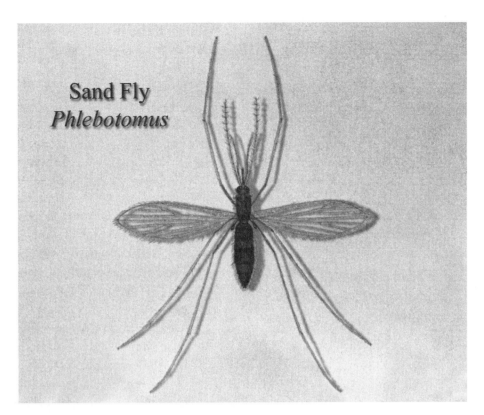

FIGURE 9-7 Phlebotomine sandfly.

Source: Courtesy of Centers for Disease Control and Prevention

subterranean areas, or homes made of adobe brick (see Figure 9-7). Leishmaniasis is associated with extreme poverty, as typically only marginalized populations live in environments that overlap with the breeding area of the sandfly. After the fly's initial bite and transmission of the parasite, the disease can manifest in four distinct ways (World Health Organization, 2012a):

- *Cutaneous.* Skin ulcers on areas exposed to bites, which heal and scar over the course of several months.

- *Diffuse cutaneous.* Widespread and long-lasting skin lesions, similar in presentation to leprosy.

- *Mucocutaneous.* Lesions in the mucous membranes, causing permanent damage.

- *Visceral.* Fever, weight loss, swelling of internal organs, and eventual death.

lesions are damaged tissue.

Leprosy

Leprosy, also referred to as Hansen's disease, is a bacterial infection caused by the bacillus *Mycobacterium leprae*, which, if left untreated, becomes a chronic disease (World Health Organization, 2010a). At the beginning of 2009, the global prevalence of Leprosy was 213,036, continuing the steady decline in reported cases of the disease since 2002, at which time there were 620,638 cases. This decline followed a dramatic decrease in the global prevalence of the disease from 1980 to 2000, which went from 21.1 per 10,000 people to less than 1 per 10,000, a 90% drop (World Health Organization, 2009c). Though leprosy cases have been documented across the globe, it is primarily found in Africa and Asia. Despite the stigma surrounding leprosy, it is difficult to contract, transmissible only in airborne droplets from the nose or mouth and typically only after close and prolonged contact with an untreated individual.

Lymphatic Filariasis

Lymphedema refers to tissue swelling.

elephantiasis consists of thickening tissue/skin on limbs.

hydrocele refers to fluid buildup.

A person is **asymptomatic** when a disease causes no visible symptoms.

More than 120 million people are infected with lymphatic filariasis, also known as elephantiasis, a parasitic disease transmitted to humans via mosquitoes (World Health Organization, 2011c). Infection occurs when a mosquito feeding on a human drops the infected larvae it carries, which then make their way into the bloodstream. These larvae are nematodes, or roundworms, which collect in a person's lymphatic system and mature, producing more larvae. The nematodes, of the family *Filariodidea*, can live in a person for years, all the while producing more parasites (World Health Organization, 2011b). In fact, most lymphatic filariasis infections occur in children, who carry their infection until it manifests later in life. Lymphatic filariasis can be a severely disfiguring disease, with acute infection involving the inflammation of the skin, lymph nodes, and lymphatic vessels, while chronic infection causes tissue swelling (**lymphedema**), thickening tissue/skin (**elephantiasis**) on limbs, and fluid buildup (**hydrocele**; World Health Organization, 2011d; see Figure 9-8). Though the majority of lymphatic filariasis infections are **asymptomatic**, quietly damaging the lymphatic system, kidneys, and immune system of their host, 40 million people are currently disfigured or incapacitated by chronic infection with the disease (World Health Organization, 2011c). Lymphatic filariasis cases occur predominantly in South-East Asia, Africa, and, to a lesser extent, in other tropical regions.

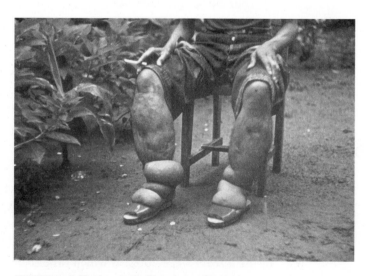

FIGURE 9–8 Elephantiasis of leg due to filariasis.

Source: Courtesy of Centers for Disease Control and Prevention

Malaria

As of 2009, the most recent data available, malaria was present in 108 countries across the globe. However, the majority of infections and deaths occur in sub-Saharan Africa, where malaria is a leading cause of child mortality (amounting to approximately 20% of childhood deaths; World Health Organization, 2011e). Vector borne, malaria is transmitted via *Anopheles* mosquitoes that are infected with *Plasmodium* parasites (see Figures 9-9 and 9-10). Nearly 20 different *Anopheles*

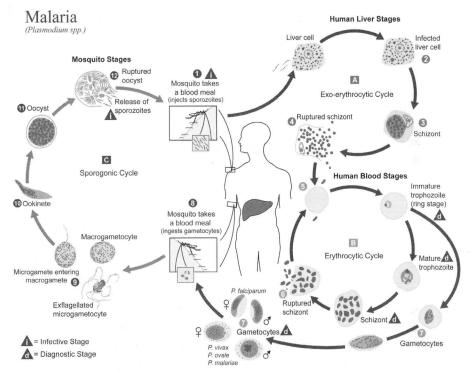

FIGURE 9–9 Malaria lifecycle.

Source: Courtesy of Centers for Disease Control and Prevention, DPDx/Alexander J. da Silva, PhD, Melanie Moser

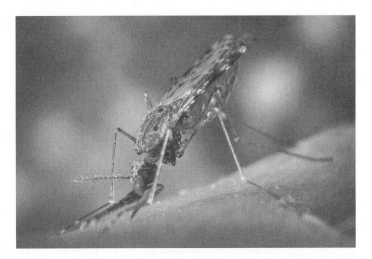

FIGURE 9–10 A female *Anopheles* mosquito, feeding on a human host.

Source: Courtesy of Centers for Disease Control and Prevention/James Gathany

mosquito species are capable of carrying malaria, responsible for 225 million cases of malaria, resulting in 781,000 deaths in 2009 (World Health Organization, 2011e). Numbers of malaria cases and deaths have fallen since the year 2000, which saw 233 million cases and 985,000 deaths, although the historically hardest-hit region, sub-Saharan Africa, still accounts for the vast majority of deaths: more than 85% (World Health Organization, 2011f). Malaria is a febrile illness, meaning that its symptoms involve fever. In a person with an immune system new to the disease, a bite from a malaria vector causes symptoms in a week and half to 2 weeks, which appear flu-like (fever, nausea, vomiting, aches, chills). The illness can rapidly progress once symptoms occur; in the case of the most virulent type of malaria, *P. falciparum*, death can occur in a matter of hours if not promptly treated (World Health Organization, 2011g). In a person with prior exposure to malaria, and thus an immune system familiar with the parasite, it is possible to be asymptomatic.

Onchocerciasis (River Blindness)

Onchocerciasis is caused by the parasitic filarial worm *Onchocerca volvulus*, which is carried from person to person in larval form via the bites of blackflies (species *Simulium*; World Health Organization, 2012b). Once inside the body, the worms grow to adulthood and mate. Female worms release upward of 1,000 larvae a day. When these larvae die, they cause several forms of illness, including blindness and skin disorders such as rashes, lesions, and loss of pigmentation. Thirty years of public–private partnerships, mostly occurring in Africa, have greatly reduced the disease burden of onchocerciasis. However, at present medications eliminate only larvae and not the adult worms, meaning yearly doses are required for populations living in endemic areas. True eradication of the disease will only occur when a safe and effective drug has been developed and distributed that kills all forms of the parasitic worm.

Schistosomiasis

Schistosomiasis is endemic in 74 countries and infects an estimated 207 million people (World Health Organization, 2010c; see Figure 9-11). A chronic disease, schistosomiasis is also parasitic, transmitted when blood flukes called schistosomes (trematode worms of the *Schistosoma* genus) burrow through the skin of a person who has come into contact with them (World Health Organization, 2010e). Blood fluke larvae live in freshwater snails, which release them into the aquatic environment. As such, schistosomiasis cases most frequently occur in rural and/or poor areas, cut off from access to safe water and sanitation. Agricultural and fishing communities are at risk, as are women who use untreated freshwater sources for daily chores, and children, who play in the same water (see Figure 9-12). Eighty-five percent of infections occur in Africa, though with increasing tourism and international travel in general, cases have been reported across the

Schistosomiasis

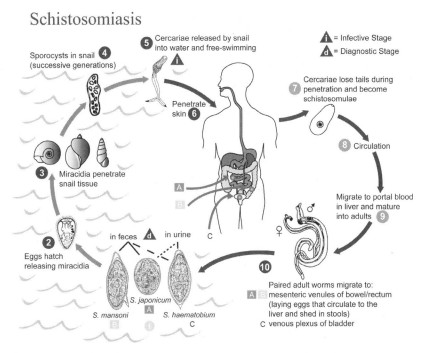

FIGURE 9–11 Schistosomiasis lifecycle.

Source: Courtesy of Centers for Disease Control and Prevention, Alexander J. da Silva, PhD, Melanie Moser

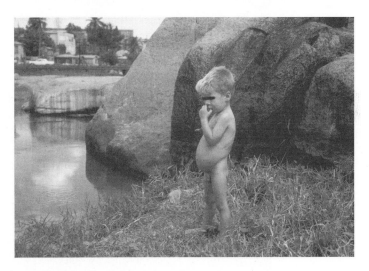

FIGURE 9–12 Boy with swollen abdomen due to schistosomiasis.

Source: Courtesy of Centers for Disease Control and Prevention

globe (World Health Organization, 2010b). Schistosomiasis can present in two forms, intestinal and urogenital. Intestinal schistosomiasis affects the intestines and related organs, such as the liver and occasionally the spleen. The urogenital form affects the urinary system and related organs, such as the bladder. Because it is a chronic disease, over time the body weakens as it tries to battle the schistosomes. If left untreated, this can result in death. There are an estimated 200,000 deaths due to this disease every year in sub-Saharan Africa (World Health Organization, 2010d).

Tuberculosis (TB)

Although nearly nine million people fell ill with TB in 2010, there has been a 40% decline in death due to the disease since 1990 (World Health Organization, 2012g). The regions most affected are South-East Asia and sub-Saharan Africa, with the former experiencing the majority of cases (40%) and the latter experiencing the most new cases per capita. TB is caused by a bacterium, *Mycobacterium tuberculosis*, which is transmitted person to person via airborne droplets from the throat and lungs. Healthy individuals can carry the bacteria without developing symptoms, reflected by approximately one third of the world's population carrying the TB bacteria (World Health Organization, 2012g). A respiratory disease, active TB lung infection manifests with coughing that sometimes carries blood, pain in the chest, and flu-like symptoms. Sadly, those with HIV are far more likely to contract TB, which is the leading cause of death among this group.

SPOTLIGHT

Special Considerations for Infectious Disease Interventions

- Global health operates according to the principles enshrined in the Universal Declaration of Human Rights, the Declaration of Alma-Ata, and the Human Rights–Based Approach. The Universal Declaration of Human Rights was adopted by the United Nations General Assembly in 1948 immediately following the end of World War II and guaranteed the right to self-determination and freedom from oppression. The Declaration of Alma-Ata, adopted in 1978, was the first formal international declaration of access to health care as a basic human right. The Human Rights–Based Approach is the culmination of efforts by United Nations agencies to integrate human rights into all programming. The approach is a framework that ensures promoting and protecting human rights is integrated into all program activities.

- Every intervention or program should exercise due diligence to conform to international, regional, national, and local laws and regulations. Though programs may be funded by an organization based in one particular country or by an organization representing the interests of multiple countries (such as the United Nations), first priority must be given to the local and national laws that apply to where operations physically take place. This approach does not sanction the ignoring of human rights abuses or responsibilities set forth in international treaties. It is an acknowledgment that successful interventions respect the local context in which they operate.

- As important as it is to respect formal laws and regulations, equally important is respect for national and local cultures and traditions. Elements of a culture can be dynamic, in that they evolve to reflect the current knowledge, attitudes, and beliefs of a population. However, other elements of a culture may be rooted in deeply held traditions that have existed for centuries. Practitioners of public health are required to respect the cultures and traditions of the populations they are serving.

This may at times lead to conflict—for example, between the responsibility of a health worker to provide evidence-based health information and the belief held by community members that a disease is caused or cured by supernatural forces. There often is no easy solution to such conflicts, though an easy way for an intervention to fail is by attempting to delegitimize the deeply held beliefs of the community it is trying to serve.

- Any public health intervention, whether taking place domestically or abroad, should include community stakeholders in its planning, implementation, and evaluation. Stakeholders include community leaders and advocates, as well as subject matter experts. There is no single right way to perform an intervention. Interventions are informed by the knowledge of public health experts but also by the knowledge of community representatives. In other words, what has worked in one community may not necessarily work in another. Transparent processes that foster dialogue are crucial to success.

Summary

This chapter provides an overview of the global environment in which infectious diseases operate, detailing the epidemiological transition, with a focus on tropical infectious diseases. Examples of specific disease-control programs were offered, focusing on diarrheal diseases, malaria and dengue and included challenges in implementing infectious disease control. Eleven specific tropical infectious diseases were described in greater detail. These diseases and their descriptions were taken from the WHO's Special Programme for Research and Training in Tropical Diseases. Finally, special considerations for infectious disease interventions were listed.

Review Questions

1. What is the definition of a tropical infectious disease?

2. Which of the following are agents of disease? (select all that apply)
    a. Virus
    b. Bacteria
    c. Parasite
    d. Bodily fluids

3. Which of the following is **not** covered in this chapter?

    a. Chagas
    b. Dengue
    c. Helminths
    d. Sexually transmitted diseases

4. Leprosy is also known as:

    a. Marburg's disease
    b. Yaws
    c. Hansen's disease
    d. Lassa fever

5. Lymphatic filariasis is caused by a:

    a. Bacterium
    b. Parasite
    c. Virus

6. (T/F): The *epidemiological transition* refers to the switch from infectious disease outbreaks occurring mostly in the developed world to the developing world.

7. Diarrheal diseases most severely affect which group?

    a. The elderly
    b. Pregnant women
    c. Children under 5 years old
    d. Adults between the ages of 20 and 35

8. What is the definition of host, as it relates to disease transmission?

9. Which strategy is mentioned in the text as being needed for wider and more effective use of insecticide-treated bed nets?

    a. Door-to-door education by community health workers
    b. Free bed net distribution
    c. Bed nets with longer-lasting insecticide built in
    d. Mobile clinics for malaria treatment

10. Oral rehydration salts (ORS) solutions treat:

    a. Fever

    b. Malaise

    c. Dehydration

    d. Stomach cramps

Web Resources

Visit the following websites to learn more about some of the topics presented in this chapter.

World Health Organization (WHO): www.who.int/en/

WHO's TDR, the Special Programme for Research and Training in Tropical Diseases: http://www.who.int/tdr/en/

The Universal Declaration of Human Rights: http://www.un.org/en/documents/udhr/

Declaration of Alma-Ata: http://www.who.int/publications/almaata_declaration_en.pdf

The UN Practitioners' Portal on Human Rights Based Approaches to Programming: http://hrbaportal.org/

References

Dowdle, W. R., & Hopkins, D. R. (1998). *The eradication of infectious diseases*. New York, NY: Wiley.

Eisele, T. P., Keating, J., Littrell, M., Larsen, D., & Macintyre, K. (2009). Assessment of insecticide-treated bednet use among children and pregnant women across 15 countries using standardized national surveys. *American Journal of Tropical Medicine and Hygiene, 80*, 209–214.

Elder, J. P., Botwe, A., Selby, A., Franklin, N., & Shaw, W. (2011). Community trial of insecticide-treated bed net use promotion in southern Ghana: the Net Use Intervention study. *Translational Behavioral Medicine, 1*(2), 341–349.

Elder, J. P., Louis, T., et al. (1992). The use of diarrhoeal management counselling cards for community health volunteer training in Indonesia: The HealthCom Project. *Journal of Tropical Medicine and Hygiene, 95*(5), 1–8.

Gubler, D. J. (1988). Dengue. 223–260. In T. P.Monath , *The arboviruses: Epidemiology and ecology* (Vol. II; pp. 223–260). Boca Raton, FL:CRC Press, Inc.

Orman, A. R. (1971). The epidemiologic transition: A theory of the epidemiology of population change. *Milbank Memorial Fund Quarterly, 49*(4), 1. Available at http://www.jstor.org/stable/3349375.

Winch, P., Lloyd, L., Godas, M. D., & Kendall, C. (1991). Beliefs about the prevention of dengue and other febrile illnesses in Mérida, Mexico. *Journal of Tropical Medicine and Hygiene, 94*(6), 377–387.

World Health Organization. (2003). *Controlling disease due to helminth infections.* Geneva, Switzerland:Author.

World Health Organization. (2009a). *Dengue and dengue haemorrhagic fever.* Fact sheet N°117. Available at http://www.who.int/mediacentre/factsheets/fs117/en/index.html.

World Health Organization. (2009b). *Dengue and dengue haemorrhagic fever, global burden of dengue.* Fact sheet N°117. Available at http://www.who.int/mediacentre/factsheets/fs117/en/index.html.

World Health Organization. (2009c). Global leprosy situation, 2009. *Weekly epidemiological record, No. 33.* Available at http://www.who.int/wer/2009/wer8433.pdf.

World Health Organization. (2010a). *Leprosy.* Fact sheet N°101. Available at http://www.who.int /mediacentre/factsheets/fs101/en/index.html.

World Health Organization. (2010b). *Schistosomiasis, epidemiology.* Fact sheet N°115. Available at http:// www.who.int/mediacentre/factsheets/fs115/en/index.html.

World Health Organization. (2010c). *Schistosomiasis.* Fact sheet N°115. Available at http://www.who.int /mediacentre/factsheets/fs115/en/index.html.

World Health Organization. (2010d). *Schistosomiasis, symptoms.* Fact sheet N°115. Available at http:// www.who.int/mediacentre/factsheets/fs115/en/index.html.

World Health Organization. (2010e). *Schistosomiasis, transmission.* Fact sheet N°115. Available at http:// www.who.int/mediacentre/factsheets/fs115/en/index.html.

World Health Organization. (2010f). *Chagas disease (American trypanosomiasis).* Fact sheet N°340. Available at http://www.who.int/mediacentre/factsheets/fs340/en/index.html.

World Health Organization. (2010g). *African trypanosomiasis (sleeping sickness), definition of the disease.* Fact sheet N°259. Available at http://www.who.int/mediacentre/factsheets/fs259/en/index.html.

World Health Organization. (2010h). *African trypanosomiasis (sleeping sickness), distribution of the disease.* Fact sheet N°259. Available at http://www.who.int/mediacentre/factsheets/fs259/en/index.html.

World Health Organization. (2011a). *Health topics. Tropical diseases.* Available at http://www.who.int /topics/tropical_diseases/en/.

World Health Organization. (2011b). *Lymphatic filariasis, cause and transmission.* Fact sheet N°102. Available at http://www.who.int/mediacentre/factsheets/fs102/en/index.html.

World Health Organization. (2011c). *Lymphatic filariasis.* Fact sheet N°102. Available at http://www.who .int/mediacentre/factsheets/fs102/en/index.html.

World Health Organization. (2011d). *Lymphatic filariasis, symptoms.* Fact sheet N°102. Available at http:// www.who.int/mediacentre/factsheets/fs102/en/index.html.

World Health Organization. (2011e). *Malaria.* Fact sheet N°94. Available at http://www.who.int /mediacentre/factsheets/fs094/en/index.html.

World Health Organization. (2011f). *Malaria, transmission.* Fact sheet N°94. Available at http://www.who. int/mediacentre/factsheets/fs094/en/index.html.

World Health Organization. (2011g). *Malaria, symptoms.* Fact sheet N°94. Available at http://www.who.int /mediacentre/factsheets/fs094/en/index.html.

World Health Organization. (2012a). *Diseases & topics. Leishmaniasis.* Available at http://www.who.int/tdr /diseases-topics/leishmaniasis/en/index.html.

World Health Organization. (2012b). *Diseases & topics. Onchocerciasis*. Available at http://www.who.int/tdr/diseases-topics/onchocerciasis/en/index.html.

World Health Organization. (2012c). *Health topics. Chronic diseases*. Available at http://www.who.int/topics/chronic_diseases/en/.

World Health Organization. (2012d). *Leishmaniasis. Burden of disease*. Available at http://www.who.int/leishmaniasis/burden/en/.

World Health Organization. (2012e). TDR. About us. Available at http://www.who.int/tdr/about/en/.

World Health Organization. (2012f). TDR. *Diseases & topics. African trypanosomiasis*. Available at http://www.who.int/tdr/diseases-topics/african-trypanosomiasis/en/index.html.

World Health Organization. (2012g). *10 facts about tuberculosis*. Available at http://www.who.int/features/factfiles/tuberculosis/en/index.html.

PART 3

HEALTH PROMOTION AND BEHAVIORAL SCIENCE RESEARCH

Chapter 10

John Pierce, PhD and Sheila Kealey, MPH, BSc

SOCIAL ECOLOGICAL FRAMEWORK AND HEALTH PROMOTION IN THE HEALTHY PEOPLE 2020 INITIATIVE

Key Terms

determinants of health

efficacy versus
   effectiveness

energy dense versus
   nutrient dense

food desert

gross rating points

healthy food
   financing initiative
   (HFFI)

low-density lipoprotein

price elasticity of
   demand

trans fats

Learning Objectives

By the end of this chapter, you should be able to:

1. Describe the role of the Healthy People 2020 initiative and objectives for health promotion/disease prevention.

2. Explain the behavioral commonalities across tobacco use, diet, physical activity, and obesity.

3. Describe the obesity trends in the last 30 years and explain how these relate to the Healthy People physical activity and diet objectives.

4. Understand the population-level interventions that influence these health behaviors such as environmental incentives, mass media and social norms, and regulation of access.

5. Give examples of the similarities in industry practices for marketing tobacco and unhealthy foods and beverages to children.

6. Understand the influence of industry marketing in promoting unhealthy behaviors, comparing and contrasting the tobacco and food industries.

7. Demonstrate the importance of establishing healthy behaviors during the school years.

Outline

Overview of Healthy People 2020
Tobacco Use
    Adult Prevalence
    Adolescent Prevalence
    Initiation
    Cessation
    Secondhand Smoke
    Interventions That Use Incentives to Decrease Tobacco Use
    Interventions That Control Access to Tobacco or Facilities Related to
        Tobacco Use
    Interventions Using Media to Discourage Tobacco Use
    Interventions That Reduce Smoking Initiation in Schools
    Interventions to Regulate Tobacco Products
Weight Status and Obesity
    Adult Prevalence
    Youth Prevalence
    Onset of Obesity
    Weight Loss
    Strategies to Reduce Overweight and Obesity
Dietary Behavior
    Adult Prevalence
    Initiation of Poor Dietary Pattern
    Strategies to Improve Dietary Behavior
Physical Activity
    Adult Prevalence
    Youth Prevalence
    Developmental Objectives for Active Transportation in Youth and Adults
    Onset of Inactivity
    Getting Sedentary People Active Again
    Strategies to Improve Physical Activity

INTRODUCTION

In 2013, the New England Journal of Medicine conducted a roundtable on the role of government in promoting health and preventing disease (Rosenthal, Farley, Gortmaker, & Sunstein, 2013). The problem, as identified in many earlier chapters in this book, is that people's lifestyles can be a strong determinant of the diseases they will suffer and the length and quality of life they will live. Tobacco use, poor diet, and physical inactivity, particularly when these lead to obesity, are causally associated with multiple diseases, and the highest treatment costs are frequently borne by the state during the senior years. According to the roundtable:

"U.S. policymakers at all levels of government are struggling to find ways to intervene and promote wellness and prevent these health problems, without overstepping the bounds of government intervention or infringing on personal liberties."

In this chapter, we will review relevant objectives from the U.S. Department of Health and Human Services Healthy People initiative. This initiative has become a critical document that focuses the health promotion priorities for professionals at the national, state, and local levels. We will limit our review to objectives that relate to tobacco use, diet, physical activity, and sedentary behavior, the latter three important to understanding the problem of obesity, a major public health challenge.

Since 1979, the Healthy People initiative has set comprehensive 10-year goals and objectives to promote health and prevent disease in the United States. Following the first publication of Healthy People (U.S. Department of Health and Human Services [USDHHS], 1979), subsequent iterations Healthy People 2000 (USDHHS, 1990), Healthy People 2010 (USDHHS, 2000), and Healthy People 2020 (USDHHS, 2011) have continued to set evidence-based objectives to provide benchmarks and monitor progress over the course of a decade. Thus, the Healthy People documents provide an important historical record of health promotion/ disease prevention in the United States. Comparing different reports enables the reader to identify the evolution in public health thinking over the past four decades while documenting successes and challenges that have faced the field. Many state and local public health departments use Healthy People to set priorities, allocate funds, measure performance, and compare state and local data. At the federal level, Healthy People helps identify high-priority health issues, critical areas of research, and needs for data collection. Healthy People is an evolving initiative, and new topics and objectives reflect changing science, societal norms, evidence-based technologies, and political or social concerns (Green & Fielding, 2011).

Each report identifies an overarching goal that guides the development of the objectives for the next decade. Table 10-1 presents the overarching goals, the number of topic areas, and the number of objectives for the four Healthy People reports. The topic areas covered have increased with each report and, most recently, number 42. The number of objectives has also increased substantially, with Healthy People 2020 identifying nearly 600 objectives with 1,200 measures to improve the health of Americans.

TABLE 10-1 Healthy People Over the Years

Target Year	1990	2000	2010	2020
Overarching Goals	Decrease mortality: infants through adults	Increase span of healthy life	Increase quality and years of life	Attain high-quality, longer lives free of preventable disease, disability, and premature death
	Increase independence among older adults	Reduce health disparities	Eliminate health disparities	Achieve health equity; eliminate disparities
		Achieve access to preventive services for all		Create social and physical environments that promote good health
Number of Topic areas	15	22	28	42
Number of Objectives/ Measures	226/NA	319/NA	467/1,000	> 580/1200

Source: Adapted from Healthy People 2020 (USDHHS, 2011)

determine health refers to the range of factors (personal, social, economic, and environmental) that influence a person's health. To improve public health, interventions should target one or more determinants of health through information, programs, and policies.

The earlier reports focused mainly on setting goals for behaviors. Healthy People 2020 is the first report to emphasize setting objectives for strategies that the Social Ecological Framework predicts will **determine health**. Thus, the overarching goal of this latest report is to create social and physical environments that promote good health. Topics covered range from cancer and diabetes to family planning and physical activity. This chapter will focus on the objectives from this most recent report and the data on progress in recent years.

OVERVIEW OF HEALTHY PEOPLE 2020

Healthy People 2020 prepared the following schematic (Figure 10-1) that demonstrates how the Social Ecological Framework informed their discussions and recommendations. It recognizes the interrelationships among the different determinants of health. An important message from this graphic is that to achieve a health outcome goal at the population level, interventions/actions will be required at multiple levels of society.

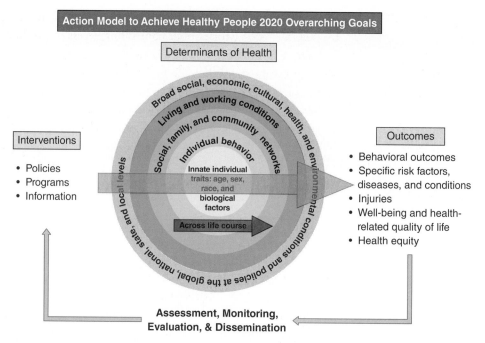

FIGURE 10–1 Action Model to Achieve Healthy People 2020 Overarching Goals.

Source: Healthy People 2020 (U.S. Department of Health & Human Services, 2011)

Further, objectives need to address population groups across the lifespan. For problem behaviors (e.g., tobacco use, sedentary behavior, overeating) and their sequelae (e.g., obesity), it is not just overall or age-specific prevalence that is important. We need to understand how and when the problem behavior develops before an intervention can successfully prevent it. Some behaviors are very difficult to change once they have become habituated (for example, tobacco use), and preventing initiation is critical. Changing habituated behaviors depends on the motivation of the individual. On a population level, both the prevalence of an expressed desire to change and the existence of recent change attempts are markers of the level of this motivation to change. A number of objectives also focus on the health system, ensuring that motivated people have access to primary prevention and other health care resources to promote adoption of healthy behaviors, and treatment to help them change unhealthy behavior.

Social norms can influence an individual's ability to change an addictive habit, as was highlighted by longitudinal studies of United States veterans of the Vietnam War. Many people had noted the serious problem of heroin use by U.S. military personnel during the waning years of the war. Heroin use was not unfamiliar to health professionals in the United States, and it was well accepted that it was extremely difficult for habituated users (addicts) to quit. Thus, health professionals in the field of addiction were astounded when Robins, Davis, and Goodwin (1974) documented that so many veterans who were heroin users in Vietnam appeared to be able to go "cold turkey" when they returned to the social environment of their former civilian life.

A focus on changing the social and environmental influences that impede performance of a healthy behavior and/or support a problem behavior is a critical approach suggested from the Social Ecological Framework. In this chapter, we will explore what Healthy People 2020 says about modifying environmental incentives for particular behaviors, about controlling access to products or healthy environs, and about the use of mass media to encourage or discourage behavioral use (including placing restrictions on business marketing to vulnerable populations). The importance of creating an environment that promotes healthy choices by youth in school settings is also an approach supported by the Social Ecological Framework and a common theme in the Healthy People initiative over the years. As the *New England Journal of Medicine* roundtable suggested, governments can also regulate products that they consider unhealthy; however, such regulations can be challenged in court if they infringe on personal liberties.

TOBACCO USE

As indicated in Chapter 6, tobacco use is the single most preventable cause of death and disease in the United States. Well over 80% of current lung cancer and respiratory diseases such as chronic obstructive pulmonary disease (COPD) are caused by excessive exposure to tobacco smoke. It is estimated that one in five deaths each year are tobacco related. A series of five papers in 1950 started the scientific quest to prove that smoking caused lung cancer (Doll & Hill; Levin, Goldstein & Gerhardt; Mills & Porter; Schrek, Baker, Ballard, & Dolgoff; Wynder & Graham), and the definitive Surgeon-General's report documenting causality was published in 1964 (USDHEW, 1964). Since then, reducing tobacco use has been a major public health priority in the United States (as depicted in Table 10-2).

TABLE 10-2 Major Healthy People 2020 Objectives for Tobacco Use Behavior

Number	Objective	Target	Baseline
TU-1.1	Reduce cigarette use by adults	12.0%	20.6%
TU-2.2	Reduce cigarette use (30 day) by adolescents	16.0%	19.5%
TU-3.2	Reduce the initiation of cigarettes among adolescents aged 12 to 17 years	4.2%	6.2%
TU-3.5	Reduce the initiation of cigarettes in 18- to 25-year-old young adults	8.8%	10.8%
TU-4.1	Increase smoking cessation attempts by adult smokers	80.0%	48.3%
TU-5.1	Increase recent smoking cessation success by adult smokers	8.0%	6.0%

(Continues)

TABLE 10-2 Major Healthy People 2020 Objectives for Tobacco Use Behavior (Continued)			
Number	**Objective**	**Target**	**Baseline**
TU-6	Increase smoking cessation during pregnancy	30.0%	11.3%
TU-7	Increase smoking cessation attempts by adolescent smokers	64.0%	58.5%
TU-11.1	Reduce the proportion of nonsmokers children (3–11 years) exposed to secondhand smoke	47.0%	52.2%

Source: Adapted from Healthy People 2020 (U.S. Department of Health & Human Services, 2011)

Adult Prevalence

In 2014, it was 50 years since the first Surgeon General's report (USDHEW, 1964) concluding that smoking caused disease and death. The decline in smoking behavior is considered one of the great public health success stories; however, the U.S. population is still a long way from a smoke-free society. The first Healthy People 2020 objective for tobacco use behavior focuses on adult use, and, for our example, we focus on the subobjective (TU-1.1) addressing cigarette use. In 2010, prevalence was 20.6% and the 2020 target is set at an ambitious 12%—indeed, this was the same target that was set for Healthy People 2010. In the previous decade (2000–2010), the prevalence of tobacco use declined significantly, with the vast majority of the decrease attributable to cigarette smoking. Cigarette smoking declined from 24% to 20.6%, at a rate of about 0.4% per year (USDHHS, 2011). Although this is a bit slower than the rate of decline seen in the 1970s and 1980s (Pierce, Fiore, Novotny, Hatziandreu, & Davis, 1989), it still indicates that progress toward a smoke-free society is continuing.

Adolescent Prevalence

The second tobacco-use objective focuses on adolescent prevalence of tobacco use and, again, our example focuses on cigarette smoking (TU-2.2). In 2009, the Youth Risk Behavior Surveillance System noted that 19.5% of adolescents self-reported smoking in the past month, and this objective sets a 2020 target of 16.6%. Again, this was the same target that was previously set for 2010. Over the past decade, there was little change in adolescent smoking rates; however, the decline in teen prevalence appears to have started again in 2011 (down to 18.1%). If the trend continues, this objective may meet its target for 2020.

Initiation

It has long been known that the initiation of smoking mainly occurs between the ages of 12 and 25 years (Gilpin et al., 1999). Without any new young smokers replacing those who quit (or die), the epidemic of tobacco use would disappear quickly. A clear example of the importance of this effect on prevalence was seen with medical students in the United States. Almost half smoked in 1964, but by 1980, the initiation rate had dropped to a very low 2% (Pierce & Gilpin, 1995). This change resulted in a major reduction in physician smoking prevalence within a very few years. Objectives TU-3.2 and 3.5 target initiation of cigarettes (experimentation with or first use) in the past year.

In 2003, the experimentation rate among 12- to 17-year-olds and 18- to 25-year-olds was equivalent at 6.6% per year (Figure 10-2). Over the next 5 years, experimentation among 12- to 17-year-olds declined to 6.2% in 2008. However, this decline was more than counterbalanced by a 25% increase in the experimentation rate among 18- to 25-year-olds, which reached 8.3% in 2008. Using 2008 as the baseline year, Objective TU-3.2 sets a target of 4.2% experimentation rate among 12- to 17-year-olds by 2020 and Objective TU-3.6 sets a target of 6.3% for 18- to 25-year-olds.

Cessation

For most smokers, quitting for good takes time and multiple quit attempts. The next set of objectives focuses on an increase of smoking cessation attempts by adult smokers (TU-4.1). In 2010, 48.3% of recent smokers reported making a quit attempt in the previous year. The target for 2020 is to increase this to 80%. However, over the decade ending in 2010, there was little change in this proportion. Between 45% and 48% of all smokers reported making such an attempt during each year in the decade.

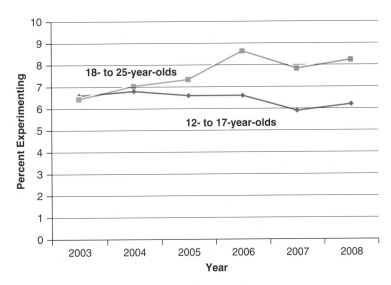

FIGURE 10–2 Trends in Experimentation with Cigarette Smoke by Age: United States

There is a priority on encouraging early-onset smokers to make a quit attempt before they ramp up their habit to a higher daily dose of nicotine. Studies suggest that quitting success is higher among motivated smokers who smoke fewer cigarettes. High school smokers were more likely than adult smokers to report making a quit attempt. In 2010, 58.4% reported making an attempt, which was slightly lower than the proportion who reported an attempt in 2003 (60%). The 2020 objective (TU-7) is to increase the proportion who make a quit attempt to 64%.

It has been argued that the proportion of recent smokers who have quit for at least 6 months is a reasonable marker of future success in staying off smoking (Hughes et al., 1992; Pierce et al., 1998), even though at least 20% will still relapse. The proportion of recent smokers who indicated that they had quit for 6 months was 6.0% in 2008 and 6.7% in 2011. The 2020 objective (TU-5.1) is to increase this further to 8.0%.

Cessation and Pregnancy

Given that maternal smoking also affects the unborn child, a separate objective (TU-6) highlights the importance of increasing cessation during pregnancy. This is assessed among women of childbearing age who had a child in the past 5 years. Smoking during pregnancy has been a huge health promotion success, with rates decreasing from 42% in 1990 to 10.7% in 2005. Of these smokers, in 2005, 11% reported stopping smoking during the first trimester of their pregnancy and staying quit for the rest of their pregnancy. By 2010, this proportion had increased to just over 18%. This excellent progress suggests optimism that the 2020 objective of 30% (same as 2010) might be reached.

Secondhand Smoke

Children and adults exposed to secondhand tobacco smoke are at increased risk for illness and chronic disease. In the early 1990s, the Environmental Protection Agency declared secondhand smoke to be a class A carcinogen. There was apparent rapid progress in the proportion of self-reported nonsmokers indicating that they were not exposed across the United States. In the decade to 2010, in-person reports of exposure to secondhand smoke among children under age 6 years decreased rapidly from 27% to 8%, while reported exposure among nonsmokers dropped by half from 84% to 41%. However, there are concerns about the validity of this self-reported measure of exposure. Fortunately, new measures of blood concentrations of key nicotine metabolites are available—and inhalation of nicotine is confined mainly to cigarette smoke. Accordingly, this measure has become the gold standard for measuring secondhand smoke exposure. Exposure is indicated by the proportion with a blood cotinine level above the accepted detection limit (0.05 ng/mL) but below 10 ng/mL (cut-point for defining smoking). Between 2005 and 2008, 52% of 3- to 11-year-olds measured in the National Health and Nutrition Examination Survey (NHANES) were categorized as exposed to secondhand smoke. The 2020 objective is to reduce this exposure level by 10%.

Interventions That Use Incentives to Decrease Tobacco Use

Healthy People 2020 has two objectives that aim to decrease tobacco use through the use of incentives (see Table 10-3).

Increasing Tobacco Taxes

Increasing the price of tobacco through higher taxes is widely thought to be the single most effective way to encourage tobacco users to quit and prevent nonsmokers from starting to smoke. Price elasticity is an estimate of how likely a population subgroup is to respond to price increases. There are consistent estimates indicating that tobacco products have a positive price elasticity, with teens being much more responsive to price than are addicted smokers. The World Health Organization recommends that the excise tax share of the final consumer price for tobacco products should be as high as 70%. In the United States, Phillip Morris currently lists all taxes, including federal, state, local, and sales taxes, as 56.6% of the total cost of a pack of cigarettes (Phillip Morris, n.d.). Thus, the average cigarette taxes in the United States would need to increase by almost 50% to reach the recommended level.

Tobacco taxes have been used for centuries by governments worldwide. Tobacco is not an essential good nor is it a great contributor to most state economies in the United States. Further, there are already taxes that are "user fees" in place, and increasing taxes can be directly tied to reducing future health consequences. Even in recent times when there is an abhorrence of raising taxes, increasing cigarette taxes are still reasonably well accepted by both the public and political leadership. The 2020 objective is to have every state increase the combined federal and state excises taxes on cigarettes by $1.50 per pack. In 2010, the average combined federal and state excise taxes on cigarettes were $2.30, so the objective is to move this to $3.80.

The level of state taxes on cigarettes varies widely. While a number of states have taxes above $2, in 2012, the following 20 U.S. states had a state cigarette excise tax of less than $1 (in descending order of state tax): Indiana, California, Colorado, Nevada, Kansas, Mississippi, Nebraska, Tennessee, Kentucky, Wyoming, Idaho,

TABLE 10-3 Healthy People 2020 Objectives That Use Incentives to Decrease Tobacco Use

Number	Objective	Target	Baseline
TU-17	Increase the number of states where the federal and state tax on cigarettes increases by $1.50	51 states	1 state
TU-8	Increase the number of states with comprehensive Medicaid insurance coverage of evidence-based treatment for nicotine dependency in states and the District of Columbia	51	6

Source: Adapted from Healthy People 2020 (U.S. Department of Health & Human Services, 2011)

South Carolina, West Virginia, North Carolina, North Dakota, Alabama, Georgia, Louisiana, Virginia, and Missouri. The lowest state tax was 0.17 cents. This tax discrepancy across states can create a significant price difference that has been associated with tax avoidance activities by smokers (e.g., driving to buy in cheaper jurisdictions), particularly by those who live close to borders. It also provides an incentive for smuggling (and tax evasion) where cigarettes are knowingly sold in jurisdictions without the requisite tax stamps. Thus, high taxes need to be accompanied by enforcement of product sales that include the state tax stamp. California led the way in 2005 when it introduced a digital tax stamp that can be easily scanned by inspectors.

Tax Avoidance Versus Tax Evasion. The price of cigarettes includes both federal and state taxes. All citizens have the right to reduce the amount of taxes they pay as long as it is by legal means. Tax avoidance/minimization is the use of legal methods to reduce cigarette taxes. Thus, visiting another state with lower state cigarette taxes to buy a pack or carton is one way to reduce the amount of state tax. Taxes can also be minimized by purchasing cigarettes on the sovereign land of Native American tribes or from duty-free stores while traveling.

Tax evasion, however, is an illegal activity. It involves the sale of cigarettes within a state jurisdiction without the state tax stamp. Those caught evading taxes are generally subject to criminal charges and substantial penalties. This usually involves some type of smuggling of cigarettes—the illicit transportation of cigarettes from an administrative division with low taxation to a division with high taxation for purposes of sale and consumption. A truckload of cigarettes smuggled into a high-tax state could be associated with a profit of as much as $2 million.

Increase Insurance Coverage for Medical Treatment

More than 45 million Americans smoke, and 70% report wanting to quit. The vast majority of quit attempts end in relapse. Overwhelming evidence from randomized trials shows that pharmaceutical treatments and state-of-the-art behavioral coaching result in almost twice the likelihood of quitting successfully compared with usual care. Based on these data, CDC recommends full coverage of all tobacco-dependence treatments (FDA–approved medications and counseling).

According to the National Center for Health Statistics, 32.6% of adult Medicaid recipients smoke, compared to 22.0% of the general population. Tobacco-related health care costs for Medicaid programs averaged $607 million per state in 2004. When health insurance covers a treatment such as smoking cessation, this is an incentive to physicians to take a much stronger role in advising smokers to quit. For smokers who have seen a physician in the past year, just over 60% report being advised to quit. Providing this as a covered service should mean that physicians may provide more than brief advice. Many are convinced that this will result in a measurable increase in use of pharmaceutical aids, which should result in greater cessation success.

However, there is still considerable controversy around the **efficacy versus effectiveness** of pharmaceutical treatment for cessation. Efficacy has clearly been demonstrated in the randomized trials. However, no study has yet been able to demonstrate that the considerable increase in usage of these aids has been associated with an increase in successful cessation (Pierce, Cummins, et al., 2012).

efficacy versus effectiveness
Efficacy refers to how an intervention produces a desired benefit. Most often, randomized clinical trials are necessary to demonstrate efficacy. Effectiveness tells us how well the intervention works in the real world. Once an intervention is shown to be efficacious in a specific population or in a specific setting, it is expected to be disseminated widely to other populations and settings. If the beneficial change accompanies such dissemination, then the intervention is said to be effective.

Indeed, some argue that the medicalization of cessation has been associated with a decline in population success (Chapman & Wakefield, 2012). Currently, only five states provide the full range of services needed to help Medicaid smokers quit, and some states provide no assistance at all.

Interventions That Control Access to Tobacco or Facilities Related to Tobacco Use

Healthy People 2020 has three objectives that focus on interventions that control access to tobacco, related to smoke-free workplaces and reducing illegal sales to minors.

Smoke-Free Workplaces

Compelling evidence shows that nonsmokers who are exposed to secondhand smoke, often at work, will have higher rates of lung cancer, heart disease, and other smoking-related diseases (Pierce, 2009). In 1992, the Environmental Protection Agency declared environmental tobacco smoke a class A carcinogen, which created the impetus for many large businesses to implement policies to limit exposure. California introduced the first statewide law mandating smoke-free workplaces, and evaluations demonstrated its effectiveness (Farkas, Gilpin, White, & Pierce, 2000; Gilpin, Farkas, Emery, Ake, & Pierce, 2002). As a result, such a requirement was also included in the WHO Framework Convention for Tobacco Control (FCTC) in 2003. Many signatories to the FCTC have implemented smoke-free workplace laws over the past decade. In 2012, 34 U.S. states had laws that prohibited smoking in public workplaces. Thirty states mandated smoke-free private workplaces and 40 required smoke-free day care centers. The 2020 objective is to get full coverage across the country.

TABLE 10-4 Healthy People 2020 Tobacco Use Objectives Focusing on Interventions That Control Access to Tobacco

Number	Objective	Target	Baseline
TU-12	Increase the proportion of persons covered by indoor worksite policies that prohibit smoking	100%	75.3%
TU-13	Increase the number of states with laws on smoke-free indoor air that prohibit smoking in public worksites	51 states	34 states
TU-19	Increase the number of states that have less than 5% illegal sales rate to minors in required compliance checks	51 states	5 states

Source: Adapted from Healthy People 2020 (U.S. Department of Health & Human Services, 2011)

Model Smoke-Free Workplace Law. A good example of a comprehensive smoke-free workplace law is the one developed by the Americans for Nonsmokers' Rights. This law has been used in hundreds of localities. Read this law at http://www .no-smoke.org.

Enforcement of "No Sales to Minors" Laws

Another issue of access is the control of sales of tobacco products to minors. Most states have had such laws since the early years of the 20th century; however, they were rarely enforced. In the mid-1990s, the federal government tied some block grant monies to states to performance on enforcement of laws banning sales to minors (called the Synar amendment; Landrine, Klonoff, & Reina-Patterson, 2000). To receive their annual Substance Abuse Prevention and Treatment (SAPT) block grant, under this amendment, states are required to report their performance on sales-to-minors compliance checks. In 2009, only five states passed this criterion for having low levels of sales to minors. However, by 2011, this had more than doubled to 12 states. Objective TU-19 aims for compliance across all states by 2020.

Compliance Checks on Sales to Minors. State attorneys general and other experts have recommended that any effort to reduce youth access to tobacco products include the following key elements:

- Designating an agency with clear responsibility for enforcement
- Providing adequate, guaranteed funding for enforcement
- Making frequent and realistic compliance checks, with a goal of sustained 95% compliance
- Meaningful penalties including graduated fines and, ultimately, prohibiting sales of tobacco products
- No preemption of local ordinances
- Education and awareness efforts for merchants and the public

There is a concern that the tobacco industry could simply pay a vendor's fine if the vendor is caught in a compliance check. To avoid this, a number of states have considered a retail license as a way to incentivize businesses that sell tobacco. If a retail license is required to sell tobacco products over the counter, then enforcement agencies could revoke the right to sell to any business not in compliance with local, state, and federal tobacco laws. For many small stores, tobacco sales make a large difference in the profitability of the business. As of June 30, 2012, 37 states require licensure for over-the-counter cigarette sales, and 29 states require licensure for smokeless tobacco product sales. The fee for licensure in the 37 states ranges from $0 in Massachusetts and Nevada to $200 in Indiana.

Interventions Using Media to Discourage Tobacco Use

Healthy People 2020 has three objectives focusing on media interventions to discourage tobacco use.

TABLE 10-5 Healthy People 2020 Tobacco Use Objectives Focusing on Media Interventions

Number	Objective	Target	Baseline
TU-14	Increase the proportion of smoke-free homes	87.0%	79.1%
TU-18	Reduce the proportion of adolescents and young adults in grades 6 through 12 who are exposed to tobacco advertising and promotion on the Internet	33.1%	36.8%
TU-20	Increase the number of states with sustainable and comprehensive evidence-based tobacco control programs	51	5

Source: Adapted from Healthy People 2020 (U.S. Department of Health & Human Services, 2011)

Smoke-Free Homes

In the United States, generally speaking, governments do not have the right to dictate policies for individuals in their own homes. What they can do is encourage individuals to take action on their own. Smoke-free homes have been shown to have a considerable influence on initiation of smoking in the young (Pierce, 2009), on the intensity of smoking among continuing smokers (Pierce, 2009), and on the likelihood of success in smokers trying to quit (Gilpin, White, Farkas, & Pierce, 1999). Accordingly, many governments use mass media to encourage people to make their homes smoke free. Such campaigns have been associated with more rapid diffusion of smoke-free homes (Gilpin, Lee, & Pierce, 2004). In the United States, in 2006 to 2007, 79% of adults reported that their homes were smoke free. The 2020 objective is to increase this to 87%.

Exposure to Tobacco Marketing Among Teens

Since the early days of the tobacco industry (late 1880s), mass media marketing has been a key strategy to encourage sales and, indeed, the tobacco industry was one of the industries that led marketing innovations (Pierce & Gilpin, 1995). Whenever there were setbacks to the industry, they increased their marketing budgets and tried new approaches. In the 1930s, when concerns about throat irritation were raised, tobacco industry campaigns used the medical profession in advertising to calm public concerns. When the first Surgeon General's report concluded that smoking caused lung cancer, the tobacco industry quickly pointed out that the studies focused only on men and introduced the first women's cigarette, the most successful being with the Virginia Slims campaign (Pierce, Lee, & Gilpin, 1994). When Congress passed a ban on broadcast media advertising of cigarettes, the tobacco industry dramatically increased expenditures and innovations using print and billboards and turned around the decline in adolescent initiation that had followed the broadcast ban (Pierce et al., 2005). Numerous countries now restrict tobacco marketing. A comparative analysis of the experience of 22 high-income countries concluded that the more comprehensive bans reduced cigarette use by up to 7.4% (Saffer & Chaloupka, 2000).

In recent times, the tobacco industry has continued its position as one of the leading innovators in marketing practice. As people have become more interested in social media and the use of the Internet, tobacco industry marketing has moved with them. This has meant that exposure to tobacco advertising and promotion among students increased from 28% to 37% over the decade to 2010 at the same time as industry expenditures on more traditional media decreased substantially. Exposure on the Internet alone increased from 36.8% to 40.6% between 2009 and 2011. The 2020 objective (TU-18) is that this exposure will decline to 33.1% by 2020.

Comprehensive Tobacco Control Programs

The first statewide counteradvertising campaigns against cigarettes were conducted in the early 1980s in Australia and were associated with a major reduction in smoking prevalence (Pierce et al., 1986; Pierce, Macaskill, & Hill, 1990). In 1988, California introduced the first comprehensive campaign that included mass media as well as training and mobilization of local activists. A major aim of the California program was to counter the tobacco industry's effective marketing. This program was also associated with a successful decline in smoking prevalence (Pierce et al., 1998) and particularly adolescent initiation (Messer & Pierce, 2010). Although many states introduced campaigns, maintaining them at effective levels proved to be difficult politically. Successful national campaigns have been conducted by the American Legacy Foundation with money from the Master Settlement Agreement between the tobacco companies and the state attorneys general and, more recently, by the federal Centers for Disease Control and Prevention (CDC). The Institute of Medicine (IOM) concluded that fully funding such comprehensive tobacco control programs is a critical component to decreasing tobacco use (IOM, 2007). Objective TU-20 targets all states to have such programs by 2020.

Part of such a comprehensive tobacco control program is mass media counter-marketing campaigns. CDC's best practices note that campaigns need to be well designed with "hard-hitting" messages. Further, they need to have sufficient reach, duration, and frequency to affect smoking behavior. In 2010, no states were able to mount a campaign that met the criteria recommended in CDC's best practices. These campaigns require sufficient funding and placement so that 80% of youth are reached with 10 exposures each (800 youth targeted rating points). However, nine states met the criterion for an effective adult campaign—80% of adults reached with an average of 15 exposures each (1,200 general audience **gross rating points**). In both 2012 and 2013, the CDC ran a national campaign meeting these requirements. Since the start of this campaign, smoking prevalence, which had been stalled at just above 20% for a number of years, dropped to 18% in 2012.

gross rating points is a measure commonly used in advertising to help assess the audience size reached by the advertisement. Gross rating points are calculated as (frequency × % reached), that is, the product of the frequency an audience sees an advertising campaign times the percentage of the audience reached. The media uses gross rating points values to compare the advertising strength of various campaigns.

Interventions That Reduce Smoking Initiation in Schools

Schools are in a uniquely powerful position to play a major role in reducing smoking initiation. Children spend almost a third of their waking time in school, or about 135 hours per month, and much of the peer pressure kids feel regarding whether to use tobacco occurs in school.

TABLE 10-6 Healthy People 2020 Tobacco Use Objectives Targeting Schools			
Number	**Objective**	**Target**	**Baseline**
TU-15	Increase tobacco-free environments in schools, including all school facilities, property, vehicles, and school events	100.0%	65.4%

Source: Adapted from Healthy People 2020 (U.S. Department of Health & Human Services, 2011)

Tobacco-Free Schools

Most current smokers started smoking before leaving high school (USDHHS, 2012). Initially, tobacco control researchers focused their efforts to reduce initiation on the school curriculum. The best programs included curriculum content on the short- and long-term negative health effects, social acceptability, social influences, negative social consequences, peer norms and peer pressure, resistance and refusal skills, and media literacy as it relates to tobacco marketing and advertising. However, the consensus assessment of these studies was that curriculum alone was not sufficient to obtain a long-term impact on initiation (Glynn, 1989).

For schools to effectively prevent and reduce youth tobacco use among their students, they must create an environment that encourages antitobacco beliefs and behaviors. The 2020 objective recognizes this and requires that schools have tobacco-free policies that are clearly and consistently communicated, applied, and enforced to reduce tobacco use among students. In 2006, two thirds of junior high schools reported to the CDC that no smoking and no smokeless tobacco use was allowed by students, staff, or visitors at or in school facilities, property, vehicles, and school events. This proportion had increased from less than half in 2000. Objective TU-15 targets to increase this to 100% by 2020.

Interventions to Regulate Tobacco Products

There are currently no 2020 objectives in this area, as this is a federal government responsibility that cannot be implemented at the state level. The enactment by Congress and the president of the Family Smoking Prevention and Tobacco Control Act in 2009 granted the Food and Drug Administration the authority to regulate the manufacturing, marketing, and distribution of tobacco products and to set performance standards for tobacco products to protect the public's health. In addition, the Tobacco Control Act grants authority to state and local governments to regulate tobacco products in certain specific respects. For example, the Tobacco Control Act partially rescinded federal preemption and now allows state and local governments to place some restrictions on the time, place, and manner of cigarette advertising and promotion. Frequently, the most stringent laws are placed at the local level where people are most affected by them. A number of states legislatures have preemption laws—these require that no city or county can have stronger laws than that of the state as a whole. Currently, 12 states preempt local community retail display laws, 13 preempt promotion laws, and 14 preempt sampling laws.

The images on cigarette packages are a major part of product marketing, and the industry has ensured that required warnings about the product are not prominent on the package and are difficult to read. Despite the evidence of the dangers of tobacco, relatively few users appear to fully understand the risks to their health. One of the first actions of the FDA under this new authority was to require that cigarette packs have much larger and more graphic warning labels, as outlined by the Framework Convention for Tobacco Control. However, the tobacco industry sued, and the courts told the FDA that it needed more evidence than was currently available on the effectiveness of such labels in reducing smoking rates before they could take such action.

Another early action of the FDA related to electronic cigarettes as potential nicotine delivery devices. Companies effectively sued to prevent the FDA taking this action, and the FDA was limited to regulating the product as a tobacco product, as long as the products were not marketed as cessation aids. Recently, the major tobacco companies have announced that they are entering the e-cigarette market with large marketing budgets. The number of Internet cigarette vendors has grown dramatically. Since early 2000, researchers have identified approximately 800 websites selling cigarettes (CDC, 2012). University of North Carolina researchers used 11- to 15-year-old teenagers in 83 attempts to purchase cigarettes online. Almost all were successful, with the cigarettes delivered to the address given. As a result, the 2010 Prevent All Cigarette Trafficking (PACT) Act (Public Law 111-154) was signed into law. Additionally, at least 33 states have passed laws regulating Internet and mail-order cigarette sales.

WEIGHT STATUS AND OBESITY

Excess body weight is linked with many health problems, including type 2 diabetes, heart disease, several types of cancer, hypertension, stroke, sleep apnea, and respiratory problems. Table 10-7 lists the Healthy People 2020 objectives dealing with weight status.

TABLE 10-7 Healthy People 2020 Weight Status Objectives

Number	Objective	Target	Baseline
NWS-8	Increase the proportion of adults who are at a healthy weight	33.9%	30.8%
NWS-9	Reduce the proportion of adults who are obese	30.6%	34.0%
NWS-10	Reduce the proportion of children and adolescents who are obese	14.6%	16.2%
NWS-11	Prevent inappropriate weight gain in youth and adults	Developmental	

Source: Adapted from Healthy People 2020 (U.S. Department of Health & Human Services, 2011)

Adult Prevalence

Healthy People 2020 sets targets for the proportion of the adult population who are at a healthy weight using body mass index (BMI). Healthy weight is defined as a BMI between 18.5 and 25, while obesity is defined as a BMI ≥ 30. The data to assess performance on these objectives come from NHANES, which includes measures of weight in an examination gown and height without shoes. Between 2000 and 2010, the proportion of adults (aged 20+) who were at a healthy weight decreased from 42% to 31% and the proportion who were obese increased from 23% to 34%. These changes reflect time trends over the past 30 years as Americans increasingly get heavier. The 2020 targets are ambitious, as they propose to turn around this trend so that the proportion of the adult population at a healthy weight is 33.9% (NWS-8) and the proportion who are obese is 30.6% (NWS-9).

Youth Prevalence

Adolescent obesity rates have also been increasing for a long time, similar to the long-term trend for adults (Wang, Orleans, & Gortmaker, 2012). The Healthy People Initiative uses the NHANES data, and obesity is assessed as the number of persons aged 2 to 19 years with a BMI at or above the sex- and age-specific 95th percentile from the CDC's Growth Charts for the United States. Among people in this age group, 16.2% were classified as obese at the 2005 to 2008 survey, and the objective (NWS-10) is to reduce this proportion to 14.6% for 2020.

Onset of Obesity

Healthy People 2020 has an objective focused on preventing inappropriate weight gain in youth and adults; however, so far the word "inappropriate" has not been defined. Even so, time periods of weight gain can be deduced from obesity prevalence at different ages. At the 2005 to 2008 assessment, the prevalence of obesity was 10.7% among 2- to 5-year-olds, 17.4% among 6- to 11-year-olds, and only slightly higher among 12- to 19-year-olds, suggesting that more than half of the onset of obesity in youth may occur during the first 5 years of life, with most of the rest occurring prior to puberty. While it is true that obese children are more likely to become obese adults (Freedman et al., 2005), many people also become obese for the first time when they are already adults. Times to look for significant weight gain are when the body's metabolic rate slows down, such as happens with menopause in women, and when levels of physical activity are decreased in both genders.

Weight Loss

Following the tobacco model, we might have expected that there would be an objective that focused on attempts to lose weight among those who were overweight or obese, as well as a focus on increasing success among such change attempts. These measures were available from the NHANES study (Duncan et al., 2011). Of the 4,784 people in the 2005 to 2008 NHANES who were measured as overweight (51%) or obese (49%), more than 80% indicated that they wanted to lose weight and 47% indicated that they had tried to lose weight in the past year. These attempt proportions are not that different from those seen among current smokers (see Objective TU-4). Just as in tobacco use, most attempts to change weight are not associated with a professional program or therapy. Best practices suggest that weight loss therapy can achieve a 10% weight loss over a 6-month period; however, without an appropriate maintenance program, the majority of that weight will be regained (USDHHS, 1998).

Strategies to Reduce Overweight and Obesity

Many organizations have put forth recommendations to address the obesity epidemic. The World Health Organization recommendations on obesity notes: "Supportive environments and communities are fundamental in shaping people's choices and preventing obesity. Individual responsibility can only have its full effect where people have access to a healthy lifestyle, and are supported to make healthy choices" (World Health Organization, 2013).

The IOM reported that addressing the obesity crisis would require a substantial increase in public- and private-sector investment (IOM, 2006) and recommended interventions that include government, industry, media, communities, schools, and families (IOM, 2005, 2006). Most of the emphasis is focused on a combination of dietary change (particularly caloric reduction) and physical activity. However, Healthy People did focus on physicians as an important source of motivation for patients (see Table 10-8).

TABLE 10-8 Healthy People 2020 Weight Status Objectives Involving Physicians

Number	Objective	Target	Baseline
NWS-5.1	Increase the proportion of primary care physicians who regularly assess body mass index (BMI) in their adult patients	53.6%	48.7%
NWS-5.2	Increase the proportion of primary care physicians who regularly assess body mass index (BMI) for age and sex in their child or adolescent patients	54.7%	49.7%
NWS-6	Increase the proportion of physician office visits made by adult patients who are obese that include counseling or education related to weight reduction, nutrition, or physical activity	31.8%	28.9%
NWS-7	Increase the proportion of worksites that offer nutrition or weight-management classes or counseling	Developmental	

Source: Adapted from Healthy People 2020 (U.S. Department of Health & Human Services, 2011)

In the background to these objectives, Healthy People notes that in 2008, physicians reported monitoring body mass index in approximately half of the patients seen. The target objective for 2020 (NWS-5.1) was to increase this by 10%. Less than one third of obese patients who saw physicians were counseled about the need to reduce weight. Again, the 2020 target (NWS-6) is to increase this by 10%. However, Healthy People was silent about how these desired increases would be achieved.

DIETARY BEHAVIOR

Many Americans eat a diet centered on refined and processed foods. This refined diet tends to have limited intake of foods like vegetables, fruits, whole grains, and legumes—foods that are nutrient rich and may play important roles in maintaining health and preventing disease. Such foods are also naturally higher in fiber, lower in fat (but contain healthy fats), and less calorically dense. On the other hand, processed foods and beverages, particularly those rich in refined carbohydrates, are often energy dense, higher in unhealthy fats and sodium, and lower in fiber and protective nutrients. Consuming large quantities of these foods increases the risk of weight gain and chronic diseases.

Traditionally, nutrition research focused on investigating the influence of intakes of specific nutrients on health, but a growing appreciation of the complex interaction among nutrients and other food components has increased interest and research into how a person's overall dietary pattern affects their health. The DASH diet (Svetkey et al., 1999) is an example of a study that demonstrated the effect of an overall dietary pattern on health consequences such as hypertension. The DASH dietary pattern emphasizes high intakes of fruits, vegetables, low-fat dairy foods, whole grains, poultry, fish, and nuts and discourages the consumption of fats, red meat, sweets, sodium, and sugar-containing beverages.

energy-dense foods are high in calories and low in nutritional value, often containing added sugars, salt, and fat.

nutrient-dense foods are typically low in calories but rich in vitamins, minerals, and other substances with potential health benefits.

SPOTLIGHT

Energy Dense versus Nutrient Dense

As explained in Chapter 4, energy-dense foods are high in calories and low in nutritional value, often containing added sugars, salt, and fat. Nutrient-dense foods are typically low in calories but rich in vitamins, minerals, and other substances with potential health benefits. These foods exclude or limit added solid fats, sugars, starches, and sodium. Examples of nutrient-dense foods include vegetables, fruits, whole grains, seafood, eggs, legumes, unsalted nuts and seeds, fat-free milk products, and lean meats and poultry. A healthful diet that emphasizes nutrient-dense foods will help Americans meet their nutrient needs without excessive calories.

TABLE 10-9 Healthy People 2020 Food and Nutrition Consumption Objectives

Number	Objectives	Target	Baseline
NWS-14	Increase the contribution of fruits to the diets of the population aged 2 years and older (cup equivalent/day)	0.9	0.5
NWS-15	Increase the contribution of total vegetables to the diets of the population aged 2 years and older (cup equivalent/day)	1.1	0.8
NWS-16	Increase the contribution of whole grains to the diets of the population aged 2 years and older (ounce per 1,000 calories)	0.6	0.3
NWS-17	Reduce consumption of calories from solid fats and added sugars (% of total calories)	29.8	34.6
NWS-19	Reduce consumption of sodium in the population aged 2 years and older	2,300 mg	3,641 mg
NWS-20	Increase consumption of calcium in the population aged 2 years and older	1,300 mg	1,118 mg

Source: Adapted from Healthy People 2020 (U.S. Department of Health & Human Services, 2011)

Healthy People 2020 sets objectives for intake of foods that would lead to better dietary habits and overall health. A number of objectives focus on increasing intake (e.g., fruits, vegetables, grains, including whole grains, and calcium) while other objectives focus on a decreasing intake (e.g., saturated fat, total fat, and total sodium; see Table 10-9).

Adult Prevalence

Food or nutrients targeted to be increased are fruits, vegetables, whole grains, and calcium. Increasing fruit and vegetable intake will increase intakes of a series of nutrients (e.g., folate, magnesium, potassium, dietary fiber, and vitamins A, C, and K) where current intakes for the average American are below recommended levels. Evidence suggests that consuming these at the higher levels should reduce the risk of chronic disease. There is also some evidence suggesting that replacing energy-dense foods with fruits and vegetables (much less energy dense) could result in weight loss (USDHHS, 2010), although this is not always the case (Saquib et al., 2008).

Fruit and vegetable intake remained stable over the 2000 to 2010 decade, well below the Healthy People 2010 targets: about 39 to 40% of Americans were consuming two fruit servings per day, and only 4% of Americans were achieving the Healthy People objective of consuming at least three daily servings of vegetables with at least one third dark green or orange. Similar to vegetable intake, only a small proportion of Americans (4%) were meeting the grain intake objective at baseline (at least six daily servings with at least three being whole grains). At the end of the decade, only 3% of Americans met the grain target. Achieving the 2020 targets will be challenging for each of these objectives and will require some powerful interventions.

Calcium is well known for its role in maintaining strong bones, but this mineral is also important for muscle contraction, blood clotting, transmitting nerve impulses, preventing hypertension, and possibly lowering the risk of colon cancer. Calcium intake is the only nutrition objective that improved over the previous decade. To achieve the 2020 target of a 16% increase (NWS-20) will require a faster rate of increase than seen in the past decade.

Food or nutrients targeted to be decreased are saturated fat, added sugars, and sodium. Objective NWS-17 aims to reduce consumption of calories from solid fats and added sugars, recognizing that these foods account for a sizable portion of the calories that Americans consume without contributing important nutrients. Solid fats include foods like butter, beef fat, and shortening that are solid at room temperature. Solid fats are high in saturated fats and/or **trans fats**, which can raise blood **low-density lipoprotein** levels. Reducing intake of these will be an important component of most weight-management interventions as well as efforts to reduce disease risk.

NHANES reported that the average American consumed 18.9% of total calories from solid fat in 2001 to 2004. The 2020 target is that solid fats will be limited to 16.7% of calories. The other component of this goal is to reduce calories from added sugars. Between 2001 to 2004, Americans consumed 15.7% of calories from added sugars, and the use of sugar-sweetened beverages to meet hydration needs was a major component of this. The 2020 goal is to reduce added sugars to 10.8% of calories—a very ambitious target, as this would require a one third reduction in the consumption of these calories from the baseline measure.

Americans consume a lot more sodium than their bodies require, which can lead to hypertension, a risk factor for heart disease and stroke (IOM, 2013). Processed foods and restaurant meals account for about three quarters of the sodium consumed. Sodium intake among Americans was 3,861 mg/day in 2003 to 2006, and this decreased by only 1.5% by the 2007 to 2010 assessment. Thus the target of 2,300 mg/d by 2020 (NWS-19) is very ambitious.

Adolescent Prevalence

On the whole, the background data for the Healthy People objectives indicates that adolescents consume similar patterns of nutrients to adults.

trans fats are created when liquid (polyunsaturated) oils are hydrogenated. Food manufacturers often add trans fats to processed foods to extend their shelf life. You'll find trans fats in foods made with "partially hydrogenated vegetable oil" (like some but not all margarines, cookies, crackers, French fries, and potato chips). Most experts consider trans fats more harmful to heart health than saturated fats.

low-density lipoprotein (LDL), also called the "bad" cholesterol, circulates in the blood and can build up in the inner walls of arteries. LDL and other substances form plaque, which is a thick, hard deposit that narrows and stiffens the arteries, increasing the risk of heart attack and stroke. Foods high in saturated fats and trans fats can increase blood LDL, while foods rich in soluble dietary fiber (e.g., oats, legumes, apples, barley, pears) may help lower LDL. Regular physical activity and a healthy weight can also lower LDL.

Initiation of Poor Dietary Pattern

Other than the evidence that young people have poor dietary patterns, there is little evidence suggesting key times that people who start with a healthy dietary pattern might change to a poorer dietary pattern or vice versa. On the other hand, people who have had a health event, such as diagnosis of cancer, become motivated to make major changes in their diet. A high proportion of women indicated that shortly after they finished treatment for cancer, they made major changes to their dietary pattern with a goal of reducing their risk of recurrence (Thomson et al., 2002).

Change in Dietary Pattern

Unlike the evidence for tobacco use and obesity, there are few data suggesting that the many people with poor-quality dietary pattern express an intention to make a major change to establish a healthy dietary pattern, nor is there any evidence of the population success rates among those who try to change. However, dietary intervention studies have shown that people can achieve major changes in dietary pattern should they be motivated to do it and have adequate support. Studies with marked changes in dietary pattern include the DASH feeding study, which achieved a dietary pattern high in vegetables, fruit and fiber, and low in energy from fat. The intervention was limited to 8 weeks; however, this was sufficient to show an impact of dietary change in reducing blood pressure levels (Conlin et al., 2000). The follow-up PREMIER study achieved and maintained a similar dietary pattern in a free-living population for 6 months, replicating the reduced hypertension effect (Appel et al., 2003). The WHEL Study tested the role of a plant-based dietary pattern in delaying cancer recurrence and death among more than 3,000 breast cancer survivors (Pierce et al., 2007). This study achieved and maintained through 6 years at least a 30% difference between intervention and comparison groups in daily intakes of vegetables, fruits, and fiber along with a reduction in energy from fat of almost 10%. These differences were achieved within 2 months of randomization and persisted throughout the study. Of importance, the patterns persisted for another 4 years after the completion of all study activities.

Strategies to Improve Dietary Behavior

The Healthy People 2020 objectives aim to improve the diets of Americans, including interventions that (1) incentivize people to improve their dietary pattern, (2) increase access to healthy foods, (3) use media to promote healthy eating, (4) promote healthy eating in schools, and (5) regulate food and beverage products.

Interventions That Incentivize People to Improve their Dietary Pattern

Healthy People 2020 includes no objectives that focus on incentivizing change in food intake patterns, but research suggests that such strategies could be effective in modifying intake. Health experts have proposed taxes for sweetened beverages because they offer no health benefits, they are associated with diabetes and obesity, and the calories may displace nutritionally superior foods and beverages. California considered implementing such a tax in 2013. Americans are consuming 250 to 300 calories more per day than they were 20 years ago, and almost half of the increase is attributable to sugar-sweetened beverage consumption (Brownell &

Frieden, 2009). One review suggested that a 10% tax on sugar-sweetened beverages could lead to an 8% to 10% reduction in soft drink purchases (Andreyeva, Long, & Brownell, 2010). More recently, Powell and colleagues (2013) found that the **price elasticity of demand** for sugar-sweetened beverages was –1.21; fast food, –0.52; fruits, –0.49; and vegetables, –0.48, suggesting that higher prices would impact sugar-sweetened beverage purchases. They also found that pricing might influence body weight: higher fast-food prices were associated with lower body weight, particularly among adolescents, and lower fruit and vegetable prices were associated with lower body weight among both low-income children and adults. A controlled field experiment showed that a 30% tax on less-healthy items (with items also labeled as less healthy) motivated people to make healthier food purchases (Elbel, Taksler, Mijanovich, Abrams, & Dixon, 2013).

price elasticity of demand is a measure that shows the responsiveness (elasticity) of the quantity demanded of a good to a change in its price; it shows us how much consumers change their purchasing behavior when prices change.

Interventions That Increase Access to Healthy Foods

Our surrounding food environment has a great influence on what we eat. People who live close to full-service grocery stores tend to eat healthier foods, including more fruits and vegetables, and have lower rates of obesity (Larson, Story, & Nelson, 2009). However, for a number of Americans, healthier food choices are not as accessible as less healthy choices. A **food desert** is a new term to describe a district with little or no access to large grocery stores that offer fresh and affordable foods needed to maintain a healthy diet. Food deserts disproportionately affect socially segregated groups in urban areas, specifically single mothers, children, and the elderly living in underprivileged urban neighborhoods. Sometimes such a food desert occurs when there has been an exodus of middle-class residents and grocery stores have either closed or relocated as well. In such places, local food choices are often restricted to inexpensive, high-calorie, nutrient-poor foods, and the local environment has been termed "obesogenic."

food deserts are areas that have poor access to affordable, healthy food. They are most often found in inner cities and were created when supermarkets abandoned the downtown core to relocate in suburbs. These areas tend to disproportionately affect socially segregated groups in underprivileged urban areas, specifically single mothers, children, the elderly, and families and individuals without a car.

Healthy People 2020 has two objectives aimed at increasing access to healthy foods (see Table 10-10).

TABLE 10-10 Healthy People 2020 Objectives to Increase Access to Healthy Foods			
Number	**Objective**	**Target**	**Baseline**
NWS-3	Increase the number of states that have state-level policies that incentivize food retail outlets to provide foods that are encouraged by the Dietary Guidelines for Americans	18 states	8 states
NWS-4	Increase the proportion of Americans who have access to a food retail outlet that sells a variety of foods that are encouraged by the Dietary Guidelines for Americans	Developmental	

Source: Adapted from Healthy People 2020 (U.S. Department of Health & Human Services, 2011)

healthy food financing initiative (HFFI)   This is a national-level initiative that supports projects through grant opportunities to increase access to healthy, affordable food in communities that currently lack these options.

Objective NWS-3 focuses on state-level policies that incentivize food retail outlets to be located within "food deserts." In 2009, eight states had such policies, and the target is to increase this to 18 by 2020. Progress on this objective looks promising, with the new national-level **Healthy Food Financing Initiative (HFFI)** that offers grant opportunities for increasing access to healthier foods in underserved communities.

SPOTLIGHT

The Healthy Food Financing Initiative (HFFI) supports projects that increase access to healthy, affordable food in communities that currently lack these options. Through a range of programs at the U.S. Departments of Agriculture (USDA), Treasury, and Health and Human Services (HHS), HFFI will expand the availability of nutritious food, including developing and equipping grocery stores, small retailers, corner stores, and farmers' markets selling healthy food.

Providing access to healthier foods for Americans at other venues can help change eating behavior: Surrounding individuals with healthy foods and limiting unhealthy foods helps make the default choice a healthy one. Workplaces, restaurants, and schools are good targets for such interventions. For example, workplaces could have cafeterias or vending machines that limit or restrict unhealthy foods and provide healthy food and beverage choices that are affordable. Some experts consider policies that help create healthy food and eating environments to be among the most effective strategies for improving the eating habits of Americans (Story, Kaphingst, Robinson-O'Brien, & Glanz, 2008).

Interventions That Use Media to Promote Healthy Eating and Discourage Unhealthy Eating

Healthy People 2020 has no objectives related to regulating food industry marketing or promotion, although the available data show that such policies could have profound influences on eating behavior. Health organizations have been urging countries to take action for more than a decade. In 2010, the World Health Organization called on governments worldwide to reduce children's exposure to food and beverage advertising and to reduce the use of powerful marketing techniques (WHO, 2010). There are lots of parallels between tobacco industry marketing and fast food and sweetened beverages marketing (Brownell & Warner, 2009; Dorfman, Cheyne, Friedman, Wadud, & Gottlieb, 2012). Nestle (2002) comments, "it is not just Big Tobacco anymore. Public health must also contend with Big Food, Big Soda, and Big Alcohol."

The United States lags behind other countries in regulating marketing directed at children, and the industry defends its right to market to whom it pleases, as it claims advertising is commercial speech protected under the First Amendment to the U.S. Constitution. The food and beverage industries have huge marketing expenditures (~$2 billion/year), and the placement of these advertisements makes it clear that children and teens are two main targets of their efforts. In 2006, the fast food industry spent approximately $5 million each day (Kovacic, 2008). As young people have migrated from television to social media, food industry expenditures have followed: Television expenditures have decreased by 19.5% and been replaced by a 50% increase in new media (online, mobile, and viral) marketing in 2009 (Federal Trade Commission, 2012). From television, Internet, social media, cell phones, interactive video games, and contests, children are surrounded by food industry messages at home, at school, and in their communities. Brand placement in movies is another prevalent and largely overlooked source of marketing (Sutherland, Mackenzie, Purvis, & Dalton, 2010).

Food marketing influences children's stated preferences, their requests to parents, and the foods that they consume (Federal Trade Commission, 2012). Almost all food ads (98%) targeting children are for products that are high in sugar, fat, or sodium; most ads (79%) are for products that are low in fiber (Larson, Story, & Nelson, 2009). And the influence of marketing may be long lasting: One study suggested that television viewing time in middle and high school predicted poorer eating habits 5 years later (Barr-Anderson, Larson, Nelson, Neumark-Sztainer, & Story, 2009). A recent study investigating the influence of fast food and sugar-sweetened beverage television advertising on elementary school children (Andreyeva, Kelly, & Harris, 2011) found that exposure to this advertising was associated with increased consumption of those foods and beverages, and that exposure to fast food advertising was significantly associated with BMI for overweight and obese children. More research demonstrating the importance of food and beverage marketing to consumption patterns is needed to support policies that limit or restrict the marketing of unhealthy foods to youth.

SPOTLIGHT
Countermarketing Campaigns

Countermarketing campaigns have been an important component of successful tobacco control programs, especially when the campaigns influenced social norms. Frieden, Dietz, and Collins (2010) recommended that nutrition countermarketing should follow tobacco's lead and focus on the harm caused by the product. Current countermarketing campaigns for nutrition are few and fragmented. The Center for Science in the Public Interest (CSPI) launched a countermarketing campaign after Coca-Cola released a series of commercials to appease growing public concern about the link between sugar-sweetened beverages and obesity. CSPI used tobacco control strategies and had Alex Bogusky create an anti–sugar-sweetened beverage video; Bogusky was the creator of the successful antitobacco "Truth®" campaign for the American Legacy Foundation, which received many awards for advertising efficacy and was praised by tobacco researchers for its ability to change smoking-related attitudes and beliefs and reduce smoking initiation (Farelly, Nonnemaker, Davis, & Hussin, 2009). CSPI's social media project features an animated music video called "The Real Bears" (www.therealbears.org). In the video, cute polar bears drink too much soda, gain weight, and the father develops diabetes, injects insulin, suffers erectile dysfunction, loses teeth, and has a paw amputated. The website campaign responds with evidence to industry quotes (called LIES) such as "There is no scientific evidence that connects sugary beverages to obesity."

In 1988, the California Department of Health Services and the National Cancer Institute (NCI) created the first 5-a-day for Better Health program, designed to encourage consumption of fruits and vegetables. A few years later (1991), NCI launched a national 5-a-Day campaign, partnering with the nonprofit Produce for Better Health Foundation, and in 2005, the CDC became the lead agency for this campaign. The current version of the campaign is called Fruits & Veggies—More Matters health initiative and encourages adults to consume at least 7 to 13 servings (3½–6½ cups) of fruits and vegetables daily. It is promoted through supermarket advertisements and brochures, on food packages, and on the Internet. Erinosho and colleagues (Erinosho, Moser, Oh, Nebeling, & Yaroh, 2012) investigated the awareness of the Fruits and Veggies—More Matters campaign and knowledge of fruit and vegetable recommendations (7–13 servings). Using data from NCI's Food Attitudes and Behaviors Survey, they found that only 2% of adults were aware of the More Matters campaign, and 6% were aware of the recommendations. In contrast, they found greater awareness of the former 5-a-Day campaign (29%) and recommendations (30%). Awareness of the 5-a-Day/ Fruits and Veggies—More Matters campaigns was associated with greater fruit and vegetable consumption. Given the food industry's clever marketing tactics and the barrage of advertisements for unhealthy foods that compete with this campaign, an emphasis on increasing awareness of the current national fruit and vegetable campaign is needed.

Interventions That Promote Healthy Eating in Schools

The school environment is an ideal setting for nutrition education and creating a healthy food environment, as children spend much of their day at school, and foods consumed at school contribute significantly to daily nutrient intake (Wechler, Devereaux, Davis, & Collins, 2000). When unhealthy foods are available, children respond to the marketing and consume less fruit and more fat and sugar (Neumark-Sztainer, French, Hannan, Story, & Fulkerson, 2005). Meals served in national lunch or breakfast programs follow federally defined nutrition standards; however, the sale of other "competitive" foods such as those sold in vending machines, a la carte, and at school stores is not strictly regulated. Vending machines are the most common provider of unhealthy foods, and, given that some of the profits go to the schools, these have become a fixture in most middle and high schools. Between 1991 and 2008, vending machines in middle schools increased from 42% to 77% and from 76% to 96% in high schools (Johnston, O'Malley, Terry-McElrath, Freedman-Doan, & Brenner, 2011; USDA, 2007). Access to vending machines increases consumption of high-fat and sugared foods and drinks (Rovner, Nansel, Wang, & Iannotti, 2011), and school policies that limit access to foods high in sugars and fat result in children and teens who are less frequent purchasers of these foods (Neumark-Sztainer, French, Hannan, Story, & Fulkerson, 2005). Healthy People 2020 recognizes that schools are important venues for reversing childhood obesity (Table 10-11).

Food preferences and dietary habits are formed early in life. Given the large numbers of children in child-care programs, this setting presents an ideal opportunity for fostering healthy eating habits. An analysis in 2009 found that there is little

TABLE 10-11 Healthy People 2020 School Policies Objectives

Number	Objectives	Target (%)	Baseline (%)
NWS-1	Increase the number of states with nutrition standards for foods and beverages provided to preschool-aged children in child care	34 states	24 states
NWS-2	Increase the proportion of schools that offer nutritious foods and beverages outside of school meals		
NWS-2.1	Increase the proportion of schools that do not sell or offer calorically sweetened beverages to students	21.3	9.3
NWS-2.2	Increase the proportion of school districts that require schools to make fruits or vegetables available whenever other food is offered or sold	18.6	6.6

Source: Adapted from Healthy People 2020 (U.S. Department of Health & Human Services, 2011)

research on the nutritional quality of foods and beverages provided in child-care settings, and studies that investigated child-care nutrition show cause for concern (Kaphingst & Story, 2009). In 2009, fewer than half of U.S. states had standards for food and beverage choices that could be provided in child-care. The target for 2020 (NWS-1) is to increase this to 34 states.

NWS Objective 2 focuses on increasing the proportion of schools that offer nutritious foods and beverages outside of school meals. In 2006, fewer than 10% of schools restricted the sale of sugar-sweetened beverages to students, and the 2020 target focuses on doubling this proportion. In 2006, only 7% of school districts required schools to make fruits or vegetables available where other food is sold. The target is to increase this to more than 18% by 2020 (NWS-2.2). Currently fewer than 25% of students are covered by such policies.

In February 2013, the U.S. Department of Agriculture proposed updated federal standards for competitive foods that would mean healthier snack foods and less junk food served to students. As adherence to such standards could influence federal grants, this could provide a much-needed incentive to change local policies. Some states have already implemented stricter food and beverage policies, providing evidence for investigators to evaluate their likely effectiveness. Taber and colleagues (2013) investigated the influence of states with policies for healthier school lunches and found that students in states with stricter standards were less likely to be obese, suggesting that new USDA standards have the potential to improve weight status among children eating school lunches. Chriqui and colleagues (2013) also reported that policies are effective: Elementary schools that had state or school district policies limiting the sale of unhealthy foods (e.g., candy, ice cream, sugar-sweetened beverages, cookies, cakes) were less likely to sell those foods.

Interventions That Regulate Food and Beverage Products

Healthy People 2020 has no objectives related to regulating food and beverage products to improve nutrition. However, there are numerous examples that such approaches are effective. Faced with demonstrated high incidence rates of diabetes and cardiovascular disease, the government of Mauritius regulated the composition of cooking oil to reduce saturated fat levels. Disease risks declined within 5 years (Uusitalo et al., 1996). In the United States, governments have encouraged voluntary industrywide changes as well as regulated usage at the local level. Recent examples include the reduction in usage of trans fat and sodium reductions in foods.

The use of trans fats in product manufacturing increased substantially in the 20th century, but evidence on the health consequences of trans fats (Mozaffarian, Katan, Ascherio, Stampfer, & Willet, 2006) and mandatory nutrition labeling in 2006 prompted many manufacturers to reduce trans fats in their products. The average trans fat exposure of Americans from food products decreased about 50% between 2000 and 2009 (Vesper, Kuiper, Mirel, Johnson, & Pirkle, 2012), but a more recent analysis suggests the pace of the decline in usage of trans fats is slowing (Otite, Jacobson, Dahmubed, & Mozaffarian, 2013). New York City took things a step further by legislating against trans fats in restaurants, and this resulted in an estimated reduction in the use of trans fats from 50% to less than 2% (Angell et al., 2009). Given that even low levels of trans fats are harmful (Mozaffarian & Stampfer, 2010), some experts recommend that the United States should follow the lead of other countries and ban any trans fats from food manufacturing (Coombes, 2011). National and local bans were more effective at removing trans fats from the food supply than was mandatory trans fat labeling, and, in countries with labeling policies but no bans, trans fat intake exceeds WHO recommendations (Downs, Thow, & Leeder, 2013).

High sodium intake can increase the risk for high blood pressure, a condition that predisposes individuals to cardiovascular disease. An Institute of Medicine report concluded that voluntary efforts to reduce sodium are ineffective and that new government standards to reduce the sodium content of the food supply should include manufacturers and restaurants (Henney, Taylor, & Boon, 2010). Experts recommend reducing sodium in the food supply gradually to allow consumers' palates time to adjust. A gradual reduction in sodium intake over 10 years has been estimated to potentially prevent more than 280,000 to 500,000 deaths in the United States each year (Coxson et al., 2013).

Some countries regulate salt, many following the UK's example. In 2003, the UK set sodium targets for key food categories and reported that the salt level in bread was reduced by 20% from 2001 to 2011 (Brinsden, Feng, Jenner, & MacGregor, 2013). The authors report that "a voluntary target-based approach works to encourage industry reductions, but the targets need to be coupled with the forceful government or quasi-government agency." Sodium is an unregulated food ingredient in the United States, although some local governments have launched efforts to reduce sodium. Because the food industry is responsible for about 80% of the sodium Americans consume, regulatory approaches could have powerful health implications.

Model for Understanding

New York City at Forefront of Public Health Policy

Cities and states are playing an important role in public health policy, with former New York City Mayor Michael Bloomberg often leading the charge and grabbing headlines for his bold and sometimes controversial initiatives. Here are some of the public health policies implemented in New York:

- New York was the first city to limit the use of trans fats in restaurants and other food vendors in 2005. Other cities followed suit, and some counties and states implemented stricter trans fat regulations.

- In 2006, the city replaced whole milk with low-fat or nonfat milk in the public school system, and in 2012, the USDA announced federal legislation that will remove whole milk from all public schools in the nation.

- In 2008, New York was the first city to legislate calorie counts on menus; now more than 20 cities or states have passed local ordinances requiring calorie counts on menus, and national restaurant chains with 20 outlets or more are now required to post calorie counts on menus.

- In 2010, Mayor Bloomberg proposed disallowing the use of food stamps to purchase sugar-sweetened beverages and tried to legislate a state soda tax—however, neither of these proposals was implemented.

- The mayor launched an initiative to reduce sodium by 25% over 5 years in packaged and restaurant foods. This initiative focused on getting an industrywide agreement to gradually reduce sodium levels in food. Recent evidence suggests that it is leading to lower sodium levels.

- In 2012, New York City's board of health approved Bloomberg's proposal banning the sale of "supersized sugar-sweetened beverages" in New York City food establishments. The American sugar-sweetened beverage industry launched a multimillion dollar campaign to block the ban and took this issue to court. A day before the law was to take effect, a state Supreme Court judge invalidated the ban. Los Angeles, California, and Cambridge, Massachusetts, have put forward similar proposals.

PHYSICAL ACTIVITY

From Chapter 5, we know that physical activity is any movement of the human body that increases energy expenditure above resting levels. Being physically active can help control weight, reduce the risk of chronic disease (diabetes, cancer, heart disease), fight fatigue, improve muscular and skeletal health, improve mental health and mood, improve sleep, and increase the chances of healthy aging. The quantity of physical activity needed to attain these benefits has been the subject of national guidelines (USDHHS, 2010). The guidelines for adults recommend two types of physical activity: at least 150 minutes of moderate-intensity aerobic activity (or equivalent) weekly, *and* muscle-strengthening activity twice weekly.

The main behavioral objectives related to physical activity are to reduce sedentary behavior in adults and to increase the proportion of adults and adolescents who meet the national guidelines for physical activity (Table 10-12).

TABLE 10-12 Healthy People 2020 Physical Activity Behavioral Objectives

Number	Objectives	Target	Baseline
PA-1	Reduce the proportion of adults who engage in no leisure-time physical activity	32.6%	36.2%
PA-2	Increase the proportion of adults who meet current federal physical activity guidelines for aerobic physical activity and for muscle-strengthening activity		
PA-2.1	Increase the proportion of adults who engage in aerobic physical activity of at least moderate intensity for at least 150 minutes/week, or 75 minutes/week of vigorous intensity, or an equivalent combination	47.9%	43.5%
PA-2.2	Increase the proportion of adults who engage in aerobic physical activity of at least moderate intensity for more than 300 minutes/week, or more than 150 minutes/week of vigorous intensity, or an equivalent combination	31.3%	28.4%
PA-2.3	Increase the proportion of adults who perform muscle-strengthening activities on 2 or more days of the week	24.1%	21.9%
PA-2.4	Increase the proportion of adults who meet the objectives for aerobic physical activity and for muscle-strengthening activity	20.1%	18.2%
PA-3	Increase the proportion of adolescents who meet current federal physical activity guidelines for aerobic physical activity and for muscle-strengthening activity		
PA-3.1	Aerobic physical activity	20.2%	18.4%
PA-3.2	(Developmental) Muscle-strengthening activity		
PA-3.3	(Developmental) Aerobic physical activity and muscle-strengthening activity		

Source: Adapted from Healthy People 2020 (U.S. Department of Health & Human Services, 2011)

Adult Prevalence

Physical inactivity is associated with greater risk for chronic diseases and early death. The first objective (PA-1) focuses on physical inactivity and uses data from the National Health Interview Survey (NHIS) to track the proportion of adults who report never doing light or moderate physical activity for at least 10 minutes and that they never do vigorous physical activity for at least 10 minutes. The baseline year for this measure was 2008, when 36.2% responded that they were physically inactive, which was down from 40% in 1997. However, this proportion of inactive Americans has been decreasing yearly since then; in 2009 and 2010 it was 32.3% and in 2011 it was 31.6%. Thus, the Healthy People 2020 target has already been achieved.

Objective PA-2 targets aerobic physical activity at the level recommended in the national guidelines. In the 2008 NHIS, 43.5% of adults reported undertaking either 150 minutes a week of light or moderate physical activity or 75 minutes a week of vigorous physical activity. Healthy People 2020 targeted a 10% increase. However, in 2008 to 2009, more than 47% reported this level of activity, and in 2011, 48.8% reported this level of activity, meeting the national guidelines. Indeed, in 2011, 33.1% exceeded the minimum national guideline recommendations and reported a level of aerobic activity associated with even greater health benefits: either light or moderate physical activity for more than 300 minutes a week or vigorous physical activity of 150 minutes a week or an equivalent combination of moderate and vigorous-intensity activity.

Strength training can help reduce body fat, control weight, and stabilize blood glucose. It can also help strengthen bones, slow age-related muscle loss, and improve balance, coordination, and mobility. Objective PA-2.3 targets the proportion of adults who report doing physical activities specifically designed to strengthen muscles at least twice per week. In 2008 (baseline), 21.9% reported some form of muscle-strengthening activities on 2 or more days per week, and the 2020 target was set for a 10% increase. However, just like the aerobic physical activity measures, this proportion increased to 22.6% in 2009 and climbed to 24.2% in 2010 to 2011, exceeding the 2020 target.

Objective 2.4 measures combined aerobic activity and strength training. This is a "leading health indicator," meaning it is part of a smaller set of objectives that communicates a high-priority health issue. In 2008, 18% of adults met the federal guidelines for aerobic and muscle-strengthening activities. Healthy People targeted that one in five American adults would meet this recommendation by 2020, but American adults exceeded this target in 2010 with 20.6% of adults meeting the combined physical activity and muscle strengthening recommendation.

However, there is some concern that the NHIS self-reported physical activity may overestimate the population's level of physical activity, particularly as the physical activity trend is in the opposite direction expected, given the clear obesity trends. To provide an objective measure of physical activity, NHANES introduced accelerometer-based assessments in 2003. Troiano and colleagues (2008) found that adherence to physical activity recommendations using these accelerometer-based measures was substantially lower than self-report measures, with only 5% of adults meeting the national guidelines. Another evaluation of NHANES physical activity measures between 2003 and 2006 focused on accelerometer-based sedentary behavior. Healy, Matthews, Dunstan, Winkler, and Owen (2011) defined sedentary time as < 100 accelerometer counts per minute (cpm) and noted that sedentary time accounted for 8.44 hours (58%) of an average of 14.6 hours/day, while time spent in light or greater activity (> 100 cpm) was .34/hours a day. The average person took nonsedentary breaks (mean = 4 minutes) approximately every half hour. Both total sedentary time and prolonged sedentary time without breaks were associated with adverse cardio-metabolic risk profiles.

Youth Prevalence

Objective PA-3.1 targets assessed aerobic activity, using data from the Youth Risk Factor Behavior Surveillance System, which asks 9th- to 12th-grade students if they were physically active for at least 60 minutes per day on 7 of the past 7 days. In 2009, 18.4% responded positively, and the 2020 target was set for 20.2%.

Recognizing the benefits of muscle-strengthening activity, Objective 3.2 will assess the proportion of adolescents who include muscle strengthening as part of their daily physical activity on at least 3 days of the week. For children, these muscle-strengthening activities will often be unstructured and part of play, for example, climbing trees or using playground equipment; for adolescents, these might involve play or be something more structured like lifting weights or using resistance bands. Healthy People 2010 did not assess muscle-strengthening activity in youth.

As with adults, Healthy People 2020 will track adolescents who engage in both aerobic physical activity and muscle-strengthening activity.

Screen Time

Time spent in front of a screen is most often sedentary and takes away from physical activity time. Also, more screen time is associated with adolescent obesity (Mitchell, Rodriguez, Schmitz, & Audrain-McGovern, 2013) and potentially adverse health outcomes (Chinapaw, Proper, Brug, van Mechelen, & Singh, 2011). Objective PA-8 focuses on amount of screen time and sets age-specific targets relative to recommendations for screen time.

These baseline estimates for children and adolescents meeting the "screen time" objectives seem high and at odds with a recent survey that reported that children and adolescents (8 to 18 years old) average more than 7.5 hours a day with media, which outweighs time spent at almost any other activity (except maybe sleeping; Kaiser Family Foundation, 2010). In the Kaiser survey, "screen time" includes all use of computer monitors, television screens, and handheld devices. Perhaps this discrepancy is due to the Healthy People data source (questions from the Youth Risk Behavior Surveillance System), which may not have addressed screen time related to phones or other handheld devices where texting, checking social media, e-mail, and so on are common and likely occupy a large percentage of children's time (see Table 10-13).

Developmental Objectives for Active Transportation in Youth and Adults

New Healthy People 2020 objectives recognize the importance of active transportation for increasing opportunities to be physically active (see Table 10-14). Walking or cycling to destinations also integrates physical activity into a daily routine, which helps overcome the time barrier that many experience. Although

TABLE 10-13 Healthy People 2020 Screen Time Objectives

Number	Objectives	Target	Baseline
PA-8	Increase the proportion of children and adolescents who do not exceed recommended limits for screen time		
PA-8.1	Increase the proportion of children aged 0 to 2 years who view no television or videos on an average weekday	44.7%	40.6%
PA-8.2	Increase the proportion of children and adolescents aged 2 years through 12th grade who view television or videos or play video games for no more than 2 hours a day		
PA-8.2.1	Children aged 2 to 5 years	83.2%	75.6%
PA-8.2.2	Children and adolescents aged 6 to 14 years	86.8%	78.9%
PA-8.2.3	Adolescents in grades 9 through 12	73.9%	67.2%
PA-8.3	Increase the proportion of children and adolescents aged 2 years to 12th grade who use a computer or play computer games outside of school (for nonschool work) for no more than 2 hours a day		
PA-8.3.1	Children aged 2 to 5 years		97.4%
PA-8.3.2	Children aged 6 to 14 years	100.0%	93.3%
PA-8.3.3	Adolescents in grades 9 through 12	82.6%	75.1%

Source: Adapted from Healthy People 2020 (U.S. Department of Health & Human Services, 2011)

walking to school used to be commonplace, this mode of active transport has decreased dramatically in the last 40 years, with only 13% of children 5 to 14 years old in 2009 usually walking or biking to school compared with 48% of students in 1969 (McDonald, Brown, Marchetti, & Pedroso, 2011). Objectives 13 and 14 focus on active transportation. There are separate subobjectives for youth and adults: the youth objectives aim to increase walking to school (if the trip is 1 mile or less) or cycling to school (if the trip is 2 miles or less). Walking or bicycling to school is an easy way for children to be physically active. This active transport is also associated with health benefits: Children and youth who walk or bicycle to school have overall higher activity levels (Dollman & Lewis, 2007) as well as better body composition and cardiorespiratory fitness (Lubans, Boreham, Kelly, & Foster, 2011).

TABLE 10-14 Healthy People 2020 Active Transportation Objectives		
Number	**Objective**	
PA-13	(Developmental) Increase the proportion of trips made by walking	Developmental Objectives lack baseline data but have a potential nationally representative data source.
PA-13.1	(Developmental) Adults aged 18 years and older, trips of 1 mile or less	
PA-13.2	(Developmental) Children and adolescents aged 5 to 15 years, trips to school of 1 mile or less	
PA-14	(Developmental) Increase the proportion of trips made by bicycling	
PA-14.1	(Developmental) Adults aged 18 years and older, trips of 5 miles or less	
PA-14.2	(Developmental) Children and adolescents aged 5 to 15 years, trips to school of 2 miles or less	

Source: Adapted from Healthy People 2020 (U.S. Department of Health & Human Services, 2011)

Onset of Inactivity

Typical Americans are active as toddlers and children, less active as adolescents, and increasingly sedentary as they move through their adult years. Technological innovations have been focused on reducing the effort and physical activity needed in daily life. Clear life events are associated with the onset of increased inactivity and sedentary behaviors. Examples include the following: when the adolescent gets a car to drive, when the adolescent or young adult stops playing competitive sports, when someone who is physically active sustains a permanent injury (e.g., knee injury for runners). A cross-sectional analysis using accelerometer-based data suggests that adolescence may be a critical period to intervene to prevent inactivity (Troiano et al., 2008). Comparing children ages 6 to 11 with those aged 12 to 15, researchers noted that adherence to physical activity recommendations decreased from 49% to 12% for boys and from 35% to 3% for girls. A focus on identifying critical periods and situations that increase the risk for inactivity will help identify potential interventions. Such a focus could also encourage people to make alternate plans to maintain their physical activity level through a substitute behavior.

Getting Sedentary People Active Again

Once a year, it is common for people who have become more sedentary than they would like to make a new year's resolution to become more active, and this may represent as many as three quarters of those who are not physically active. Many purchase gym memberships. However, by February the enthusiasm has waned and it's just the "regulars" in the gym. Of those who intend to increase their physical activity, approximately half achieve a meaningful increase. Very few of those who say they have no intention to change will actually increase their activity level (Rhodes & De Bruijn, 2013). Many programs help coach people to increase their physical activity level. Indeed, increasing physical activity is seen as a necessary component in most weight loss programs and has been identified as an essential ingredient in successful weight loss programs.

Strategies to Improve Physical Activity

Healthy People strategies to improve physical activity among Americans include objectives to improve access to physical activity facilities and promoting physical activity in schools.

Provide Incentives for Physical Activity

Although there are no objectives in Healthy People 2020 that focus on providing incentives to increase physical activity, it has been proposed in the literature (Hill, Peters, & Wyatt, 2007). Some countries are considering tax incentives to promote physical activity. Canada was the first country to institute a Children's Fitness Tax Credit in 2007 (parents can claim up to $500 per child on their annual income tax returns for registration in sport and recreation activities). In the United States, a proposed Personal Health Investment Today (PHIT) Act would allow tax deductions for athletic activities (for example, health club memberships or youth sports programs; PHIT, 2009).

Currently there are limited data to suggest that income tax incentives change health behaviors. Criticisms are that the benefit is likely to be small (the Canadian credit is only around $75 per child), and isn't a significant incentive. The substantial public funds for such programs might have greater influence if they were directed toward more immediate rewards (i.e., sales tax exemptions, rebates at point of sale, subsidized programing) or used to improve recreational facilities or physical activity programs in schools (von Tigerstrom, Larre, & Sauder, 2011).

Interventions That Improve Access to Facilities Related to Physical Activity

Using the Social Ecological Framework, Healthy People 2020 recognizes the importance of access to facilities within the community that would make it easier to be physically active. Three objectives focus on this area (Table 10-15).

	TABLE 10-15 Healthy People 2020 Objectives That Improve Access to Physical Activity Facilities		
Number	**Objective**	**Target**	**Baseline**
PA-10	Increase the proportion of the nation's public and private schools that provide access to their physical activity spaces and facilities for all persons outside of normal school hours (that is, before and after the school day, on weekends, and during summer and other vacations)	31.7%	28.8%
PA-12	(Developmental) Increase the proportion of employed adults who have access to and participate in employer-based exercise facilities and exercise programs		
PA-15	(Developmental) Increase legislative policies for the built environment that enhance access to and availability of physical activity opportunities, specifically, (15.1) community-scale policies; (15.2) street-scale policies; and (15.3) transportation and travel policies		

Source: Adapted from Healthy People 2020 (U.S. Department of Health & Human Services, 2011)

Most schools have playgrounds, tracks, playing fields, gyms, and pools that could provide opportunities for community members to be active, but most remain vacant beyond school hours. Joint use policies are a way for schools and communities to share spaces and facilities, but unfortunately, often there are no policies to encourage use of school facilities. Objective PA-10 focuses on joint use policies. In 2006, 28.8% of schools provided access to their physical activity spaces after hours: Healthy People 2020 targets 31.7% of schools accessible by 2020.

Because many American adults spend most of their waking hours at work, workplaces are another setting that can play an important role in encouraging physical activity. Some research suggests that employment that encourages sitting for long hours may be contributing significantly to the high rates of obesity (Church et al., 2011). Objective PA-12 addresses the need for occupational settings to encourage physical activity in workers and aims to increase the proportion of employed adults who have access to and participate in employer-based exercise facilities and exercise programs. Workplaces could also consider "flextime" to give employees opportunities to be physically active while maintaining their work hours.

Although providing greater access to opportunities for aerobic or strength-based activities in the workplace is important, the workplace is also an ideal setting for implementing strategies to reduce sitting time, or sedentary behavior. Workplace architectural design has not been well studied but may provide another venue for discouraging sedentary behavior (McGann, Jancey, & Tye, 2013). For example, many buildings have prominently displayed elevators, with shiny and inviting doors that open with a finger touch to good lighting, music, and carpeting; in contrast, stair entrances are harder to find, behind doors labeled as fire or emergency, that often open to uninviting concrete structures. Reducing sitting with workstations such as "standing" desks (height-adjustable workstations) or treadmill desks (employees work while walking at slow speed) is another new area of research targeting sedentary behavior that shows promise (Koepp et al., 2013). Behavior modification strategies are likely more feasible and could include "walk-and-talk" meetings instead of conference room meetings, moving trash cans out of cubicles to make people walk to throw out garbage, or promoting standing when it is possible (for example, when talking on the telephone).

Objective 15 aims to increase legislative policies for the built environment that enhance access to and availability of physical activity opportunities and will focus on community-scale, street-scale, and transportation and travel policies. Policies that influence the design of a community can encourage physical activity. Policies that enhance access to physical activity opportunities include the following design elements: street crossings, lighting, parks, sidewalks, cycling lanes, walking trails, recreational facilities, and playgrounds. Several studies show that community, street, and transportation design can positively influence activity: people are 65% more likely to walk when sidewalks are available (Giles-Corti & Donovan, 2002); residents with safe places to walk were more likely to meet physical activity recommendations than those without safe places to walk (Powell, Martin, & Chowdhury, 2003); and residents of walkable neighborhoods report more weekly aerobic physical activity and are less likely to be overweight than residents of low-walkable neighborhoods (Sallis et al., 2009).

Transportation and travel policies are another way to encourage physical activity as part of a daily routine through active transportation. Examples of such policies could be (1) discouraging or reducing access to motor vehicle use (taxes, tolls, congestion pricing in downtown areas; reduce parking availability); (2) enhancing infrastructure to support bicycling (bike lanes, shared-use paths, bike racks); (3) enhancing infrastructure supporting walking (sidewalks, trails, pedestrian crossings); (4) improving access to public transportation (this could encourage physical activity as transit users walk or cycle to transit points); and (5) enhancing traffic safety in areas where people could be physically active. Encouraging active transport to school for youth is another critical area that could benefit from policies. National funding through the Federal Highway Administration National Safe Routes to School Program should help the success of these policies and programs.

Using Media to Promote Physical Activity

Promoting physical activity through media campaigns is a way to encourage children or adults to become more active. An example of such a campaign in the $339 million VERB™ campaign to "help children develop habits to foster good health over a lifetime." The campaign ran from 2002 to 2006 and targeted 9- to 13-year-olds using marketing strategies popular within this age group, with the goal of successfully competing with the multitude of other marketing directed at these children. The campaign positively influenced physical activity, built lasting awareness of the VERB brand with effects that persisted through teen years (Huhman et al., 2010), and was considered a great success on many fronts. Unfortunately, funding for the campaign ended in 2006. Healthy People has no objectives related to using media to promote physical activity.

Promoting Physical Activity in Schools

The Healthy People 2020 emphasis reflects research and expert opinions that targeting the school environment to increase physical activity in youth should be a key strategy in health promotion (National Research Council, 2013; Pate et al., 2006). The objectives in Table 10-16 address time for recess, regularly scheduled

TABLE 10-16 Healthy People 2020 Objectives to Promote Physical Activity in Schools

Number	Objective	Target	Baseline
PA-4	Increase the proportion of the nation's public and private schools that require daily physical education for all students		
PA-4.1	Elementary schools	4.2%	3.8%
PA-4.2	Middle and junior high schools	8.6%	7.9%
PA-4.3	Senior high schools	2.3%	2.1%
PA-5	Increase the proportion of adolescents who participate in daily school physical education	36.6%	33.3%
PA-6	Increase regularly scheduled elementary school recess in the United States		
PA-6.1	Increase the number of states that require regularly scheduled elementary school recess	17 states	7 states
PA-6.2	Increase the proportion of school districts that require regularly scheduled elementary school recess	62.8%	57.1%
PA-7	Increase the proportion of school districts that require or recommend elementary school recess for an appropriate period of time	67.7%	61.5%
PA-9	Increase the number of states with licensing regulations for physical activity provided in child care		
PA-9.1	Require activity programs providing large-muscle or gross motor activity, development, and/or equipment	35 states	25 states
PA-9.2	Require children to engage in vigorous or moderate physical activity	13 states	3 states
PA-9.3	Require number of minutes of physical activity per day or by length of time in care	11 states	1 state

Source: Adapted from Healthy People 2020 (U.S. Department of Health & Human Services, 2011)

school recess, daily physical education in elementary schools, and physical activity policies in child-care settings.

Children and youth spend more time in schools than almost any other setting—with the exception of their homes—and if the child's home environment does not encourage physical activity, the school may be the only chance for a child to be active. Another factor to consider is that much of the time at school is spent sitting, which is increasingly being recognized as a contributing factor to health problems, even in active individuals (Owen, Bauman, & Brown, 2009). Counteracting the effects of these extended periods of sedentary behavior in the school environment is critical. Increased time for recesses and regular physical education classes are strategies that can help improve physical activity in schools, and Healthy People 2020 will monitor these measures.

Low levels of physical activity are common in child-care settings, and levels of sedentary behavior are very high (Reilly, 2010). Healthy People 2020 recognizes that the child-care environment is an ideal opportunity to promote physical activity, with objectives specifically related to the child-care setting (Objective PA-9).

The lack of improvement in school physical activity in the last decade is cause for concern, since this venue has the potential to have a dramatic influence on physical activity in youth, hopefully establishing habits they will sustain through adulthood. Although schools have been faced with increasing pressure to focus on test scores and academic achievement since 2001's No Child Left Behind Act (U.S. Department of Education, 2001), reducing resources and time allocated to physical activity might not be in the best interest of children or schools. Besides the health consequences, youth who spend more time in physical education classes do not have lower test scores than youth who spend less time in physical education classes (Sallis et al., 1999), and some evidence suggests that being physically active can improve youth's concentration, memory, and classroom behavior (Strong et al., 2005) and possibly promote higher levels of academic performance (Carlson et al., 2008).

The latest IOM report (National Research Council, 2013) calls on the U.S. Department of Education to develop a consistent nationwide policy to help reverse the trend that has had schools reduce recess and physical education time to focus on standardized testing.

Summary

Government has an important interest in promoting health and preventing disease and strives to accomplish this interest without infringing on personal liberties. In the United States, the Healthy People initiative is the key document that addresses disease prevention and health promotion issues of public health significance. The Healthy People Initiative sets objectives for the decade and provides benchmarks to monitor progress for various health areas. An overarching goal of Healthy People 2020 is to create social and physical environments that promote good health, highlighting the importance of the Social Ecological Framework that informed the development and objectives of Healthy People 2020. This chapter reviewed progress on the Healthy People objectives for the areas of tobacco use, diet, physical activity, and by extension weight status, and examined how policies can influence these lifestyle behaviors and their consequences.

The influence of tobacco control policies on cigarette smoking has been a health promotion success story, with smoking rates continuing to decline over time. Although much progress still needs to be made (for example, more than 50% of 3- to 11-year-olds were still exposed to secondhand smoke between 2005 and 2008), tobacco control efforts provide examples of strategies that can be used to influence change in other lifestyle behaviors. This chapter provided examples of policies that (1) provide incentives for healthy behaviors and disincentives for unhealthy behaviors, (2) control access to either products or facilities related to the behavior, (3) use media to promote healthy behaviors or discourage unhealthy behaviors and regulate industry marketing and promotion, (4) promote healthy behaviors in schools, and (5) regulate behavior-related products.

Obesity has been increasing among adolescents and adults for at least the past 30 years, and there is little sign that the peak has been reached. To change the overweight/obesity proportion requires reductions in calorie intake and increases in physical activity. Clearly, improvements in these behaviors have not been sufficient to influence the prevalence of overweight/obesity in the desired direction.

Overall, Americans are not consuming a health-promoting diet, and Healthy People set objectives focusing on increasing fruits, vegetables, whole grains, and calcium and decreasing intakes of solid fats, added sugars, and sodium. Healthy People has no objectives that focus on incentivizing change in dietary habits or limiting advertising of unhealthy foods, although the evidence suggests such policies would be effective.

Self-reported physical activity has remained stable or increased slightly over the past decade, and progress toward Healthy People 2020 targets has already been achieved for several objectives, although there is worrying evidence of significant overreporting. New objectives reflect the importance of the Social Ecological Framework for physical activity and target environmental changes to make physical activity more accessible to all.

It can be expected that the Social Ecological Framework will play an even bigger part in the next Healthy People initiative. Also, the strategies that have been so well implemented in the tobacco control field will likely be increasingly used as a model for novel strategies to improve health in other major topic areas.

Review Questions

1. How often does the federal government set goals and objectives with the Healthy People initiative?

    a. Every 10 years
    b. Every 5 years
    c. Every 20 years
    d. They do it on an as-needed basis.

2. _____ is the single most preventable cause of death and disease in the United States.

    a. Tobacco use
    b. Obesity
    c. Inactivity
    d. Sedentary behavior
    e. High-fat diet

3. Which of the following has NOT been associated with the decline in smoking prevalence seen in the United States?

    a. Smoking cessation workshops
    b. Increasing the price of tobacco through higher taxes
    c. Comprehensive tobacco control programs
    d. Smoke-free workplaces

4. Which of the following is most important to success in reducing tobacco initiation among school-aged youth?

    a. Tobacco control curriculum in all school grades
    b. Tobacco control curriculum at least every other year of middle and high school
    c. Encouraging teachers not to smoke
    d. Implementing a smoke-free campus

5. Obesity rates have been increasing over the last 30 years in which groups of Americans?

    a. Children in the first 5 years of life
    b. Young people prior to puberty
    c. Adults aged 18 to 45 years
    d. Adults over the age of 45 years
    e. All of the above

6. Which of the following is *not* recommended to be increased to achieve a healthy dietary pattern in the United States?

    a. Vegetable servings
    b. Fruit servings
    c. Whole grain servings
    d. Percentage energy from solid fats
    e. Calcium intake
    f. All of the above

7. Which of the following did Healthy People focus on as a strategy to improve the dietary pattern of Americans?

    a. Increasing price on unhealthy foods
    b. Conducting mass media campaigns to motivate healthy eating
    c. Improving access to healthy food choices
    d. Regulating the types of food that can be sold
    e. All of the above

8. What proportion of Americans report getting no physical activity at all?

    a. 52%
    b. 32%
    c. 22%
    d. 12%

9. Which strategies does Healthy People 2020 focus on to increase physical activity?

    a. Limiting screen time for young people
    b. Increasing active transportation
    c. Improving community access to already available facilities for physical activity
    d. Increasing daily physical activity requirement in schools
    e. All of the above

10. What are the weekly physical activity guidelines for adults?

    a. Time spent on aerobic activity
    b. Muscle strengthening activity
    c. A combination of both of the above
    d. Guidelines are limited to moderate intensity walking

Web Resources

Visit the following websites to learn more about some of the topics presented in this chapter.

Healthy People 2020 http://www.healthypeople.gov/2020/default.aspx

The Centers for Disease Control and Prevention: Overweight and Obesity http://www.cdc.gov/obesity/

The Centers for Disease Control and Prevention: Smoking and Tobacco Use http://www.cdc.gov/tobacco/

The Centers for Disease Control and Prevention: Physical Activity http://www.cdc.gov/physicalactivity/

The Centers for Disease Control and Prevention: National Health and Nutrition Examination Survey (NHANES) http://www.cdc.gov/nchs/nhanes.htm

The U.S. Department of Agriculture and U.S. Department of Health and Human Service's Dietary Guidelines for Americans: http://www.cnpp.usda.gov/dietaryguidelines.htm

The U.S. Department of Agriculture and U.S. Department of Health and Human Service's Physical Activity Guidelines for Americans: http://www.health.gov/paguidelines/

References

Andreyeva, T., Kelly, I. R., & Harris, J. L. (2011). Exposure to food advertising on television: Associations with children's fast food and soft drink consumption and obesity. *Economics and Human Biology, 9*(3), 221–233.

Andreyeva, T., Long, M. W., & Brownell, K. D. (2010). The impact of food prices on consumption: A systematic review of research on the price elasticity of demand for food. *American Journal of Public Health, 100*(2), 216–222.

Angell, S. Y., Silver, L. D., Goldstein, G. P., Johnson, C. M., Deitcher, D. R., Frieden, T. R., & Bassett, M. T. (2009). Cholesterol control beyond the clinic: New York City's trans fat restriction. *Annals of Internal Medicine, 151*(2), 129–134.

Appel, L. J., Champagne, C. M., Harsha, D. W., Cooper, L. S., Obarzanek, E., Elmer, P. J., et al. (2003). Effects of comprehensive lifestyle modification on blood pressure control: Main results of the PREMIER clinical trial. *JAMA, the Journal of the American Medical Association, 289*(16), 2083–2093.

Barr-Anderson, D. J., Larson, N. I., Nelson, M. C., Neumark-Sztainer, D., & Story, M. (2009). Does television viewing predict dietary intake five years later in high school students and young adults? *International Journal of Behavioral Nutrition and Physical Activity, 6*(1), 7.

Brinsden, H. C., Feng, J. He, Jenner, K. H., & MacGregor, G. A. (2013). Surveys of the salt content in UK bread: Progress made and further reductions possible. *British Medical Journal Open, 3*(6). Retrieved from http://www.ncbi.nlm.nih.gov/pubmed/23794567.

Brownell, K. D., & Frieden, T. R. (2009). Ounces of prevention—the public policy case for taxes on sugared beverages. *New England Journal of Medicine, 360*(18), 1805–1808.

Brownell, K. D., & Warner, K. E. (2009). The perils of ignoring history: Big tobacco played dirty and millions died. How similar is big food? *Milbank Quarterly, 87*(1), 259–294.

Carlson, S. A., Fulton, J. E., Lee, S. M., Maynard, L. M., Brown, D. R., Kohl, H. W., & Dietz, W. H. (2008). Physical education and academic achievement in elementary school: Data from the early childhood longitudinal study. *American Journal of Public Health, 98*(4), 721–727.

Centers for Disease Control and Prevention (CDC). (2012). Internet cigarette vendors study prompts policy changes in government and industry. Retrieved from http://www.cdc.gov/prc/prevention -strategies/internet-cigarette-vendors-study.htm.

Chapman, S., & Wakefield, M. (2012). Smoking cessation strategies. [Comment Editorial]. *British Medical Journal, 344*, e1732.

Chinapaw, M. J., Proper, K. I., Brug, J., van Mechelen, W., & Singh, A. S. (2011). Relationship between young people's sedentary behaviour and biomedical health indicators: A systematic review of prospective studies. *Obesity Reviews, 12*(7), e621–e632.

Church, T. S., Thomas, D. M., Tudor-Locke, C., Katzmarzyk, P. T., Earnest, C. P., Rodarte, R. Q., et al. (2011). Trends over 5 decades in U.S. occupation-related physical activity and their associations with obesity. *PLoS one, 6*(5). Retrieved from http://www.plosone.org/article/info%3Adoi%2F10.1371%2Fjournal .pone.0019657.

Chriqui, J. F., Turner, L., Taber, D. R., & Chaloupka, F. J. (2013). Association between district and state policies and U.S. public elementary school competitive food and beverage environments. *JAMA Pediatrics, 167*(8), 714–722.

Conlin, P. R., Chow, D., Miller, E. R., Svetkey, L. P., Lin, P. H., Harsha, D. W., Moore, T. J., et al. (2000). The effect of dietary patterns on blood pressure control in hypertensive patients: Results from the Dietary Approaches to Stop Hypertension (DASH) trial. *American Journal of Hypertension, 13*, 949–955.

Coombes, R. (2011). Trans fats: Chasing a global ban. *British Medical Journal, 343*. doi: http://dx.doi .org/10.1136/bmj.d5567.

Coxson, P. G., Cook, N. R., Joffres, M., Hong, Y., Orenstein, D., Schmidt, S. M., & Bibbins-Domingo, K. (2013). Mortality benefits from U.S. population-wide reduction in sodium consumption: Projections from 3 modeling approaches. *Hypertension, 61*(3), 564–570.

Doll, R., & Hill, A. B. (1950). Smoking and carcinoma of the lung; preliminary report. *British Medical Journal, 2*(4682), 739–748.

Dollman, J., & Lewis, N. R. (2007). Active transport to school as part of a broader habit of walking and cycling among South Australian youth. *Pediatric Exercise Science, 19*(4), 436–443.

Dorfman, L., Cheyne, A., Friedman, L. C., Wadud, A., & Gottlieb, M. (2012). Soda and tobacco industry corporate social responsibility campaigns: How do they compare? *PLoS Medicine, 9*(6), e1001241.

Downs, S. M., Thow, A., & Leeder, S. R. (2013). The effectiveness of policies for reducing dietary trans fat: A systematic review of the evidence. *Bulletin of the World Health Organization, 91*, 262–269H. doi: http://dx.doi.org/10.2471/BLT.12.111468.

Duncan, D. T., Wolin, K. Y., Scharoun-Lee, M., Ding, E. L., Warner, E. T., & Bennett, G. G. (2011). Does perception equal reality? Weight misperception in relation to weight-related attitudes and behaviors among overweight and obese U.S. adults. *International Journal of Behavioral Nutrition and Physical Activity, 8*(1), 20.

Elbel, B., Taksler, G. B., Mijanovich, T., Abrams, C. B., & Dixon, L. B. (2013). Promotion of healthy eating through public policy: A controlled experiment. *American Journal of Preventive Medicine, 45*(1), 49–55.

Erinosho, T. O., Moser, R. P., Oh, A. Y., Nebeling, L. C., & Yaroch, A. L. (2012). Awareness of the Fruits and Veggies—More Matters campaign, knowledge of the fruit and vegetable recommendation, and fruit and vegetable intake of adults in the 2007 Food Attitudes and Behaviors (FAB) Survey. *Appetite, 59*(1), 155–160.

Farkas, A. J., Gilpin, E. A., White, M. M., & Pierce, J. P. (2000). Association between household and workplace smoking restrictions and adolescent smoking. *JAMA, 284*(6), 717–722.

Farrelly, M. C., Nonnemaker, J., Davis, K. C., & Hussin, A. (2009). The influence of the national truth campaign on smoking initiation. *American Journal of Preventive Medicine, 36*(5), 379–384.

Federal Trade Commission (FTC). (2012). *A review of food marketing to children and adolescents follow-up report.* Retrieved from http://www.ftc.gov/os/2012/12/121221foodmarketingreport.pdf.

Freedman, D. S., Khan, L. K., Serdula, M. K., Dietz, W. H., Srinivasan, S. R., & Berenson, G. S. (2005). The relation of childhood BMI to adult adiposity: The Bogalusa Heart Study. *Pediatrics, 115*(1), 22–27.

Frieden, T. R., Dietz, W., & Collins, J. (2010). Reducing childhood obesity through policy change: Acting now to prevent obesity. *Health Affairs (Project Hope), 29*(3), 357–63.

Giles-Corti, B., & Donovan, R. J. (2002). Relative influences of individual, social environmental, and physical environment determinants of physical activity. *Social Science and Medicine, 54*, 1793–1812.

Gilpin, E. A., Choi, W. S., Berry, C., & Pierce, J. P. (1999). How many adolescents start smoking each day in the United States? *Journal of Adolescent Health, 25*(4), 248–255.

Gilpin, E. A., Farkas, A. J., Emery, S. L., Ake, C. F., & Pierce, J. P. (2002). Clean indoor air: Advances in California, 1990–1999. *American Journal of Public Health, 92*(5), 785–791.

Gilpin, E. A., Lee, L., & Pierce, J. P. (2004). Changes in population attitudes about where smoking should not be allowed: California versus the rest of the USA. *Tobacco Control, 13*(1), 38–44.

Gilpin, E. A., White, M. M., Farkas, A. J., & Pierce, J. P. (1999). Home smoking restrictions: Which smokers have them and how they are associated with smoking behavior. *Nicotine & Tobacco Research, 1*(2), 153–162.

Glynn, T. J. (1989). Essential elements of school-based smoking prevention programs. *Journal of School Health, 59*(5), 181–188.

Green, L. W., & Fielding, J. (2011). The U.S. Healthy People initiative: Its genesis and its sustainability. *Annual Review of Public Health, 32*, 451–470.

Healy, G. N., Matthews, C. E., Dunstan, D. W., Winkler, E. a H., & Owen, N. (2011). Sedentary time and cardio-metabolic biomarkers in U.S. adults: NHANES 2003-06. *European Heart Journal, 32*(5), 590–597.

Henney, J. E., Taylor, C. L., & Boon, C. S. (Eds.). (2010). *Committee on strategies to reduce sodium intake.* Institute of Medicine. Washington, DC: National Academies Press.

Hill, J. O., Peters, J. C., & Wyatt, H. R. (2007). The role of public policy in treating the epidemic of global obesity. *Clinical Pharmacology and Therapeutics, 81*(5), 772–775.

Huhman, M. E., Potter, L. D., Nolin, M. J., Piesse, A., Judkins, D. R., Banspach, S. W., & Wong, F. L. (2010). The influence of the VERB campaign on children's physical activity in 2002 to 2006. *American Journal of Public Health, 100*(4), 638–645.

Hughes, J. R., Gulliver, S. B., Fenwick, J. W., Valliere, W. A., Cruser, K., Pepper, S., Shea, P., Solomon, L. J., & Flynn, B. S. (1992). Smoking cessation among self-quitters. *Health Psychology, 11*(5), 331–334.

Institute of Medicine (IOM). (2005). Committee on Prevention of Obesity in Children and Youth. Preventing Childhood Obesity: *Health in the Balance.* Washington, DC: National Academies Press.

Institute of Medicine (IOM). (2006). *Progress in preventing childhood obesity: How do we measure up?* Washington, DC: National Academies Press.

Institute of Medicine (IOM). (2007). *Ending the tobacco problem: A blueprint for the nation.* Washington, DC: National Academies Press.

Institute of Medicine (IOM). (2013). *Sodium intake in populations: Assessment of evidence.* Washington, DC: National Academies Press.

Johnston, L. D., O'Malley, P. M., Terry-McElrath, Y. M., Freedman-Doan, P., & Brenner, J. S. (2011). *School policies and practices to improve health and prevent obesity: National secondary school survey results, school years 2006–07 and 2007–08. Volume 1.* Ann Arbor, MI: Bridging the Gap Program, Survey Research Center, Institute for Social Research. Retrieved from http://www.bridgingthegapresearch .org/_asset/984r22/SS_2011_monograph.pdf

Kaiser Family Foundation. (2010). *Generation M²: Media in the lives of 8- to 18-year-olds.* Menlo Park, CA: Henry J. Kaiser Family Foundation.

Kaphingst, K. M., & Story M. (2009). Child care as an untapped setting for obesity prevention: State child care licensing regulations related to nutrition, physical activity, and media use for preschool-aged children in the United States. *Preventing Chronic Disease, 6*(1). Retrieved from http://www.ncbi .nlm.nih.gov/pubmed/19080017.

Koepp, G. A., Manohar, C. U., McCrady-Spitzer, S. K., Ben-Ner, A., Hamann, D. J., Runge, C. F., & Levine, J. A. (2013). Treadmill desks: A 1-year prospective trial. *Obesity, 21*(4), 705–711.

Kovacic, W. E. (2008). *Marketing food to children and adolescents: A review of industry expenditures, activities, and self-regulation.* A Federal Trade Commission report to Congress. Washington, DC: Federal Trade Commission. Retrieved from http://www.ftc.gov/sites/default/files/documents/reports /marketing-food-children-and-adolescents-review-industry-expenditures-activities-and-self -regulation/p064504foodmktingreport.pdf.

Landrine, H., Klonoff, E. A., & Reina-Patton, A. (2000). Minors' access to tobacco before and after the California STAKE Act. *Tobacco Control, 9* (suppl 2: ii15–ii17).

Larson, N. I., Story, M. T., & Nelson, M. C. (2009). Neighborhood environments: Disparities in access to healthy foods in the U.S. *American Journal of Preventive Medicine, 36*(1), 74–81.

Levin, M. L., Goldstein, H., & Gerhardt, P. R. (1950). Cancer and tobacco smoking. *JAMA, 143,* 2.

Lubans, D. R., Boreham, C. A., Kelly, P., & Foster, C. E. (2011). The relationship between active travel to school and health-related fitness in children and adolescents: A systematic review. *International Journal of Behavioral Nutrition and Physical Activity, 8*(1), 5.

McGann, S., Jancey, J., & Tye, M. (2013). Taking the stairs instead: The impact of workplace design standards on health promotion strategies. *Australasian Medical Journal, 6*(1), 23–28.

Messer, K., & Pierce, J. P. (2010). Changes in age trajectories of smoking experimentation during the California Tobacco Control Program. *American Journal of Public Health, 100*(7), 1298–1306.

Mills, C. A., & Porter, M. M. (1950). Tobacco smoking habits and cancer of the mouth and respiratory system. *Cancer Research, 10,* 3.

Mitchell, J. A., Rodriguez, D., Schmitz, K. H., & Audrain-McGovern, J. (2013). Greater screen time is associated with adolescent obesity: A longitudinal study of the BMI distribution from Ages 14 to 18. *Obesity, 21*(3), 572–575.

Mozaffarian, D., Katan, M. B., Ascherio, A., Stampfer, M. J., & Willett, W. C. (2006). Trans fatty acids and cardiovascular disease. *New England Journal of Medicine, 354*(15), 1601–1613.

Mozaffarian, D., & Stampfer, M. J. (2010). Removing industrial trans fat from foods. *British Medical Journal, 340.* Retrieved from http://www.ncbi.nlm.nih.gov/pubmed/20395265.

National Institutes of Health. (1998). Clinical guidelines on the identification, evaluation, and treatment of overweight and obesity in adults: The evidence report. *Obesity Research, 6* (suppl 2), 51S–209S. Retrieved from http://www.nhlbi.nih.gov/guidelines/obesity/ob_gdlns.pdf.

National Research Council. (2013). *Educating the student body: Taking physical activity and physical education to school.* Washington, DC: National Academies Press.

McDonald, N. C., Brown, A. L., Marchetti,L. M., & Pedroso, M. S. (2011). U.S. school travel, 2009 an assessment of trends. *American Journal of Preventive Medicine, 41*(2), 146–151.

Neumark-Sztainer, D., French, S. A., Hannan, P. J., Story, M., & Fulkerson, J. A. (2005). School lunch and snacking patterns among high school students: Associations with school food environment and policies. *International Journal of Behavioral Nutrition and Physical Activity, 2*(1), 14.

Nestle, M. (2002). *Food politics: How the food industry influences nutrition and health.* Los Angeles: University of California Press.

Otite, F. O., Jacobson, M. F., Dahmubed, A., & Mozaffarian, D. (2013). Trends in trans fatty acids. Reformulations of U.S. supermarket and brand-name foods from 2007 through 2011. *Preventing Chronic Disease.* 120198. doi: http://dx.doi.org/10.5888/pcd10.120198.

Owen, N., Bauman, A., & Brown, W. (2009). Too much sitting: A novel and important predictor of chronic disease risk? *British Journal of Sports Medicine, 43*(2), 80–81.

Pate, R. R., Davis, M. G., Robinson, T. N., Stone, E. J., McKenzie, T. L., & Young, J. C. (2006). Promoting physical activity in children and youth: A leadership role for schools: A scientific statement from the American Heart Association Council on Nutrition, Physical Activity, and Metabolism (Physical Activity Committee) in collaboration with the Councils on Cardiovascular Disease in the Young and Cardiovascular Nursing. *Circulation, 114*(11), 1214–1224.

Pierce, J. P. (Working Group Chair). (2009). *Evaluating the effectiveness of smoke-free policies.* Handbook of Cancer Prevention, Tobacco Control, Vol. 13. Lyon, France: IARC (International Agency for Research on Cancer Prevention).

Pierce, J. P., Caan, B. J., Parker, B. A., Greenberg, E. R., Flatt, S. W., Rock, C. L., et al. (2007). Influence of a diet very high in vegetables, fruit, and fiber and low in fat on prognosis. *JAMA, 298*(3), 289–298.

Pierce, J. P., Cummins, S. E., White, M. M., Humphrey, A., & Messer, K. (2012). Quitlines and nicotine replacement for smoking cessation: Do we need to change policy? [Research Support, Non-U.S. Gov't Review]. *Annual Review of Public Health, 33,* 341–356. doi: 10.1146/annurev-publhealth -031811-124624.

Pierce, J. P., Dwyer, T., Frape, G., Chapman, S., Chamberlain, A., & Burke, N. (1986). Evaluation of the Sydney "Quit. For Life" anti-smoking campaign. Part 1. Achievement of intermediate goals. *Medical Journal of Australia, 144*(7), 341–344.

Pierce, J. P., Farkas, A. J., & Gilpin, E. A. (1998). Beyond stages of change: The quitting continuum measures progress towards successful smoking cessation. *Addiction, 93*(2), 277–286.

Pierce, J. P., Fiore, M. C., Novotny, T. E., Hatziandreu, E. J., & Davis, R. M. (1989). Trends in cigarette smoking in the United States. Projections to the year 2000. *JAMA, 261*(1), 61–65.

Pierce, J. P., Gilmer, T. P., Lee, L., Gilpin, E. A., de Beyer, J., & Messer, K. (2005). Tobacco industry price-subsidizing promotions may overcome the downward pressure of higher prices on initiation of regular smoking. *Health Economics,14*, 1061–1071.

Pierce, J. P., & Gilpin, E. A. (1995). A historical analysis of tobacco marketing and the uptake of smoking by youth in the United States: 1890–1977. *Health Psychology, 14*(6), 500–508.

Pierce, J. P., Gilpin, E. A., Emery, S. L., White, M. M., Rosbrook, B., Berry, C. C., & Farkas, A. J. (1998). Has the California Tobacco Control Program reduced smoking? *JAMA, 280*(10), 893–899.

Pierce, J. P., Lee, L., & Gilpin, E. A. (1994). Smoking initiation by adolescent girls, 1944 through 1988. An association with targeted advertising [see comments]. *JAMA, 271*(8), 608–611.

Pierce, J. P., Macaskill, P., & Hill, D. (1990). Long-term effectiveness of mass media led antismoking campaigns in Australia. *American Journal of Public Health, 80*(5), 565–569.

Powell, K. E., Martin, L. M., & Chowdhury, P. P. (2003). Places to walk: Convenience and regular physical activity. *American Journal of Public Health, 93*(9), 1519–1521.

Phillip Morris USA Inc. (n.d.) http://www.philipmorrisusa.com/en/cms/Responsibility/Government _Affairs/Legislative_Issues/default.aspx?src=top_nav, Accessed June 26, 2013.

PHIT. (2009). *Personal Health Investment Act of 2009*. HR 2105, 111th Cong.

Reilly, J. J. (2010). Low levels of objectively measured physical activity in preschoolers in child care. *Medicine and Science in Sports and Exercise, 42*(3), 502–507.

Rhodes, R. E., & De Bruijn, G. J. (2013). How big is the physical activity intention-behaviour gap? A meta-analysis using the action control framework. *British Journal of Health Psychology, 18*(2), 296–309. Robins, L. N., Davis, D. H., & Goodwin, D. W. (1974). Drug use by U.S. Army enlisted men in Vietnam: A follow up on their return home. *American Journal of Epidemiology, 99*(4), 235–249.

Rosenthal, M. B., Farley, T., Gortmaker, S., & Sunstein, C. R. (2013). Health promotion and the state. *NEJM* perspective roundtable. *New England Journal of Medicine, 368*(25), e34.

Rovner, A., Nansel, T., Wang, J., & Iannotti, R. (2011). Food sold in school vending machines is associated with overall student dietary intake. *Journal of Adolescent Health, 48*(1), 13–19.

Saffer H. & Chaloupka, F. (2000). The effect of tobacco advertising bans on tobacco consumption. *Journal of Health Economics, 19*(6), 1117–1137.

Sallis, J. F., McKenzie, T. L., Kolody, B., Lewis, M., Marshall, S., & Rosengard, P. (1999). Effects of health-related physical education on academic achievement: Project SPARK. *Research Quarterly for Exercise and Sport, 70*(2), 127–134.

Sallis, J. F., Saelens, B. E., Frank, L. D., Conway, T. L., Slymen, D. J., Cain, K. L., Chapman, J. E., et al. (2009). Neighborhood built environment and income: Examining multiple health outcomes. *Social Science & Medicine, 68*(7), 1285–1293.

Saquib, N., Natarajan, L., Rock, C. L., Flatt, S. W., Madlensky, L., Kealey, S., & Pierce, J. P. (2008). The impact of a long-term reduction in dietary energy density on body weight within a randomized diet trial. *Nutrition and Cancer, 60*(1), 31–38.

Schrek, R. S., Baker, L. A., Ballard, G. P., & Dolgoff, S. (1950). Tobacco smoking as an etiological factor in disease. *Cancer Research, 10*, 9.

Story, M., Kaphingst, K. M., Robinson-O'Brien, R., & Glanz, K. (2008). Creating healthy food and eating environments: Policy and environmental approaches. *Annual Review of Public Health, 29*(1), 253–272.

Strong, W. B., Malina, R. M., Blimkie, C. J. R., Daniels, S. R., Dishman, R. K., Gutin, B., Hergenroeder, A. C., et al. (2005). Evidence based physical activity for school-age youth. *Journal of Pediatrics, 146*(6), 732–737.

Sutherland, L. A., Mackenzie, T., Purvis, L. A., & Dalton, M. (2010). Prevalence of food and beverage brands in movies: 1996–2005. *Pediatrics, 125*(3), 468–474.

Svetkey, L. P., Sacks, F. M., Obarzanek, E., Vollmer, W. M., Appel, L. J., Lin, P. H., et al. (1999). The DASH Diet, Sodium Intake and Blood Pressure Trial (DASH-sodium): Rationale and design. DASH-Sodium Collaborative Research Group. *Journal of the American Dietetic Association, 99:* S96–S104.

Taber, D. R., Chriqui, J. F., Powell, L., & Chaloupka, F. J. (2013). Association between state laws governing school meal nutrition content and student weight status: Implications for new USDA school meal standards. *JAMA Pediatrics, 167*(6), 513–519.

Thomson, C. A., Flatt, S. W., Rock, C. L., Ritenbaugh, C., Newman, V., & Pierce, J. P. (2002). Increased fruit, vegetable and fiber intake and lower fat intake reported among women previously treated for invasive breast cancer. *Journal of the American Dietetic Association, 102*(6), 801–808.

Troiano, R. P., Berrigan, D., Dodd, K. W., Masse, L. C., Tilert, T., & McDowell, M. (2008). Physical activity in the United States measured by accelerometer. *Medicine & Science in Sports & Exercise, 40*(1), 181–188.

USDHEW. (1964). *Smoking and health.* Report of the Advisory Committee to the Surgeon General of the Public Health Service. Washington, DC: U.S. Dept. of Health, Education, and Welfare, Public Health Service, Center for Disease Control.

U.S. Department of Agriculture (USDA). (2007). School nutrition dietary assessment study—III. Retrieved from http://www.fns.usda.gov/school-nutrition-dietary-assessment-study-iii.

U.S. Department of Agriculture, U.S. Department of Health and Human Services (USDHHS). (2010). *Dietary Guidelines for Americans, 2010* (7th ed.). Washington, DC: U.S. Government Printing Office.

U.S. Department of Education. (2001). No Child Left Behind Act of 2001. Retrieved June 26, 2013, from http://www2.ed.gov/policy/elsec/leg/esea02/index.html.

U.S. Department of Health and Human Services (USDHHS). (1979). *The Surgeon General's report on health promotion and disease prevention.* Washington, DC. U.S. Government Printing Office, DHEW (PHS) Publication No. 79-55071.

U.S. Department of Health and Human Services (USDHHS), National Institutes of Health (1998). *Clinical guidelines on the identification, evaluation, and treatment of overweight and obesity in adults: The evidence report.* Washington, DC. NIH Publication NO. 98-4083. http://www.nhlbi.nih.gov /guidelines/obesity/ob_gdlns.pdf.

U.S. Department of Health and Human Services (USDHHS) Office of Disease Prevention and Health Promotion. (1990). *Healthy People 2000: National health promotion and disease prevention objectives.* Washington, DC: U.S. Government Printing Office Publication No. 017-001-00474-0.

U.S. Department of Health and Human Services (USDHHS) Office of Disease Prevention and Health Promotion. (2000). *Healthy People 2010.* Washington, DC: U.S. Government Printing Office.

U.S. Department of Health and Human Services (USDHHS). (2011). *Healthy People 2020.* Washington, DC: Retrieved from http://www.healthypeople.gov/2020/default.aspx.

U.S. Department of Health and Human Services (USDHHS). (2012). *Preventing tobacco use among youth and young adults: A report of the Surgeon General.* Atlanta, GA: U.S. Department of Health and Human Services, Centers for Disease Control and Prevention, National Center for Chronic Disease Prevention and Health Promotion, Office on Smoking and Health.

Uusitalo, U., Feskens, E. J., Tuomilehto, J., Dowse, G., Haw, U., Fareed, D., et al. (1996). Fall in total cholesterol concentration over five years in association with changes in fatty acid composition of cooking oil in Mauritius: Cross sectional survey. *BMJ British Medical Journal, 313*(7064), 1044–1046.

Vesper, H., Kuiper, H., Mirel, L., Johnson, C., & Pirkle, J. (2012). Levels of plasma trans-fatty acids in non-Hispanic White adults in the United States in 2000 and 2009. *JAMA, 307*(6), 2012–2013.

Von Tigerstrom, B., Larre, T., & Sauder, J. (2011). Using the tax system to promote physical activity: Critical analysis of Canadian initiatives. *American Journal of Public Health, 101*(8). Retrieved from http://www.ncbi.nlm.nih.gov/pubmed/21680912.

Wang, Y. C., Orleans, C. T., & Gortmaker, S. L. (2012). Reaching the Healthy People goals for reducing childhood obesity: Closing the energy gap. *American Journal of Preventive Medicine, 42*(5), 437–444.

Wechsler, H., Devereaux, R. S., Davis, M., & Collins, J. (2000). Using the school environment to promote physical activity and healthy eating. *Preventive Medicine, 31*(2), S121–S137.

World Health Organization (WHO). (2010). *Set of recommendations on the marketing of foods and non-alcoholic beverages to children.* Geneva, Switzerland: World Health Organization. Retrieved from http://whqlibdoc.who.int/publications/2010/9789241500210_eng.pdf.

World Health Organization (WHO). (2013). *10 facts of obesity.* Geneva, Switzerland: World Health Organization. Retrieved from http://www.who.int/features/factfiles/obesity/en/.

Wynder, E. L., & Graham, E. A. (1950). Tobacco smoking as a possible etiologic factor in bronchogenic carcinoma. *JAMA, 143,* 329–336.

Chapter 11

John Pierce, PhD

CONCLUSIONS

Chapter Outline

INTRODUCTION TO GOOD HEALTH PROMOTION PRACTICE

The World Health Organization has the most widely used definition of health promotion, which is "the process of enabling people to improve their health." Initially, this was perceived as a task focused on the individual; however, over time, we began to recognize the crucial role that the environment plays in determining almost all behaviors that can influence health. The current emphasis includes a focus on organizations, communities, and the policies they have in place that influence healthy behaviors.

This definition assumes that health promotion practice begins with the identification of a problem that is limiting the health potential of a group of people.

Thus, before conducting an intervention, a planning process determines why an intervention is needed. This planning process has been codified into a number of models that practitioners can use, such as PRECEDE-PROCEED, PATCH, APEX-PH, MAPP, and CDCynergy, as well as a number that fit under the rubric of logic models. While application of these models has worked in a number of different health promotion settings, undoubtedly there will be settings in which practitioners need to use the basic six steps of program planning: (1) needs assessment, (2) priority setting, (3) setting goals and objectives, (4) methods and implementation, (5) evaluation, and (6) budgeting.

The importance of evaluation to effective health promotion practice cannot be overemphasized. CDC has developed an excellent framework for evaluation, which also includes six steps: (1) engage stakeholders, (2) describe the program, (3) focus the evaluation design, (4) gather credible evidence, (5) justify conclusions, and (6) ensure use and sharing of lessons learned. Some of the health promotion challenges mentioned later in this chapter can be directly traced back to not keeping key community stakeholders engaged in the process. To avoid misunderstandings and mishaps, health promotion practitioners should use *process evaluation* strategies from the beginning through the delivery of a specific program, *impact evaluation* strategies to assess the program's immediate effect on participants, stakeholders, and settings, and *outcome evaluation* to assess how well the intervention in achieved the program goal.

THE IMPORTANCE OF THEORY

Kurt Lewin, often considered the father of social psychology, had an oft-quoted epigram: "There is nothing so practical as a good theory" (Lewin, 1951, 169), which has been interpreted as saying that the best theories are those that can be used to solve social or practical problems, and the best way to improve current practice in an area like health behavior is to design interventions using such a theory. Ideally, applied research that tests such a theory should have a feedback loop that leads to an improvement of the theory that can then inform the next intervention.

There is not one single health behavior theory that health promotion practitioners should use. However, promoting health and preventing disease can require behavior change at the individual, organizational, and community level, and this has resulted in a preference for theories that fit within the Social Ecological Framework. The targeted changes for a health promotion intervention may involve a simple behavior, (e.g., voting for policy change) or more complex behavior (e.g., changing well-established habits), or they could involve restricting the behavior of others at an organizational or societal level (e.g., workplace policies, options for purchasing).

TRANSMISSIBLE DISEASES

Life expectancy increased dramatically during the 20th century. Although the life expectancy of a newborn in 1900 was less than 50 years, it now exceeds 80 years in several countries. While the gains were mainly in higher-income countries in the early half of the 20th century, in the latter half of the century, rapid gains were seen also in East Asian countries, where life expectancy at birth increased from less than 45 years in 1950 to more than 74 years by 2010. These dramatic gains in life expectancy have been accompanied by a shift in the leading causes of mortality and morbidity from infectious and parasitic diseases to noncommunicable diseases and chronic conditions. With this shift has come an increasing emphasis on changing modifiable risk factors.

However, transmissible diseases are still responsible for one in three deaths worldwide and, except for sexually transmitted diseases, are particularly problematic in low-income and tropical countries. These include diarrheal diseases, malaria, and dengue. Diarrheal diseases are most often related to limited access to clean water and are a major health promotion problem in a number of countries. Dehydration and loss of nutrients associated with diarrheal disease can be fatal but can be prevented with rehydration treatments (either home remedies or oral rehydration solutions). Educating communities about oral rehydration is a major role for health promotion practitioners in these countries. The malaria parasite is transmitted by mosquitoes, and in affected countries, it can be the leading cause of illness and death, particularly in children. Health promotion practice of disseminating use of insecticide-treated bed nets (ITNs) to prevent mosquito bites has reduced deaths by 20%. Mosquitoes also transmit up to four dengue viruses, and this is a leading cause of mortality and morbidity in many tropical countries. The most effective recommended prevention strategies involve sustainable community-based mosquito control. However, health promotion efforts to control diarrhea through oral rehydration and malaria through ITNs have been more successful than health promotion efforts to control dengue fever. Health promotion efforts for these and other tropical diseases are usually overseen by global health organizations. Given that health promotion practitioners are often not from the culture, additional issues are critical to the success of these efforts, including ensuring that interventions respect the cultures, traditions, and laws of the communities and that community stakeholders have a critical say in designing, implementing, and evaluating the health promotion activity.

The large economic and health consequences of human immunodeficiency virus infection and acquired immune deficiency syndrome (HIV/AIDS) and other sexually transmitted diseases became obvious to the world with the rapid increase of AIDS in the United States and many other parts of the world in the early 1980s. HIV is transmitted primarily via unprotected sexual intercourse (including anal and oral sex), contaminated blood transfusions, hypodermic needles, and from mother to child during pregnancy, delivery, or breastfeeding. For people who already have the infection, the emphasis is on ensuring access to medication and medication adherence and reducing the possibility of disease transmission. The main HIV–prevention efforts include strategies to keep uninfected individuals from becoming infected (primary prevention) and programs to educate those living with HIV to encourage optimal care and reduce transmission (secondary prevention). The Centers for Disease Control recommends focusing on routine HIV testing with immediate treatment, as such a policy has had success at lowering the circulating virus in the population, thus reducing transmission. Many health promotion practitioners are focused on removing known obstacles to getting testing, including a reluctance of affected individuals to disclose the problem or discuss sexual health issues openly because of HIV– and STD–related stigma and the lack of symptoms in some 20% of individuals living with HIV who don't know they're infected (some who have been diagnosed as HIV positive are in denial). The Social Ecological Framework has provided a good basis for identifying activities to remove these obstacles, as changes are needed at the individual level (increased knowledge), the interpersonal level (family or sexual partner perceptions), community/societal level (e.g., social norms and community perceptions about HIV), and environmental/policy-level (e.g., structural-location, organizational—hours or operation, and policy—for example, teenagers may require a parent's permission).

A FOCUS ON DISEASES WITH MODIFIABLE RISK FACTORS FOR CHRONIC DISEASES

Increasingly, noncommunicable chronic diseases, including type 2 diabetes, cardiovascular disease, and cancer, present the greatest disease risk to the health of people of all nations. Such diseases are the leading cause of death and disability in the United States, and disease treatment consumes approximately 75% of health care expenditures.

An individual's risk of these diseases includes heritable factors but also factors that are eminently under our own control, including what and how much we eat (nutrition), how much physical activity we do, and whether we inhale combustible biological products such as tobacco. Obesity is increasing rapidly in many nations, which is a consequence of the consumption of more energy (food) than the body expends (physical activity).

Tobacco

Europeans discovered tobacco use when they colonized the Americas, and it was quickly disseminated around the globe. However, it was not until the 20th century that manufactured cigarettes became readily available and marketed so that they became the dominant form of tobacco use. By midcentury, the first evidence of the harmful consequences of cigarette smoking was published in both the United States and the United Kingdom, and the evidence quickly grew so that, by the early 1960s, both countries had accepted that cigarette smoking was a major public health problem. More than 80% of lung cancer and chronic obstructive pulmonary disease are caused by cigarette smoking, and lung cancer can be modeled adequately using only two variables: the duration of smoking and the intensity of exposure. In addition to lung cancer and heart disease, this behavior has been associated with numerous other diseases and is widely recognized as the single most preventable cause of death and disability in the world today. Not only does it affect the health of the smoker, it also affects the health of individuals exposed to the toxic chemicals produced by burning tobacco (secondhand smoke or environmental tobacco smoke).

Health promotion goals are to prevent smoking initiation and help addicted smokers quit. However, a large obstacle to their efforts is the powerful force and influence of tobacco industry advertising and promotion. Since the start of the public health campaign against cigarette smoking, there has been an evolution of health promotion strategies that have successfully reduced the problem behavior. In 2003, these were codified when the World Health Organization implemented the first-ever international treaty on a health behavior: the Framework Convention for Tobacco Control. Although much progress still needs to be made to reduce smoking behaviors, the accomplishments of health promotion approaches to tobacco control provide examples of strategies that could be adopted to change other lifestyle behaviors. Using the Social Ecological Framework, these include programs at the individual level (e.g., tobacco use education), interpersonal level (e.g., family and peer influences, interventions by health care providers or health coaches), organizational level (e.g., workplace smoking policies), community level (e.g., laws to regulate tobacco, restricting youth access to tobacco products), and public policy level (e.g., smoking bans, taxation of tobacco products, public passive smoking interventions, advertising bans). Healthy People 2020 outlines the following important policy strategies that have been shown to be effective: (a) provide incentives for healthy behaviors and disincentives for unhealthy behaviors; (b) control access to either products or facilities related to the behavior; (c) use media to promote healthy behaviors or discourage unhealthy behaviors and regulate industry marketing and promotion; (d) promote healthy behaviors in schools, and (e) regulate behavior-related products.

Nutrition

Health promotion efforts are focused not just on how much food but on what type of food is eaten. Despite problems with measurement, researchers have been able to demonstrate that broad food patterns such as plant-based dietary patterns and Mediterranean diets are associated with lower risks of many chronic diseases, whereas high-fat Western dietary patterns have been associated with increased risks particularly of cardiovascular disease.

However, the measurement of dietary intake has not been optimal and offers a significant challenge to the field. There are thousands of food items, each of which is composed of many component nutrients. Further, the nutrients per food item (e.g., a carrot) vary depending on where it was grown. Current measurement methods include food frequency questionnaires and food diaries or dietary recalls. These approaches rely on memory, and there is substantial participant burden involved in collecting this dietary information.

Repeated measures show substantial systematic bias (people answering in the same pattern), and many individuals report less intake than would be needed to maintain their weight (under normal assumptions on metabolic rate). Further, people seem to take shortcuts so that the second and third measures are completed in shorter time periods and result in lower estimates of caloric consumption, even when there was no recorded change in weight. On the Healthy People 2020 objectives, neither the weight status nor the nutrition intake of the United States population improved in the previous decade, and this is a growing concern for the health of Americans. It suggests the need for more comprehensive strategies, modeled on those used to combat tobacco use, if we are to start to make progress in the near future.

Physical Activity

The importance of physical activity to health is becoming increasingly apparent as individuals become more sedentary. In fact, many experts now claim that being active is one of the best things individuals can do for their health. Health promotion efforts to improve physical activity are critical, as physical activity helps individuals live longer and healthier lives, protecting them from heart disease, stroke, high blood pressure, type 2 diabetes, and some cancers while improving mental health, sleep, heart, lung, bone health, and muscle function. Being physically active can also help reduce excess weight, which significantly decreases the risk of numerous diseases and clinical disorders. Despite the many health benefits of being physically active, the proportion of the population who engage in regular physical activity is small and has not changed over the past decade.

Technological advances are improving the objective measurement of physical activity, allowing researchers to gather more detailed and accurate information on daily activity and sedentary behavior and providing individuals with motivational feedback about their activity levels. These advances are increasing the quality of the research focused on individual and interpersonal influences. However, to increase physical activity to the recommended levels will require interventions at all levels of the Social Ecological Framework. This is particularly the case for policies that will help create an environment that is much more supportive of an active lifestyle. Such policies have been made into objectives in the Healthy People 2020.

MUSINGS ON CHALLENGES AND OPPORTUNITIES

As public health professionals look toward the future, a number of trends indicate challenges and opportunities for research and practice to improve the health of populations.

Challenges to Vaccination: The Polio Story

Polio is an acute, viral, infectious disease spread from person to person, primarily via the fecal-oral route. In about 1% of cases, the virus preferentially infects and destroys motor neurons, leading to lower-limb paralysis. Vaccines were developed in the early 1950s, at which time, in the United States, there were approximately 29,000 new polio cases each year, mainly among children. After two doses of the injectable vaccine, 90% or more of individuals develop protective antibodies to all three serotypes of poliovirus, and at least 99% are immune to poliovirus following three doses (Atkinson, Hamborsky, McIntyre, & Wolfe 2009). The World Health Organization made the eradication of polio a priority, and more than 2.5 billion children have been immunized worldwide—a great health promotion success story. Polio cases dropped precipitously.

However, recently, in war-torn regions, it has been impossible to vaccinate children, and polio cases have begun to reappear in Syria and Somalia. Worse, the public health community has not been able to convince all stakeholders of the importance of vaccination to prevent polio. In 2003, in northern Nigeria—a country that at that time was considered provisionally polio free—a religious fatwa was issued declaring that the polio vaccine was a conspiracy by the United States and the United Nations against the Muslim faith and that the vaccination could sterilize true believers (UNICEF, 2009). Following this, health workers administering polio vaccine were targeted and killed. Subsequently, polio reappeared in Nigeria and spread from there to several other countries. On May 5, 2014, the World Health Organization (WHO) declared a public health emergency of international concern. There appears to be a need to go back to health promotion basics and ensure that critical stakeholders become engaged and participate in the vaccination program rather than target it for removal.

The Clean Water Story and Climate Change

Along with other rapid changes associated with global population and economic growth, the recent evidence of rapid climate change means increased risks of extreme weather, such as heat waves, floods, and storms, as well as shifts to long-term drought conditions in many regions, melting of glaciers that supply fresh water to large population centers, and sea-level increases leading to salination of sources of agriculture and drinking water. These events could have a serious impact on infectious disease dynamics (EPA, 2014), with the effect most marked in many of the poorest nations who are already struggling to control malaria, diarrhea, and protein-energy malnutrition (Campbell-Lendruma, Corvalána, & Neira, 2007).

The Increasing Sedentary Epidemic

A Simon Fraser University health sciences professor, Scott Lear (Lear et al., 2014), looked at data from more than 150,000 adults from 17 different countries of varying income levels. These included Canada, Sweden, and United Arab Emirates (high income); Argentina, Brazil, Chile, Malaysia, Poland, South Africa, and Turkey (upper-middle income); China, Columbia, and Iran (lower-middle income); and Bangladesh, India, Pakistan, and Zimbabwe (low income). Participants were queried about the type of technology they owned, as well as their physical activity and eating habits. Participants who owned technology items such as TVs, desktop or laptop computers, and automobiles were compared to those who did not. More than three quarters of all households (78%) owned at least one television, while 34% owned a computer and 32% owned a car. The researchers reported that ownership of all three devices increased from low- to high-income countries (4–83%). Specific to participants from low-income countries, those who had multiple technology items (especially when one was a television) were four times more likely to be obese and more than twice as likely to have diabetes. Owning all three technologies was associated with a 30% decline in physical activity and a 20% increase in time spent in a sedentary position.

Worldwide mobile phone penetration is projected to reach 70% by 2017 (eMarketer, 2014), and almost half of these users (2.2 billion people worldwide) will go online via mobile at least monthly. A Nielson study (Halleck, 2014) reported that, in three developed countries (United States, UK, and Italy), more than one quarter of the mobile time was social—however, this increasingly does not involve an actual face-to-face communication; rather, it is text messaging, tweeting, and so on. Very little of the mobile time is spent on gathering information or educational materials, exploring places to go, or even investigating news. Further, there is a strong association of increased use with younger ages. For both boys and girls, each additional hour of weekday TV watching was linked with an increase in the risk of poor family functioning (such as the child not getting along well with parents; Hinkley et al., 2014). A second study reported that higher media use, when combined with less monitoring by the mother, was linked with a higher body mass index (BMI) in the child at age 7.

References

Atkinson W., Hamborsky J., McIntyre L., & Wolfe, S. (Eds.). (2009). Centers for Disease Control and Prevention. Poliomyelitis. In *Epidemiology and prevention of vaccine-preventable diseases. The pink book* (11th ed.; pp. 231–244). Washington, DC: Public Health Foundation.

Campbell-Lendrum, D., Corvalána, C., & Neira, M. (2007). Global climate change: Implications for international public health policy. *Bulletin of the World Health Organization, 85*(3), 161–244.

eMarketer. (2014). Smartphone users worldwide will total 1.75 billion in 2014. Retrieved from eMarketer.com.

EPA. (2014). Climate change and water. Accessed from water.epa.gov.

Halleck, T. (2014). We spend more time on smartphones than traditional PCs: Nielsen. *International Business Times.* Retrieved from http://www.ibtimes.com/.

Hinkley T., Verbestel V., Ahrens W., Lissner L., Molnár D., Moreno L. A., et al. (2014). Early childhood electronic media use as a predictor of poorer well-being: A prospective cohort study. *JAMA Pediatrics, 168*(5), 485–492.

Lear, S. A., Teo, K., Gasevic, D., Zhang, X., Poirier, P. P., Rangarajan, S., et al. (2014). The association between ownership of common household devices and obesity and diabetes in high, middle and low income countries. *Canadian Medical Association Journal, 186*(4), 258–266.

Lewin, K. (1951). *Field theory in social science: Selected theoretical papers* (D. Cartwright, Ed.). New York, NY: Harper & Row.

UNICEF. (2009). Polio eradication efforts in Nigeria and India. Accessed from www.unicef.org.

Glossary

A

access to health care is used to describe the degree to which individuals are able to obtain health care services when needed, measured by the presence of resources that facilitate health care use, such as insurance coverage, having had a recent physician's visit, and adequate economic resources.

acquired immune deficiency syndrome (AIDS) is a term used to indicate when HIV has impacted an individual's immune system to the extent that their CD4+T-cell count falls below a certain threshold. It is an advanced stage of HIV infection, when a person's immune system is damaged and has difficulty fighting diseases and certain cancers.

action stage is when the person is performing the desired behavior or not performing the undesirable behavior for at least 30 days.

activities of daily living are activities that are performed or completed throughout an individual's day.

An **agent** is an organic or nonorganic factor that causes disease, otherwise known as a pathogen.

appraisal support refers to the type of support that involves helping with decisions, providing appropriate feedback, or helping decide which course of action to take.

A person is **asymptomatic** when a disease causes no visible symptoms.

audience segmentation is dividing the target audience into groups based on certain characteristics, like behaviors, personal preferences, and values.

B

bacteria are one-celled (unicellular) microorganisms, some of which are harmful to humans.

bacterial infections are the invasion of bacteria into the body and subsequent growth/multiplication of the bacteria.

basal metabolic rate (BMR) is the amount of energy required to maintain the basic biological processes for life.

A **baseline measure** is the initial measure of a behavior or health outcome at the start of a health program. Put simply, it provides information about the health problem at the beginning of the program.

basic activities of daily living are self-care responsibilities, including bathing, dressing, feeding, toileting, and walking, that are performed by individuals themselves or with the aid of a caregiver.

behavior refers to performing the desired action.

behavioral capability is a person's *knowledge* and *skill* to enact the desired behavior.

behavioral intentions represent a person's likelihood to engage in the behavior.

A **biomarker** is a biological molecule sampled from an individual that reflects a specific metabolic process or biological state.

C

carcinogens are cancer-causing agents or substances. Tobacco products contain a wide array of carcinogens that are damaging to the human body.

A **caregiver** is an individual, often a friend or family member, who assists and supports another individual through management and treatment of an illness.

CD4 cells or **T-cells** are specialized white blood cells in the human immune system that help fight infections. These cells send signals to activate the body's immune response when they detect a virus (like HIV).

The **chronic care model** is a framework designed to increase positive health outcomes among chronically ill individuals by ensuring the patient and the health provider work in partnership and utilize a series of community and health system elements, including self-management support, resources and policies, delivery system design, organization of health care, decision support, and clinical information systems.

A **chronic disease developmental pathway** is a pathway to explain the link among social determinants such as income, education, access to resources, air pollution, and morbidity or mortality.

chronic disease management includes the actions and behaviors taken by health providers, caregivers, and patients to reduce the complications and impact of a chronic disease.

chronic diseases are long-term, noncontagious, and irreversible diseases that are often related to unhealthy behaviors such as physical inactivity, poor eating habits, and cigarette smoking, as well as other factors such as family history and age.

clinical information systems refer to the organization of patient medical records and other information sources within a health care setting.

cognitive-behavioral therapy are interventions that address thoughts and behaviors associated with problems.

A **community** is a group of individuals who share common values and beliefs and provide a sense of belonging to the members of the group.

community health workers are members of the community they are trying to reach who are trained to provide various forms of support to promote health and reduce risk of illness.

community-level tobacco interventions include laws to regulate tobacco, enforcement of restrictions on tobacco access, and efforts on the part of community leaders and institutions to influence community behavior.

community mobilization strategies involve a process through which community members, groups, or organizations design, implement, and evaluate public health programs for the purpose of improving the overall quality of life of the community.

community resources and policies are linkages between the community and the health care organization.

comorbidities are the presence of more than one disease or condition in the same person at the same time. Conditions described as comorbidities are often chronic or long-term conditions. Other names to describe comorbid conditions are coexisting or co-occurring conditions. For example, tuberculosis could be a comorbid condition among individuals living with HIV.

A **comparison group** is the group of participants in a program who do not receive the health intervention.

compatibility is the consistency between the innovation and current processes.

competitive foods are foods and beverages including snacks, meals, and sodas sold on campus that are not funded under school-based meal programs. Competitive foods are also referred to as a la carte items and include foods sold by outside vendors such as fast food companies and also foods sold by school groups as part of fundraisers.

complexity is how difficult the innovation is to understand or accomplish.

conceptual models are physical depictions of causal relationships between constructs.

consciousness raising is using new information to become more aware of a problem.

constructs are the main concepts of a theory.

contemplation is a stage in which the person is intending to change in the near future (usually defined as 6 months). The person is often weighing the pros and cons of performing the action.

contingency management is a type of behavioral conditioning that frames behavior change as motivated through reinforcements for healthy behavior.

cost objectives include a predetermined budget set for each program component.

counterconditioning involves replacing one behavior with another. Rather than changing a behavior by eliminating it and leaving a void, one replaces the unhealthy behavior with a healthy behavior.

cues to action are "triggers" for the targeted health behavior.

cultural competency describes an individual's or organization's level of awareness, familiarity, and comfort with the values, traditions, and behaviors of a specific cultural, ethnic, or racial group.

D

decisional balance   is the perception of the relative benefits and disadvantages of performing the behavior.

decision support   means having a set of clear practice guidelines for the treatment and management of chronic diseases.

delivery system design   refers to creating an ideal division of labor. This includes defining where specific medical staff (i.e., physicians vs. nurses) are needed and dividing the tasks accordingly.

determinants of health   refers to the range of factors (personal, social, economic, and environmental) that influence a person's health. To improve public health, interventions should target one or more determinants of health through information, policies, and programs.

dietary behaviors   include food and beverage purchasing behaviors, meal, snack, and beverage preparation behaviors, and what people and situations cue the consumption of certain foods and beverages, which all ultimately influence what foods and beverages are consumed.

A **dietary pattern**   describes an individual's usual dietary intake of foods and beverages.

domain-specific activity   is the grouping of physical activities into distinct environments where they occur throughout the day, such as work and home.

The **dose**   of a health behavior intervention represents the level of exposure that individuals who are enrolled in the program have to the behavior change material and activities, such as the number of educational sessions or support groups attended. For programs implemented at the family level, dose could be counted as number of home visits completed.

dramatic relief   is an emotional reaction to the problem behavior. Taking action to improve the behavior reduces the negative emotions.

drug addiction   is a chronic disease characterized by the compulsive use of a substance (e.g., alcohol or drug) despite negative or dangerous personal or societal impact.

drug resistance   occurs when microorganisms such as bacteria, viruses, fungi, and parasites change in ways that reduce the medication's effectiveness to cure or treat the health problem. HIV drug resistance may occur if antiretroviral treatment is not taken as prescribed (e.g., when medication doses are missed).

duration   is the length of time, usually in minutes, an individual engages in physical activity.

E

early adopters   are the 13.5% of the population, after the innovators, to accept the innovation and are more socially integrated than the innovators.

early majority   are the 34% of the population, after the early adopters, to accept the innovation.

economic interventions   are interventions that rely on economic factors as their primary tactic. These include increasing tax rates on tobacco, which can decrease sales and tobacco use, especially in areas where disposable income is limited.

efficacy versus effectiveness   efficacy refers to how an intervention produces a desired benefit. Most often, randomized clinical trials are necessary to demonstrate efficacy. **Effectiveness** tells us how well the intervention works in the real world. Once an intervention is shown to be efficacious, it is expected to be disseminated widely. If the beneficial change accompanies such dissemination, then the intervention is said to be effective.

elephantiasis   consists of thickening tissue/skin on limbs.

emotional arousal management   refers to how a person addresses and copes with the negative or positive emotions surrounding the performance of a behavior.

emotional support   is showing love, compassion, and care and incorporates behaviors like listening and physical affection. It refers to the amount of sympathy, care, and understanding provided by others.

endemic   refers to a disease regularly found in a particular geographic area or population.

energy-dense foods   energy dense foods and beverages high in calories and low in nutritional value, often contain added sugars, salt, and fat. They include candy, snack foods such as chips and cookies but can also include other foods consumed as meals, such as packaged sweetened breakfast cereals and frozen or prepared meals such as pizza.

entomological surveillance   involves monitoring the location and number of disease vectors, such as mosquitoes, as well as eradication effectiveness.

environmental change strategies   are techniques used to alter factors external to an individual or in the community.

An **environmental food audit**   is a precise measurement of physical or social aspects of that environment that can influence the quality, accessibility, and availability of various food items. Environmental food audits are typically completed with standardized forms; examples include audits that measure the physical environments of institutions, food retail outlets, workplace organizations, and even communities. Additional resources on environmental food audits can be found on the National Institutes of Health website for the NCCOR initiative.

environmental reevaluation   is assessing how the behavior impacts others and society and can include both mental and emotional strategies.

environmental tobacco restrictions   are restrictions placed on where tobacco can be advertised, sold, or used. These can include designated areas for smoking and outright smoking bans.

equivalence   frames social proximity as similarity. Specifically, two people are equivalent if their social networks are similar.

evaluation   is the process of assessing the quality and effectiveness of a program.

exchange   is the idea that self-interest, or the desire to maximize benefits and minimize costs, drives behavior.

excise taxes   are taxes on the sale or production of a specific good or product.

exercise   is structured or planned participation in physical activities in order to improve or maintain physical fitness.

An **experimental design**   is a study design in which participants are randomly assigned to one or more study groups, the case and control groups.

F

food deserts   are areas that have poor access to affordable, healthy food. They are most often found in inner cities and were created when supermarkets abandoned the downtown core to relocate in suburbs. These areas tend to disproportionately affect socially segregated groups in underprivileged urban areas, specifically single mothers, children, the elderly, and families and individuals without a car.

food security   refers to the minimum level of socially acceptable access to food required to sustain normal functioning. Food security also includes access to healthy foods items required for proper nutrition.

formal networks   are networks of individuals that have formal structures (e.g., sporting or recreational clubs, and political parties).

framework   provides a way of viewing the behavior but does not explain relationships between constructs.

frequency   is the rate of participation in physical activity, or how often one engages in physical activities.

functionality   describes an individual's mental and physical ability to perform activities of daily living.

G

generalization   refers to whether a behavior will occur in a new physical or social context.

A **goal**   is a broad statement of intention that describes the expected effects of a program.

gross rating points   is a measure commonly used in advertising to help assess the audience size reached by the advertisement. Gross rating points are calculated as (frequency × % reached), that is, the product of the frequency an audience sees an advertising campaign times the percentage of the audience reached. The media uses gross rating points values to compare the advertising strength of various campaigns.

H

A **health behavior**   is a way of looking at how people behave in relation to their health, including nutrition, exercise, and accessing preventative medicine. Understanding and influencing health behavior is a key way of improving health.

health behavior models   or theories are frameworks that help us explain and predict human behavior and are especially helpful when planning health promotion programs.

The **health belief model**   theorizes that health-related behavior change depends on having sufficient motivation, a belief of a perceived health threat, and belief that the intended behavior will reduce the perceived threat.

health care organization   includes the organization's values, policies, training, and orientation toward patients.

health communication strategies   are a set of techniques used to inform individuals or groups of topics pertaining to health.

health disparity   is a difference in the incidence, prevalence, mortality, or burden of disease that is observed in specific subgroups when compared to the health status of the general population.

health education   is a combination of planned learning experiences based on theories that provide individuals, groups, and communities the opportunity to acquire information and the skills needed to make informed health decisions.

health education strategies   are formal scholastic techniques used to increase the knowledge and skills of an individual or group pertaining to a health topic.

health literacy   is an individual's ability to find, process, and understand information and services relevant to medical and health needs and to perform essential health functions such as reading and comprehending health information and communicating with health care providers.

health policy/health enforcement strategies   are the application and enforcement of mandated regulations pertaining to health behaviors or factors that could influence health such as laws banning smoking in public areas to protect nonsmokers from second-hand smoke.

health promotion   is a process of enabling others to improve their health.

health-related community service strategies   include health-related services, tests, and programs offered to the community.

health-related quality of life   includes an individual's perceived mental and physical health, as well as the perceived experience the individual has of his or her illness and activity limitations.

healthy food financing initiative (HFFI)   This is a national-level initiative that supports projects through grant opportunities to increase access to healthy, affordable food in communities that currently lack these options.

healthy people 2020   is a set of goals and objectives with 10-year targets designed to guide the public health efforts of the United States.

helping relationships   emphasizes the role of trusting, nurturing relationships in promoting change.

HIV–related stigma   is a socially driven negative attitude toward or response to individuals living with HIV. This type of attitude may build upon and reinforce other negative attitudes about marginalized behaviors, such as sex work, drug use, and homosexual and transgender sexual practice. Stigma can have negative repercussions on the health and well-being of individuals who are stigmatized.

The **host**   is the organism a parasite attaches itself to or lives within.

human immunodeficiency virus (HIV)   is the virus that impacts an individual's immune system by destroying specific blood cells (see *CD4 cells* definition) that are crucial to helping the body fight disease.

hydrocele   refers to fluid buildup.

I

impact evaluation   involves assessing the short-term effects of a program on behavior change.

An **impact objective**   is a statement that describes the effect of a program or intervention on behavior within 1 to 5 years following program initiation.

in-kind contributions   are nonmonetary support, such as goods and services, provided by external sources.

infectious diseases   are illnesses that are caused by an organism such as a virus, bacteria, parasite, or fungus (otherwise known as pathogens).

informal networks   are social networks of individuals and/or groups without formal structures, linked together by one or more social relationships, such as kinship and friendship.

informational support   is providing helpful, relevant facts and information.

informational support   refers to the provision of advice or information related to the need.

innovators   are the first individuals to adopt the new idea.

instrumental activities of daily living   include tasks that are not considered self-care responsibilities and are thus supplemental activities, including personal financial management, preparing and cooking meals, shopping, and using communication devices.

instrumental support   is defined as the help, aid, or assistance with material resources like providing a ride to a gym, paying bills, and cleaning.

instrumental support   is offering tangible help like money for a gym membership or a ride to the physician's office.

intensity   is the effort required to perform physical activity.

interdisciplinary/multidisciplinary care   is the collaboration of health care specialists from various fields who come together to effectively and efficiently treat a patient.

interpersonal networks   are spheres of association composed of influences from a personal social network of peers, family members, and health care providers, among others. Interpersonal networks can be drawn on to address tobacco behaviors and initiate interventions.

interpersonally focused interventions   can increase intangible (e.g., coping) and tangible (e.g., money) resources that lead to positive health behaviors (e.g., physical activity) and health outcomes.

A health **intervention**   is an effort to modify health-related behaviors. Interventions can take many forms, including individual, organizational, social, economic, and political.

An **ITN** is an insecticide-treated bed net.

K

The **knowledge-attitude-behavior (K-A-B)** approach assumes that either on an individual level or via mass communication, changing knowledge and attitudes may result in risk factor reduction and other forms of behavior change.

L

laggards are the final 16% of the social system's population to accept the innovation.

large-scale programs consist of efforts at the state and city level. These programs create a synergistic, collaborative strategy that taps readily available resources, bolstering them with funds and a coordinated effort to gather input across a broad demographic.

late majority are the 34% of the population that accepts the innovation after the early majority and before the laggards.

A **learning objective** is a statement that describes the changes in knowledge, attitudes, skills, or awareness as a result of a program or intervention within 1 year of program initiation.

lesions are damaged tissue.

low-density lipoprotein (LDL), also called the "bad" cholesterol, circulates in the blood and can build up in the inner walls of arteries. LDL and other substances form plaque, which is a thick, hard deposit that narrows and stiffens the arteries, increasing the risk of heart attack and stroke. Foods high in saturated fats and trans fats can increase blood LDL, while foods rich in soluble dietary fiber (e.g., oats, legumes, apples, barley, pears) may help lower LDL. Regular physical activity and a healthy weight can also lower LDL.

lymphedema is the name for tissue swelling.

M

maintenance is the stage in which the person has incorporated the change into daily life (usually for at least 6 months).

A **market basket** is defined by the USDA as the sum of a variety of food and beverage items that will allow an individual to follow the recommended dietary guidelines for 1 week. Market baskets can also be computed for households. The USDA creates a series of recommended market baskets based on four income levels to help individuals and households maintain a healthy diet while considering price (Carlson, Lino, Juan, Hanson, & Basiotis, 2007).

marketing involves publicizing the program to raise awareness and is performed prior to and during program implementation.

marketing mix or the "four Ps" (i.e., product, price, place, and promotion), is a foundational concept in commercial marketing and has been appropriated by social marketers to promote behavior change.

medication adherence involves following a recommended medication regimen closely every day: taking the correct dose of a medication and at the correct time as prescribed by a clinician. High medication adherence to HIV treatment is critical to the health of the individual and can contribute to decreased HIV transmission at the community level.

messages both media and cultural, are communications from television, radio, Internet, and cultural groups that promote or inhibit healthy behavior.

The **metabolic equivalent (MET)** is a unit used to describe physical activity intensity by measuring or estimating the amount of oxygen consumed relative to body weight.

migration is the movement of a person or a group of persons, either across an international border or within a country. This population mobility could encompass any kind of movement of people, regardless of the length of time they move, the composition of mobile groups, and causes of mobility. Migration includes refugees, victims of natural disasters, economic migrants, and persons moving for other purposes such as for family reunification.

ministries of health are government bodies in charge of public health nationally.

A **model** presents and explains relationships between constructs.

multilevel interventions use a mix of programs, interventions, and other efforts designed to address all levels of the socio-ecological model. When tackling small, specific aspects of a larger problem, it is important that multiple levels of influence complement already existing approaches to understanding tobacco initiation and any possible measure of intervention to postpone uptake and dependency, if not prevent them altogether.

N

A **needs assessment** is the initial step in program planning in which the priority population and the health issues within the population are identified to determine what is needed to improve health outcomes.

nicotine is the stimulant in tobacco that is responsible for its addictive nature.

nitrosamines are among the most harmful carcinogens found in tobacco products.

nutritional epidemiology is the study of how dietary intake and nutritional status impact the distribution of disease and mortality among humans.

O

An **objective** is a specific statement that describes incremental effects of a program or intervention leading toward achieving the program goal.

observability is how much others can perceive the effects of the innovation.

An **observational design** is a study design in which there is only one group of participants that is observed independently.

observational learning maintains that a person often learns by seeing others model the behavior and receiving a positive consequence as a result of its enactment.

An **occasional smoker** is someone who smokes less frequently than daily.

organizational interventions are interventions performed in the workplace, school, church, or other community locations.

outcome evaluation involves assessing the long-term effect of a program on the target health issue.

outcome expectancies are how much a person values the particular outcome.

outcome expectations are what a person thinks will happen as a result of enacting the behavior.

An **outcome objective** is a statement relating to the long-term effect of the program on the target health problem, usually achieved 5 to 10 years following program initiation.

P

passive smoking also known as secondhand smoking or environmental tobacco smoking, occurs when a person other than the individual smoking a tobacco product inhales tobacco smoke.

patient education is a process of improving patients' knowledge and skills with the purpose of influencing specific attitudes and behaviors required to maintain or improve health.

patient empowerment is a method to help individuals to increase their self-efficacy and take control of their health by obtaining skills and knowledge necessary to make informed and educated behavioral decisions.

patient-centered care is health care that is respectful and delivered in a way that is responsive to the patient's preferences, needs, and values.

patient–provider communication affects a patient's satisfaction, level of disclosure, and adherence to treatment regimens and physician recommendations, which all increase as patients feel communication levels with providers are improved.

perceived barriers are obstacles to performing the recommended health behavior.

perceived behavioral control is one's belief regarding how much power one has over the enactment of the behavior.

perceived benefits of taking action interact with perceived susceptibility and perceived severity. Specifically, if a person views a particular action as reducing susceptibility or severity, the individual will view the action as beneficial.

perceived severity is a person's belief in the extent of negative consequences of contracting the disease, condition, or negative health outcome.

perceived susceptibility is the belief that one is likely to contract a particular disease, condition, or negative health outcome.

physical activity is the movement of the human body that increases energy expenditure above resting levels.

physical activity energy expenditure (PAEE) is the energy expenditure needed by biological processes necessary for participating in physical activity.

physical environments are environments that are human modified, including homes, schools, workplaces, air pollution, the transportation system, highways, urban sprawl, and other design features that may provide opportunities for travel and physical activity.

physical fitness is the body's ability to carry out physically active tasks.

physical structures are the attributes of products, neighborhoods, and all other environmental objects that promote or inhibit healthy behavior.

pilot testing   is the process of trying out certain components of the intervention, such as surveys or written materials, on a small group of people before starting the intervention to make sure that they can be used and interpreted as intended.

policy   refers to the legislative, regulatory actions taken by local, state, or federal governments that are meant to influence behavior by demanding specific behaviors or inhibiting others; policies may be implicit (e.g., informal policy at work) or explicit and policy interventions require public support.

positivism   is a school of thought in which only phenomena that can be directly and reliably assessed through sensory observation are of interest to science.

post-exposure prophylaxis   involves taking antiretroviral medication as soon as possible after exposure to HIV to decrease the chance that a newly exposed person will become infected.

precontemplation   stage is when the person is not considering making a change.

pre-exposure prophylaxis (PrEP)   is an HIV–prevention strategy for individuals who are at high risk for acquiring HIV. PrEP involves taking one combination antiretroviral pill every day to reduce the risk of becoming infected with HIV.

preparation   stage is when the person is intending to change in the near future (usually defined as 1 month) and has done small actions to get ready for change.

price elasticity of demand   is a measure that shows the responsiveness (elasticity) of the quantity demanded of a good to a change in its price; it shows us how much consumers change their purchasing behavior when prices change.

primary data   are information collected via direct observation, interviews, or surveys from the priority population to inform a health program.

priority setting   involves selecting the key health issue the program will target based on the importance and changeability of that health issue.

process evaluation   provides information on whether the program is implemented the way it was originally proposed.

A **process objective**   is a statement that describes the completion of program tasks during the implementation of a program.

program management   is the continuous organization of program resources including staff, materials, and funds throughout a program.

program planning   is the process of designing a public health program through implementation and evaluation.

promotores/as de salud   Similar to a community health worker or lay health advisor, **promotores/as de salud** are individuals who are part of the Hispanic/Latino community and who provide outreach, education, and support to individuals of similar background.

public education campaigns   are efforts to educate the public about the health effects of smoking and increase awareness of cessation resources.

public policy interventions   are interventions at the policy level. These include smoking bans, taxation of tobacco products and raising the price of such products, advertising bans, regulated portrayals of smoking in popular media, and FDA product regulations regarding package warnings.

Q

quality of life   is the subjective measurement of categorical factors such as income and socioeconomic status, environmental quality, or educational attainment.

A **quasi-experimental design**   is a study design in which participants are assigned to one of two study groups, the case and comparison groups.

R

recall bias   is a description of the error that occurs when individuals use memory to describe past experiences or behaviors.

reciprocal determinism   refers to the dynamic relationship among the self, behaviors, and the environment, both social and physical.

recreational tobacco consumption   involves ingesting tobacco for its intoxicating effects rather than for medicinal or religious purposes.

A **regular smoker**   is someone who smokes daily.

reinforcement   originates from operant conditioning and includes positive reinforcement (i.e., rewards following the enactment of a behavior) and negative reinforcement (i.e., removal of unpleasant stimulus following the enactment of the behavior).

relative advantage   is how much the new idea, or innovation, is superior to the current idea.

resource development   is the identification and organization of program components.

risk behaviors   are behaviors that place a person at risk for poor health. For HIV, this includes activities in which people engage that place them at risk for acquiring HIV (e.g., using drugs and/or alcohol before having sex, having unprotected sex, and using contaminated syringes).

S

sales restrictions   are restrictions placed on where and to whom cigarettes can be sold. These can include other ways of limiting access to tobacco products, including a consideration of advertising.

secondary data   are preexisting information not collected for the priority program.

segmentation   is a process of dividing a large population into smaller subgroups based on personal characteristics such as ethnicity, religion, age, or education.

self-efficacy   is an individual's confidence in her or his own ability to perform certain actions or behaviors.

self-efficacy,   within the context of health behavior, is one's perceived confidence in performing a specific health behavior.

self-liberation   is the belief that change is possible and the person has a personal commitment to follow through with the change.

self-management   includes the actions and behaviors taken by patients to successfully manage and control the effects and symptoms of their illness on a routine basis.

self-management support   involves teaching patients with a chronic disease how to care for themselves.

self-monitor   is a technique individuals often use to track behaviors in an effort to document patterns of behavior and to use those patterns to effect behavior change. For example, individuals may use collected data to identify barriers to behavior change (e.g., time of day, emotional state, physical location). Selfmonitoring is also a method to empower individuals with a way to monitor progress toward a behavior-change goal.

self-reevaluation   is conceptualizing the self with the problem behavior and without the problem behavior and then differentiating between these two possible identities to make a decision about which type of person to be.

smokeless tobacco   is tobacco that is chewed or held in the mouth rather than smoked.

smokeless zones   also known as smoke-free spaces, are combinations of intervention levels (organizational, policy, community, etc.) that aim to ban smoking in certain areas.

smoking bans   involve outlawing smoking in a particular environment, such as indoors, at restaurants, at work, and the like.

smoking cessation   means ceasing to use or quitting tobacco products. Cessation programs can take many forms, including quitting "cold turkey," cutting down, or replacing tobacco products with a variety of substances such as patches, gums, electronic cigarettes, and so on.

social environments   include environments of economic relations, power relations, social inequalities, cultural practices, religious institutions, and political or societal forces that shape the availability and choices for physical activity.

social liberation   refers to changing social norms to promote healthy behaviors.

social networks   refer to the social structure composed of individuals (or organizations) called "nodes," which are tied (connected) by one or more specific types of interdependency, such as friendship, kinship, common interest, financial exchange, dislike, intimate relationships, or relationships involving specific beliefs, knowledge, or prestige.

social proximity   is how close you are to someone else in your network.

social support   is a social network function (as it provides aid and assistance) given by members in a social network.

social structures   are policies and laws that promote or inhibit healthy behavior.

stimulus control   refers to the removal of factors associated with unhealthy behaviors.

structural cohesion   frames social proximity in "terms of the number, length, and strength of the paths that connect actors in networks" (Marsden & Friedkin, 1994, p. 7).

structural intervention   is an action or a series of actions designed to reduce or remove barriers to health or health behavior. In terms of HIV prevention, structural interventions may address physical, social, cultural, organizational, community, economic, legal, or policy barriers that contribute to HIV transmission.

subjective norms   are the pressure one feels from others to engage in the behavior.

T

The **target** is the final measure of a behavior or health outcome a health promotion program aims to reach. Put simply: where we want to be at the end of the program.

termination is the stage when a person has incorporated the change and is not tempted to relapse.

tobacco advertising is media messaging that creates specific cultural perceptions and attitudes about smoking. It is of particular concern in relation to youth smoking.

total energy expenditure (TEE) is the sum of the three main components of energy expenditure during waking and nonwaking hours. This includes the basal metabolic rate, thermic effect of food, and energy expenditure associated with physical activity.

trans fats are created when liquid (polyunsaturated) oils are hydrogenated. Food manufacturers often add trans fats to processed foods to extend their shelf life. You'll find trans fats in foods made with "partially hydrogenated vegetable oil" (like some but not all margarines, cookies, crackers, French fries, and potato chips). Most experts consider trans fats more harmful to heart health than saturated fats.

trialability is how much one can "experiment" with the innovation before fully adopting it.

tropical infectious diseases are diseases that occur solely or principally in the tropics.

V

A **vector** is any living thing that carries an infectious agent.

A **vector-borne disease** is a disease that is transmitted to humans via a carrier of a different species.

vertical control programs are focused on a specific disease, health issue, or population.

viral infection is the invasion of a virus into the body and subsequent replication of the virus.

A **virus** is an infectious pathogen many times smaller than bacteria that replicates inside an organism's cells.

visioning is a process of structured brainstorming by program stakeholders that culminates in a statement of vision and values for a program.

vulnerable populations are populations who may be at increased risk for HIV acquisition by virtue of conditions such as their socio-economic status, gender, age, disability status, and risk status related to low access to condoms or other effective prevention of HIV.

W

WHO stands for the World Health Organization, the United Nations public health arm.

Index